The Austr Health Care System

SECOND EDITION

S.J. Duckett

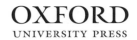

OXFORD

UNIVERSITY PRESS

OXFORD
UNIVERSITY PRESS

253 Normanby Road, South Melbourne, Victoria 3205, Australia

Oxford University Press is a department of the University of Oxford.
It furthers the University's objective of excellence in research, scholarship,
and education by publishing worldwide in

Oxford New York

Auckland Cape Town Dar es Salaam Hong Kong Karachi
Kuala Lumpur Madrid Melbourne Mexico City Nairobi
New Delhi Shanghai Taipei Toronto

With offices in

Argentina Austria Brazil Chile Czech Republic France Greece
Guatemala Hungary Italy Japan Poland Portugal Singapore
South Korea Switzerland Thailand Turkey Ukraine Vietnam

OXFORD is a trade mark of Oxford University Press
in the UK and in certain other countries

National Library of Australia
Cataloguing-in-Publication data:

Duckett, S.J. (Stephen John), 1950–.
The Australian health care system.

2nd ed.
Bibliography.
Includes index.
For health sciences students.
ISBN 0 19 551745 8.

1. Public health—Australia. 2. Medical care—Australia.
3. Medical policy—Australia. I. Title

362.10994

Typeset by OUPANZS
Printed through Bookpac Production Services, Singapore

Contents

List of Tables

List of Figures

List of Acronyms and Abbreviations

ACAS	Aged Care Assessment Service
ACCC	Australian Competition and Consumer Commission
ACHS	Australian Council on Healthcare Standards
AHEC	Australian Health Ethics Committee
AHMAC	Australian Health Ministers' Advisory Council
AHWAC	Australian Health Workforce Advisory Committee
AHWOC	Australian Health Workforce Officials Committee
AIHW	Australian Institute of Health and Welfare
AMWAC	Australian Medical Workforce Advisory Committee
DALY	disability adjusted life years
DRG	Diagnosis Related Group
DVA	Department of Veterans' Affairs
FRACP	Fellowship of the Royal Australasian College of Physicians
GDP	Gross Domestic Product
GST	Goods and Services Tax
HACC	Home and Community Care program
ICF	International Classification of Functioning, Disability and Health
MBS	Medicare Benefits Scheme
MDC	Major Diagnostic Category
NH&MRC	National Health and Medical Research Council

NHS	National Health Service
NOHSC	National Occupational Health and Safety Commission
NPHP	National Public Health Partnership
OECD	Organization for Economic Cooperation and Development
PBAC	Pharmaceutical Benefits Advisory Committee
PBS	Pharmaceutical Benefits Scheme
PHERP	Public Health Education and Research Program
PHIAC	Private Health Insurance Administration Council
PHOFA	Public Health Outcome Funding Agreements
PYLL	potential years of life lost
SCCSISA	Standing Committee of Community Services and Income Security Administrators
SF-36	short form, 36 questions, National Health Survey
SMR	standardised mortality ratio
SWPE	Standardised Whole Patient Equivalent
TGA	Therapeutic Goods Administration
VACS	Victorian Ambulatory Classification System
WHO	World Health Organization
YLD	years of life lived with a disability
YLL	years of life lost

Acknowledgments

This edition could not have been written without the same two extremely important forms of structural assistance which facilitated the first edition. First, the Australian Institute of Health and Welfare provides a range of data relevant to the Australian health care system. This book is characterised by extensive use of data from the Institute and the Institute's existence has made this style of book possible. I have also greatly benefited from formal and informal assistance given to me by staff of the Institute.

Secondly, the book would not have been able to be written in the absence of the Outside Studies Program (sabbatical leave) granted to me by La Trobe University. Sabbatical leave has historically been an extremely important part of Australian academic life and continues to be so. During my leave I was a Visiting Scholar at the Health Economics Unit of Monash University (thanks to Professor Jeff Richardson, Head of that Unit).

Permission to publish earlier versions of various chapters and sections of chapters and material from other authors is gratefully acknowledged:

Figure 1.2 is produced from Dror, D. M. and A. S. Preker, Eds. (2002) and is published with permission of the publisher.

Figure 2.9 is produced from Mathews (1997) and is published with permission of the author and publisher.

The following have been reproduced with the permission of the Australian Institute of Health and Welfare:

Table 8.3 is from Residential aged care in Australia 2000–01: A statistical overview, AIHW Aged Care Series No. 11, AIHW Cat. No. AGE 22

Appendix 1 is from Health expenditure Australia 2001-02. Canberra, Cat no. HWE24,

Figure 2.6 is from The burden of disease and injury in Australia (Cat. No. PHE 17).

Data used in Figures 7.5 and 7.6 were provided by the Communicable Diseases Network, Australia and New Zealand.

The following have been produced, with permission, from Australian Bureau of Statistics data. Copyright in ABS data resides with the Commonwealth of Australia and is used with permission:

Figure 2.4 is reproduced from Australian Social Trends (Cat. No. 4102.0) 1997.

Tables 2.3, 4.1 and 4.2 are the result of special tabulations.

Thanks also to Anne Mulvaney who provided excellent editorial comment, Dr Terri Jackson who contributed through collegial and personal support, and Sarah Duckett who contributed by suffering an occasionally grumpy dad.

The health care system in Australia changes rapidly and consequently a book of this kind can date relatively quickly. Comments on the first edition have helped me prepare this edition. It is my intention to produce a third edition of this book if time and publisher permit. Accordingly, I would welcome any suggestions from readers as to sections of the book which are unclear, or could warrant further explication. Similarly, suggestions are welcome for issues that have been left out of the book.

Stephen Duckett
December 2003

Introduction

The Australian health care system is, in part, a contested terrain characterised by conflict over values and policy choices. So pervasive is this
conflict that Sax entitled his 1984 book about health services *A Strife of
Interests*. As with many areas of society there is no neutral description of the
structure or functioning of the relevant institutions and processes. What is
described or analysed is selected, emphasised, and written up within a
particular framework or from a particular perspective.

There are many ways of looking at health care systems and of decompos-
ing their constituent parts. Grant (1985), for example, has analysed the
operation of hospitals from an organisation perspective, emphasising the
organisational structures and the interrelationships within hospitals. Willis
(1994), Lupton and Najman (1995), George (1998), and Germov (2002)
have emphasised sociological perspectives on health and health care in
Australia, looking at how sociological structures and institutions affect the
operation of a system and the impact of the health care system on particular
groups within society. Mooney and Scotton's book (1998) adopts an
economic approach to analysing the health care system. A number of books
focus on a specific component of the health care system such as public health
(Baum 1998), occupational health and safety (Mayhew and Peterson 1999),
and aged care (Gibson 1998). Crichton (1990) and Gillespie (1991) review
the historical evolution of government's role in health care in Australia.
Palmer and Short (1994), Gardner (1995, 1997), Bloom (2000), and Gardner
and Barraclough (2002) focus on aspects of Australian health policy.

This book adopts a systems approach to analysing Australian health
services structured around the inputs and processes of the system and the
associated outputs and outcomes (see figure 1.1). It is, however, written by
an economist, and economic and policy issues will tend to be the emphasis,
an emphasis common in health policy making in Australia (Lewis and
Considine 1999).

Following this introduction, chapter 1 provides frameworks that are used throughout the book especially outlining the criteria that will often be used in assessing policies: equity, efficiency, quality, and acceptability. Chapter 2 describes the health of the Australian population and the factors that have an impact on health. The principal focus of this book, however, relates to the inputs and institutions of the health system. Chapters 3 and 4 focus on inputs: finance in chapter 3, and the health workforce in chapter 4. Chapters 5 to 9 deal with institutional structures of the health system. Chapter 5 outlines the structures of governance and cooperation, analysing the organisational structures of state health departments and the relative roles of Commonwealth and state governments and the relations between these two levels of government. Chapter 6 focuses on hospitals; chapter 7 on public health activities, including health protection and health promotion; chapter 8 on community-based services, including residential services and medical practice; and chapter 9 on pharmaceuticals. Chapter 10 concludes by outlining some of the challenges facing the Australian health care system.

Importantly, the 'health care system' as described in this book can more accurately be described as an 'illness care system' because the vast majority of institutions and personnel are devoted to caring for people with illness rather than promoting health. The relative contribution of illness care to gross measures of improvement in health status and length of life—compared with the role of adequate housing, income, an environment free of pollution, the availability of clean air and water—has been questioned (see chapter 2). However, the term 'illness care system' should not be regarded as a pejorative one, as hospitals and other care providers can, and do, make a major contribution to restoring individuals to health and providing appropriately supportive environments for those in need of care.

This book focuses on the institutions of care provision, including the structure and funding of health care organisations. Equally important are the processes that take place within those institutions, and patients' experience of these institutions (Waitzkin 1991). Consumers' experiences will be affected by their race, gender, ethnicity, and class: health professionals employed in the institutions will usually not be from the same background as their clients or patients and this has negative consequences for the processes of health care.

Interactions between doctor and patient (and between other health professionals and clients or patients) are complex. They are essentially relations of power, but are often presented paternalistically as being entirely about 'caring' for the patient's interest. Health professionals may make their own judgment about what treatment is in the patient's best interest rather than allowing patients to make such decisions themselves. Complaints lodged against doctors are often about the way in which the patient was treated, not in the medical sense of the word but in terms of the respect shown by the doctor to the patient. This lack of respect shows itself both in terms of the dignity with which the patient is treated (for example, not inviting all and sundry to examine the patient without providing an explanation or seeking permission) and also the information given to the patient about the course of his or her treatment and the likely outcome. Increasingly, patients are questioning the content of the doctor–patient interaction, and lodging complaints or taking legal action when not satisfied with the processes or outcomes of care, calling into question the premises of paternalism in health.

The functioning of health care institutions reflects both the organisational structures of these institutions, and the myriad interactions between patients and the health care providers working within the organisations. It has been argued that the internal processes of hospitals and nursing homes are structured to protect health professionals, not consumers (Millman 1977). Changing this balance is going to be one of the most difficult issues for managers, professionals, consumer advocates, and health policy makers in the future.

Shifting the balance back to consumers will require opening 'the black box' of the institutions. There are hopeful signs that this will occur as government-sponsored patient satisfaction surveys and other strategies to involve consumers are implemented. In the USA it is common for government to publish score cards of case fatality rates by hospital, and in some states, by surgeon. The professions have, of course, opposed this exposure. In the long term, however, consumer confidence in the professions and continued support for professional training (and for the high incomes that health professionals generally enjoy) will be facilitated by opening up the processes and demonstrating that action is taken where processes and outcomes do not meet patients' expectations of dignity, compassion, information provision, and involvement when they are ill.

The 'black box' of the processes of care is one of the most dynamic aspects of the health system. The health professions in Australia, especially the medical profession, are exposed to the developments and innovations in diagnosis, treatment, and management that occur throughout the world. Health professionals in teaching hospitals, especially doctors, regularly travel to international conferences and develop professional relationships with their colleagues in other countries. This means that they are able to act as conduits for the rapid transmission of innovations in diagnosis and treatment. Similarly, global companies are keen to market their new diagnostic, treatment, and management technologies in Australia.

Diagnostic and treatment technologies are changing rapidly. New anaesthetic agents and microsurgery have transformed surgical practice in Australia and internationally. This has led to substantial reductions in the average length of stay in hospital for most surgical procedures, and changed

the nature of risk of many surgical operations, thus expanding the population who might safely undergo a surgical procedure. There has also been a
transformation in the way patients are diagnosed and treated. Diagnosis is
now typically complete before a hospital admission, and most hospital
treatment can now be done on a 'same day' basis. The increase in the
proportion of patients who can be treated on a day-only basis has major
implications for the design and operation of hospitals. This day procedure
trend is continuing and is likely to have a further impact over the next few
decades, reducing the demand for overnight stays in hospital and reducing
the hospital capacity required to meet population needs.

Hospitals will also be affected by the development of genetic technologies, not only through the identification of genetic predisposition to certain
diseases and thus possibly affecting opportunities for prevention; but also
through the development of a new generation of pharmaceuticals that will
enable medical rather than surgical treatment of diseases and tailoring of
medication to the specific genetic make-up of individual patients and their
specific response to the medication. New pharmaceuticals may also reduce
the demand for hospital admission for medical treatment because highly
targeted drugs may not require the same level of supervision during their
delivery.

Management technologies are also changing the processes of care. The
most notable development of management technology has been an
improved ability to describe patients through development of casemix
measures (see chapter 6), and the introduction of casemix funding. Casemix
funding has changed the nature of incentives for hospitals and has often led
to changes in the organisational structure of hospitals.

Information technology is also having a profound impact on the health
care system (Goldsmith 2000). Information technology and the development of the Internet are leading to a more informed patient clientele,
because consumers are able to access information about their disease both
directly on the Internet and through information exchanges with other
people with similar conditions through disease-related chat groups. In many
cases consumers may thus be more informed about the latest development in
treatment technologies than their treating practitioners. Web-based
technologies are also empowering consumers in their interaction with
hospitals, for example, by allowing patients to book their own outpatient
clinic appointments.

Although it is unlikely that an integrated electronic record will achieve
all the benefits identified by its advocates (Mount et al. 2000), it does have
the potential to change the nature of health care provision. The new
information technology brings with it certain challenges, not least being the
need to ensure that the patient record is just that, namely, a record owned by
the patient with access to the information in the record controlled by the

patient rather than providers and/or companies involved in selling drugs and other services to the patient (Carter 2000). Information technology has the ability not only to transform the relationship between the consumer and the provider, but also relationships between providers through facilitating changed payment arrangements; longitudinal or episode of care payment is only feasible with records linking the number and type of interactions between a consumer and/or providers. New information technology may also improve efficiency in terms of reducing duplication of diagnostic work-ups and assessments.

These changes in information technology, pressure from consumers, research advances, and demographic changes in the population impact on health systems. This means that the Australian health care system as outlined in this book, is hopefully not the same as the system will be in five or 10 years. However, the basic building blocks of the system will be recognisable; this book attempts to outline sources of data so that checking facts and new structural arrangements is facilitated. Also relatively enduring are some of the health system design choices, the subject of the first chapter.

1

Frameworks for Analysis

All organisations can be described in terms of a system, with inputs, processes, outputs, and outcomes (Kast and Rosenzweig 1972). Figure 1.1 shows a general outline of the organisation of health services as a system. This framework is used to describe the Australian health care system in this book. A similar systems framework has been used by the World Health Organization (WHO) as part of its framework for evaluating health systems (WHO 2000).

The underpinning of any set of inputs into the health care system is the ability to pay for those inputs, and hence costs or financing is critical to

Figure 1.1 Organisation of health services: a systems perspective

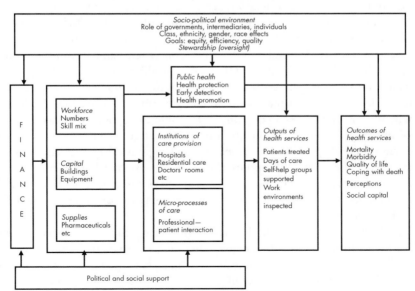

creating or obtaining the other inputs: the workforce, capital, and supplies. A qualitatively different type of input is 'political and social support'. This derives from Easton's (1979) conceptualisation of the political process as a system. The extent of political or social support for the health system is reflected in the trust people have in the system and the ability of the system to garner additional resources, either from taxation or individual contributions.

The inputs allow the provision of care through a variety of processes. In figure 1.1 these processes of care are divided into two major components: the institutions of care provision and microprocesses of care.

The principal outputs vary across the different types of health services and processes and include patients treated, days of care, and so on. There are also 'intermediate' outputs such as pathology tests that are also inputs into care processes. The principal outcomes are of two kinds. The health system impacts on health status, usually measured in terms of length and quality of life. There are also other outcomes of the health system and individual interactions with it. At the individual level, the outcomes include perceptions of the quality of the interaction, for example the extent to which a person felt their dignity had been protected or infringed, and the extent of information provided. More broadly, the outcomes include the contribution of the system to building 'social capital', for example does the health system help to build a stronger community or to enhance equity in society.

It is important to stress that the Australian health care system is not some free-floating entity existing in a social vacuum. The health care system exists in a socio-political environment that has particular characteristics: the place of women, racial discrimination and discrimination against people from a non-English speaking background, and the role of class divisions. These characteristics affect the health care system both in its interaction with other aspects of society (for example the education system) and also in the modus operandi of the system itself. Choices in health care system design have equity implications in terms of which groups are winners and which are losers. Decisions about the relative role of government versus individuals and whether or not there is a government response to needs are not taken solely within the bounds of the health care system. The wider political environment shapes the choices that are on the political agenda, and these in turn shape the outcome of political debates. The political environment can, of course, change over time, which can affect the nature of what health system design choices are seen as appropriate or viable politically (Schlesinger 2002).

The health care system also has an impact on the wider social system. Australia's health insurance scheme, Medicare, is designed to ensure that all Australians have equal access to care in a public system. This attribute means that all Australians have a stake in ensuring that the public system functions effectively. Medicare thus contributes to social cohesion and social solidarity. The more Medicare is relegated to being a system for the 'poor' and the more middle class or wealthy individuals seek to opt out of a public system to rely on private insurance and private services for their care, the more social solidarity will be weakened and government expenditure on Medicare and the public system will be questioned by those groups who do not see themselves benefiting from that expenditure.

The WHO has identified 'stewardship' as an important component of the health care system and its environment (Saltman and Ferroussier-Davis 2000). The stewardship function provides the oversight and overall governance of the health system as a whole. Stewardship is about designing the regulatory framework for the system and ensuring compliance; establishing the roles of the agencies and authorities; and adjusting the system on the basis of monitoring and feedback systems. Although 'stewards' may be participants in the health system, they can and do change the shape of the overall health care system and so have been placed as part of the environment in figure 1.1.

The final aspect of a system, not shown in the diagram, is feedback. A system adapts and changes in response to its environment, and through evaluation of the adequacy of the processes and outcomes. Feedback processes can be formal (committees of review, research studies) or informal. Feedback can work through political processes to change major aspects of the system or at local levels, bringing research results or feedback from consumers to bear on choice about treatment or organisational processes.

A number of authors have proposed frameworks for describing or evaluating a health care system. One of the early frameworks was that of the American Public Health Association (Myers 1965), which proposed evaluating health care systems in terms of accessibility, quality, continuity, and efficiency. Aday et al. (1998), in a more contemporary approach, have suggested three main criteria: equity, efficiency, and effectiveness.

This book uses a two dimensional approach to evaluation. On one dimension are quality, efficiency, and acceptability. Equity is a fourth and special criterion. It is an objective (or evaluation criterion) in itself; it is also a qualifier or second dimension to both quality and acceptability. Both of these latter criteria need to be assessed in terms of their level of attainment and the equity of that attainment. A focus on equity requires analysis of health status or health care differences in geography, class, race, ethnic origin, gender, and so on with the aim of reducing such differences. Which groups are analysed is a matter of value choice and is always limited by data availability. The relative emphasis placed on equity versus efficiency issues (to the extent that they are trade-offs) will also in part depend on one's value position. A policy focus on equity can be cast in a number of different ways. The system difference or attribute being analysed is critically important: whether the measurement of equity is in terms of outputs (usually described as 'equity of access', highlighted by Myers as the separate criterion of accessibility) versus a much stronger, but more difficult to achieve focus on equity of outcomes.

Overall system efficiency has three key contributing factors: technical, dynamic, and allocative efficiency. Technical efficiency can be defined as efficiency in production; normally operationalised as inputs, such as costs, divided by outputs (for example patients treated). Dynamic efficiency is the extent to which a system is able to adapt to change. Allocative efficiency can be defined as ensuring that there is an optimum allocation of resources so that the marginal dollar spent on any program yields the same level of marginal benefit as the last dollar spent in any other program. Allocative efficiency thus involves a focus on outcomes (such as improved quality of life) relative to inputs. A simple decomposition shows that allocative efficiency (inputs per outcome) incorporates technical efficiency (inputs per output) and moves beyond it to incorporate a focus on effectiveness (outputs per outcome). Improving allocative efficiency (reducing inputs per outcome or increasing outcomes per input) can thus be achieved by improving technical efficiency (reducing inputs per output) or improving effectiveness (reducing outputs needed to achieve a given outcome or increasing outcomes for each output).

Clearly understanding efficiency requires us to measure the clinical outcomes of programs. This can be done using specific clinical measures (for example, scales developed for specific diseases or conditions), but more generic measures, such as quality of life measures, are required for comparisons of outcomes across different programs.

Effectiveness has two components: efficacy (the maximum extent to which a given output can contribute to outcome, usually achieved under controlled research conditions) and the extent to which a particular service or program is able to approach that 'ideal' efficacy. This latter component is essentially a measure of the clinical quality of the service while other aspects of quality measure patient acceptability, regardless of clinical quality. Systematic measurement of quality using outcome measures has been handicapped by lack of agreement on appropriate means to standardise for casemix, an essential prerequisite for any comparison of effectiveness (Iezzoni 1994). Outcomes have many dimensions, from short-term clinical changes to longer-term changes in a patient's quality of life. (Chapter 6 includes a more comprehensive discussion of measurement of quality of care, focusing on measurement of quality of hospital care.)

The final criterion for evaluating health systems is acceptability of the system from the perspective of patients, communities, and providers. This criterion is especially relevant in publicly funded health systems where political and social support for the system is an important determinant of the level of resourcing. Conversely, changes in the health system not seen as acceptable may impact adversely in the wider political environment.

A key element of acceptability is that the health care system should be seen to be fair and should be seen to operate ethically. Beauchamp and Childress (2001) have distilled the key principles that contribute to the acceptability of the health care system or contribute to an ethical health care system. They identified four key ethical principles for health care systems. The first principle is respect for autonomy, from which concepts of informed consent derive. The second principle is non-maleficence, the obligation not to inflict harm intentionally, from which is derived the obligation on health services to ensure that health care systems provide safe environments and that adverse events associated with care are minimised. The third principle is beneficence, which in contrast to the previous principle is a positive one about doing good; this principle also requires that the benefits and drawbacks of care be balanced. The fourth and final principle is justice in health care, which requires that treatment is allocated fairly, equitably, and appropriately.

Some of these principles involve contentious elements; for example the principle of non-maleficence may conflict with the role of the medical profession in assisted death for people who are chronically ill and in continuing pain not amenable to alleviation. Justice is also contentious as there are different conceptions of what fairness means, for example about whether it requires equal states of health (fairness in outcomes) or about whether those in the same state of health can access care equally (fairness in access or processes). Although most health care providers would agree with these principles, they may not be fully operationalised. Designing a system that fully accepts autonomy would require a much better understanding of consumer wishes and would present information to enable choice in ways different to the current norm (Lubalin and Harris-Kojetin 1999).

Choices in health system design

There are some common design issues that are relevant to the design of any health and community care program. Essentially, every such program is designed to respond to a 'need'. The choices as to which needs are recognised and how those needs are framed are important ones in terms of both social policy debates and the design of service systems to respond to those needs. Which 'needs' are seen as important and the priority accorded to them is a value choice (Shiell 1997; James 1999). Funding and policy arrangements for social service systems have some common elements. Except to the extent the service system has been internationalised, all the funds for operation of the system arise in the household sector (this issue is discussed further in chapter 3). The way in which funds flow from households to providers reflects the key programmatic choices in the design of the service system response to 'needs'.

The concept of need is one that has been the subject of much debate. Who defines needs? Are needs that are identified by professionals more relevant in social policy terms than those identified by consumers? Has society identified some 'basic needs' that must be met and funded by taxpayers? Translation of some illnesses into needs is self-evident and obvious: a person with a broken leg would clearly benefit from medical care and such a person clearly has a need for health care. The situation of a person with a headache is much more complex. Different people react to a headache differently: some do nothing; some simply take pain relievers; some take a day off work; and some immediately go to a doctor. Thus the very recognition of a need for action varies between individuals.

Needs are framed in different ways by consumers, providers, and policy makers (Donabedian 1973). There is rarely any external, objective 'needometer' which enables needs to be empirically determined and measured without regard to a social context. Rather, needs are best understood as being determined and framed within a social and political context (Braybrooke 1987).

Just as needs must be considered within a social and political context, so too with the nature of the service system response: the personal, social, and political environment will determine what needs are seen as deserving of a societal or government response and what needs will be seen as being the responsibility of individuals or the market. A similar range of environmental factors, together with economic factors, will affect the extent to which needs are translated into demands for services.

Figure 1.2 Schematic description: interaction of needs, demand, and supply

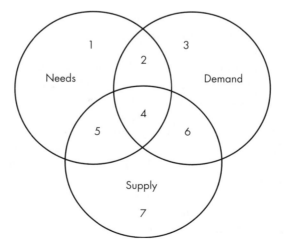

Needs, supply, and demand are three distinct concepts that Dror et al. (2002) have portrayed as three overlapping circles (see figure 1.2) that generate seven distinct zones:

Table 1.1 Intersections between need, supply, and demand in health care

1 Extant but unmet needs	Examples might include improving water or air quality beyond designated thresholds, where the costs are high, but there is a benefit.
2 Needs in demand but no supply	For example immunisation against vaccine-preventable disease where the immunisation program has not been established.
3 Demand, for services of low need, but no supply	Demand for unnecessary surgery not met by supply.
4 Adequate supply to meet priority needs, for which individuals or society will pay	Aim to maximise this zone
5 Needs and supply but no demand	Unpopular preventive measure (e.g. some types of vaccinations)
6 Supplier induced demand for low priority needs	Supply of unnecessary diagnostic services
7 Excess supply; neither need nor demand	Inappropriately located, poor quality services, or services responding to needs that have passed

The impact of different policy mixes can be considered in terms of their effect on the different zones of need, supply, and demand. The balance of social and 'private' service or policy response to needs and demand will change over time. This balance will differ between cultures, reflecting political factors relating to the power of the relevant interest groups, the contemporary economic situation of the country, history, culture, dominant 'values', and other factors (Gibson 1998). Table 1.2 (which extends a schema developed by Hacker and Marmor 1999) describes a number of dimensions on which different national health systems make different choices.

Further, there may be differences on these dimensions within a given country for different elements of the health system.

The extent to which there is mutualisation of funding is probably the critical component of system design. Mutualisation in the health sector is necessary, as health care costs can be large and unpredictable (Arrow 1963), and these are the very circumstances where insurance arrangements are the most appropriate. Mutualisation can cover the whole population for a broad range of services or it can be relatively limited (either to population segments or to a defined range of activities). Most developed countries have recognised the importance of mutualisation of funding, principally on equity

Table 1.2 Key dimensions of choice in health system design

Dimension	Explanation/Options
Mutualisation of funding (including scope; eligible population; and type of financing)	Degree to which funding is shared across consumers. Ranges from pooling across whole populations (e.g. compulsory insurance or government tax-funded provision), through part-population (e.g. voluntary insurance or targeted programs) to no insurance (individual payment). Insurance may or may not be subsidised by government.
	Also affected by the extent of co-payments (i.e. patient contribution): the greater the level of co-payment, the lower the level of mutualisation.
	Whole population pooling can be undertaken via tax-funded arrangements, compulsory 'savings' programs, or 'social insurance'. The latter two involve individuals making designated contributions to a fund pool.
	The extent of mutualisation also involves determining what is the scope of services included in a scheme or 'covered' by the insurance or other arrangements (how this is effected may vary; see the fourth point under constraints on provider choices in this table).
Service provision and administration	Choices include direct government provision or regulation/subsidy of non-government provision with a subsidiary choice of whether nongovernment providers can only be not-for-profit or whether for-profit providers are allowed.
	Administration of the program can be by a government department, separate statutory authority, or through private intermediaries.
Constraints on provider choices	The extent to which providers' choices are constrained. Options include:
	Constraint on treatment choices (a number of managed care programs in the USA limit providers in this way, through utilisation review or requirements for adherence to approved treatment protocols). Formal rules and regulations can be used, or strategies based on information including feedback about relative performance.
	Constraints on ability to charge co-payments or determine client eligibility; co-payments may be proscribed or only able to be charged in accordance with guidelines or can be provider-determined; co-payments may supplement or offset funded payments.
	Constraints on consumer prioritisation: priority setting processes may be according to specific guidelines or providers may have autonomy in prioritisation.
	Constraints on service scope: the range of funded services may effectively vary with local autonomy on scope of provision or services funded may be tightly specified.
Constraints on consumer choices	Consumers may have free choice of any (registered) provider or be limited to seek treatment/care from a subset of providers. Consumers may also be restricted in access to some services (e.g. secondary care) without prior authorisation ('gatekeeping'). The restriction may be absolute or in the form of a financial incentive (e.g. a higher rebate if prior approval has been obtained).

Table 1.2 Key dimensions of choice in health system design (cont.)

Dimension	Explanation/Options (cont.)
Risk pooling with providers	The extent to which the funder shares (cost) risk with providers. Risk pooling can be national; by state/region or specialty; in a specific plan; or by individual providers.
Payment arrangements	A variety of payment methods can be used, each creating different incentives:
	Historical/political
	Input related (e.g. number of staff, hours of provision).
	Output or volume related (normally according to a designated schedule with different prices for different types of services). Output/volume-related funding may also require specification of a volume cap. The fee schedule can be predetermined or may vary in response to bids or tenders.
	Population or 'capitation' payment, usually weighted for population attributes (e.g. age, sex).

grounds, to ensure that financial barriers do not inhibit access to needed care. However, compulsory insurance programs have also enhanced efficiency (Evans 1995). The USA is the single outstanding exception to this pattern among OECD countries. In the USA mutualisation of funding only occurs for segments of the population: the elderly under the US 'Medicare' program and the poor (as defined differentially in the different states) under the US 'Medicaid' program. Most of the rest of the American population receive health insurance cover through employment-based arrangements. This leaves a significant proportion of the American population without any form of health insurance with resulting problems in access to care.

In Australia, hospital, pharmaceutical, medical, and residential aged care services have very high degrees of mutualisation of funding while dental services, for example, are primarily funded by individuals.

The extent of mutualisation of funding does not predetermine the organisational structure of provision as there are four distinct functions within the health care system: funding, purchasing, provision, and ownership.

The purchasing function involves a range of management and policy choices which, in turn, involve decisions about four of the dimensions in table 1.2. Purchasers may make decisions on service scope (that is, what services will be within the mutualisation framework), aspects of constraining provider choices, and they may also limit the availability of providers thus constraining consumer choices. Different purchasers will structure payment arrangements and risk pooling with providers in different ways (see Hacker and Marmor 1999 for a discussion of the use of the three dimensions of constraints on provider choices, risk pooling, and constraints on consumer choices in the US context).

Chernovsky (1995) argues it is important that there are at least two separate structures involved across the broad functions of funding, purchasing ('organisation and management of care consumption' in his parlance), and provision. In particular, he argues that the structure of the system is more efficient if there is either:

- separation of funding from purchasing and provision (the most notable examples of this form of organisation are the traditional Health Maintenance Organisations in the USA); or
- funding and purchasing functions are separated from provision (commonly referred to as a purchaser–provider split, exemplified in the early 1990s structural reforms of the United Kingdom's National Health Service and New Zealand and in hospital casemix funding arrangements in most Australian states).

The identification and development of the purchasing function principally occurred from the early 1990s. Prior to then, there were few explicit efficiency constraints on consumer or provider choices in most health care systems. The evolution of the purchaser function has in part occurred because of a breakdown of an 'implicit bargain' between the medical profession and government funders that gave the medical profession autonomy in treatment policy (Evans 1995). This breakdown of the 'bargain' was a reaction to accelerated cost escalation in the health sector but also may be attributed to increasing public scepticism that the profession is able to ensure effective priority setting without some form of independent purchaser oversight.

Interventionist purchaser roles can bring risks in terms of accountability to consumers (see Rodwin 1995) and in terms of ensuring that priority setting is done with the objective of promoting high quality care rather than simply to contain costs. The more a purchasing organisation is motivated by commercial considerations, the more it risks being influenced by short-run cost containment and profit maximisation rather than goals of maximising access for patients and quality of care.

In most countries consumers are also involved in choices about health systems: at the macro level, their choices are exercised through political processes, at the micro level they make choices about providers and treatments. However, consumer choice research suggests that:

> not all consumers have choices; those that do have access to information needed to contribute to their decisions do not necessarily have the information they most want or need; consumers cannot necessarily understand or use the information they are given; consumers do not necessarily want to make certain types of decisions about their health care, preferring instead to trust knowledgeable representatives to choose for them; choices may conflict depending on who is choosing, and representatives may have conflicting forces affecting their decis-

ions that may not necessarily benefit the consumer; and health plans and providers, in particular, that are judged to be higher cost or lower quality appear to survive (at least so far).

Bernstein and Gauthier 1999, pp. 19–20

The choices that are made about each of the dimensions in table 1.2 vary within cultures and over time. This book assumes that the criteria for choice should be the impact on equity, efficiency, quality, and acceptability of the system. Inevitably there are trade-offs among these attributes. The more there are constraints on provider choices, for example, the lower will be the acceptability to providers. On the other hand, constraints on provider choices may promote efficiency and, in some cases, equity.

It is sometimes argued that equity and efficiency are intrinsically in conflict. Efficiency should be used in the economic sense of technical, allocative, and dynamic efficiency. There is little evidence that there is any trade-off between equity and efficiency in these terms. Indeed, equity is most often achieved through mutualisation of funding which has been shown to bring with it efficiency improvements (including reduced administrative costs of one funding source rather than many; see also Evans 1990b, 1995, 1997).

There may be a trade-off, however, between equity and cost containment, as providing increased access (by eliminating financial barriers) inevitably results in expanded provision, which comes at a cost. This cost has benefits and decision makers need to assess the cost–benefit trade-off. (Note that this trade-off is about cost containment or expenditure, not efficiency.)

The various choices made in health care systems also have an impact on the overall health status and access to adequate and comprehensive care for people in need. The success of the Australian health care system in this regard is discussed in chapter 2.

2

The Australian Population and its Health

Australia's population at the 2001 Census was just under 19 million people, double the 1947 population. The population aged over 65 almost trebled in this period. The population is unevenly distributed: over half (10 million) people live in a state or territory capital, or in Canberra, the national capital. The 10 biggest cities account for two-thirds of the population. Despite its image of being the great 'outback', Australia is one of the most urbanised countries in the world. New South Wales has slightly over one-third of the total population, Victoria slightly under one-quarter, Queensland about one-fifth, Western Australia about one-tenth, and the remaining states account for under one-eighth (South Australia 8 per cent, Tasmania 2 per cent, and the Northern Territory and Australian Capital Territory 1 per cent each).

The age–gender composition of the population is a very important determinant of utilisation of health services. For example, children between five and 14 years of age use far fewer hospital days than the aged (75+ years). Gender is also an important determinant. In the younger age groups, females tend to have much higher hospitalisation rates, partly because of maternity admissions. At older ages, males have higher rates of hospitalisation. Age and gender also influence utilisation of other health services. Since use of the health care system varies considerably between age and gender groups, analysis of population utilisation patterns must take into account age and gender composition.

The health of Australians

'How are you?' and 'How are you going?' are probably the most commonly asked questions in Australia. Although they normally do not elicit detailed information on the health status of the respondents, they do illustrate a concern with our health.

There are many different ways in which health can be conceptualised. Traditionally, health has been defined by its obverse, namely the absence of disease or disability. Larson (1999) described this approach as the 'medical model' because it ignores factors related to social well-being. A further weakness is that one can have a disease without being ill, if the disease is at the pre-symptomatic stage.

The most commonly used definition of health is that of the WHO, adopted in 1947: 'health is a state of complete physical, mental and social well-being and not merely the absence of disease or infirmity'. While the breadth of this definition serves a useful political end in drawing attention to the positive nature of health, that same breadth may handicap measurement and, in turn, accountability for moving towards improvement in health status.

In 2001 the WHO introduced a new system for classifying health status known as the International Classification of Functioning, Disability and Health, or ICF (WHO 2001). The conceptual framework of the ICF is a useful advance in that it facilitates recording of all factors that impact on functioning. The ICF includes systems for classifying body functions (such as voice functions, heart functions) and body structures (such as the eye, endocrine system). The classification system allows assignment of 'qualifiers' (ranging from zero for none to four for complete) to indicate whether a person has an impairment in either body function or structure. The classification system also includes systems for classifying activities and participation (such as communication, self-care). Again qualifiers record the extent of difficulty in activity or participation.

An important contribution of the ICF is that it also provides a classification for environmental factors (such as products or technology, attitudes, services) that can either be barriers or facilitators. This element of the ICF thus highlights that the effects of impairment are in part the result of factors within a person's environment and that the environment can be modified. The ICF does not adopt a 'sickness' or 'medical model' of classification, but rather attempts to focus on the whole person, the consequences of their impairment in functioning and the environmental factors that impact on them.

The main source of information on health status is population-based, household interview surveys, the most recent such survey in Australia being the Australian Health Survey 2001 (ABS 2002). Although data on illness (or 'morbidity') can be obtained from hospital or general practice records, these sources do not provide information on population patterns (incidence or prevalence) of disease, as only those who use health services are captured in the data.

Information from population surveys also conveys only a partial picture of health. Broadhead (1985, 1987) highlighted some of the relevant issues in his analysis of an earlier Australian Health Survey. Apart from problems relating to the validity of the data (for example can people accurately recall what was happening to their health last week, or is person A's perception the same as person B's), Broadhead notes that the conceptualisation (and hence interpretation) of health interview surveys is confused. Citing Twaddle's distinction between disease, illness, and sickness (Twaddle 1980), Broadhead argues that health interview surveys can only be used to analyse illness (subjective, self-identified dimensions of non-health) and sickness (the social dimension; the consequences of the decisions of society). Health interview surveys cannot provide information on disease that is a biologically defined and measured entity. Thus interview survey data need to be complemented by data from other sources to provide a complete picture of a population's health. It is also important to be clear about the source of health data in order to understand its strengths and limitations.

Overview of health status in the community

In broad terms, the Australian population rates its health highly: over 80 per cent of adults in the 2001 survey reported good to excellent health. Table 2.1 summarises key data on health status for 2001.

Table 2.1 Summary of the health of the Australian population, 2001

Overall evaluation of health	81.2 per cent of adults aged 18 years and over reported their health was good, very good or excellent
Long-term conditions	78 per cent were experiencing a long-term condition (six months or more)
	The prevalence of long-term conditions varied with age:
	0–14 years 43.5 per cent
	15–24 years 71.0 per cent
	25–34 years 78.0 per cent
	35–44 years 84.7 per cent
	45–54 years 96.0 per cent
	55–64 years 99.0 per cent
	65–74 years 99.4 per cent
	75 and over 99.0 per cent
	The most common long-term conditions were: long or short-sighted (29.7 per cent of population); back pain (20.8 per cent); hayfever (15.5 per cent); asthma (11.6 per cent)

Source: ABS 2002

Despite the relatively high ranking of reported health, 78 per cent of the population (females 79 per cent, males 76 per cent) experienced a long-term condition, some of which were easily rectifiable (for example, the eyesight conditions experienced by about 30 per cent of the population are largely rectifiable by glasses).

As would be expected, illness increased with age. Even young adults (25 to 34 years old) reported high levels (78 per cent) of long-term conditions. Over 95 per cent of the population over 45 report some form of illness.

Mortality

It is ironic that early measures of 'health' status were based on death. This was primarily because deaths have had to be recorded for legal reasons. The availability of mortality statistics, the complexity of collecting alternative health measures, and the relative absence of definitional problems have led to the widespread use of these data. Often underpinning the use of mortality statistics is the questionable assumption that death is a good surrogate indicator of health; that mortality moves in the same direction as morbidity or disability (see Murray et al. 2002 for a review and critique of various summary measures of health status).

The simplest statistic used to compare mortality is the crude death rate: the number of deaths (in a given time interval) per 1000 population. Because death rates vary substantially with age, it is more appropriate to use age (or age and gender) standardised death rates or a standardised mortality ratio (SMR) defined as the death rate of the population group under study relative to the population average. Another summary measure used for comparison is life expectancy (at birth or some later date, such as 65 years of age). Figure 2.1 shows the historical trends in life expectancy for Australia.

Newborn Australians can now expect to live just over twenty years

Figure 2.1 Australia: Trend in life expectancy (years) by gender, 1881–2000

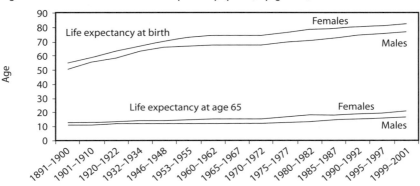

Source: Office of the Australian Government Actuary, 1995 and ABS 1999e

longer than those born a century ago (22 years longer for males, 24 years for females); at age 65, males have on average an additional six years of life, females, eight years. Life expectancy has steadily increased since the last century for all age and both gender groups, but the increase has been much greater for females. A century ago a newly born girl could expect to live about four years longer than her brother. The 65-year-old woman could expect to live to 78, a year-and-a-half longer than her brother. By the early 1990s, the female–male gap at birth was six years, with the woman expecting to live to 80. The life expectancy gap at 65 is now five years.

The 1950s and 1960s saw little increase in life expectancy. However, as shown in figure 2.1, beginning in the early 1970s there was a resurgence in the improvement in life expectancy. The all cause standardised death rate was 689.3 per 100,000 population in 1991 (885.1 for males, 537.3 for females); the rate declined to 542.2 in 2001 (680.8 for males, 430.0 for females). Improvements in mortality rates occurred across almost all causes (for example circulatory declining from 306.7 to 197.5; neoplasms from 182.9 to 165.1).

In international terms, the life expectancy of Australians is comparable to that of residents in other developed countries (see table 2.2).

Table 2.2   Comparative expectation of life (years), selected countries, 2000

Country	At birth, total population	At 65, females	At 65, males
Australia	79.3	20.4	16.9
Austria	78.3	19.6	16.2
Belgium	77.7	19.5	15.5
Canada	79.4	20.5	16.9
Czech Republic	75.1	17.1	13.7
Hungary	71.5	16.3	12.6
Japan	81.2	22.4	17.5
Mexico	74.1	18.3	16.8
Netherlands	78.0	19.2	15.3
New Zealand	78.3	19.8	16.4
Norway	78.7	19.7	16.0
Poland	73.8	17.3	13.6
Slovak Republic	73.3	16.5	12.9
Turkey	68.1	14.2	12.6
United Kingdom	77.8	18.9	15.6
USA	76.8	19.2	16.3

Data Source: OECD 2003

In 2000, residents of most developed countries could expect to live around 80 years (slightly longer in Japan, about 77 years in the USA) and females to live about 20 years at age 65. Former Eastern Bloc countries have a life expectancy at birth about five years shorter than the rest of Europe. There have been significant shifts over the last 40 years. Life expectancy at birth is now over 20 years longer in Japan than it was in 1961; Australian life expectancy is about eight years longer, and this is the pattern in a number of other countries (Canada, Austria, New Zealand, the United Kingdom). Life expectancy in the former Eastern Bloc countries has increased about three years over this period.

Causes of death

Figure 2.2 shows the principal causes of death in 2001.

Almost 40 per cent of deaths are associated with circulatory disorders with just over a quarter of all deaths being associated with cancer. No other cause of death accounts for more than 10 per cent of mortality.

The principal causes of death vary substantially with age; for example, transport accidents account for over one-third of the deaths of males in the 15- to 24-year-old group, and is the leading cause of death for this group (see table 2.3). In later age groups, the so-called 'degenerative diseases' predominate. Causes of death also vary with gender, the most notable distinction being the different patterns of suicide ('intentional self-harm') between males and females of all ages.

Figure 2.2 Australia: Cause of death by diagnostic category, 2001

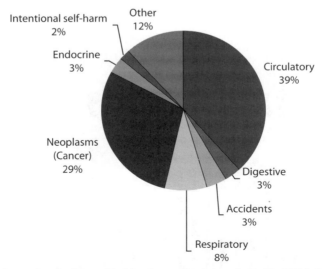

Data Source: Australian Bureau of Statistics, *Causes of Death, Australia*, Cat. No. 3303.0, Canberra: ABS

Table 2.3 Australia: Death rates(a) by selected underlying cause of death by gender by age at death

		Age Group									
Cause of Death	Gender	Under 1 year(b)	1–14 years	15–24 years	25–44 years	45–54 years	55–64 years	65-74 years	75-84 years	85 years and over	Total(c) and over
Malignant neoplasms	Males	—	4	5	20	105	366	968	1848	3008	208
Malignant neoplasms	Females	—	2	4	23	108	253	565	981	1489	127
Ischaemic heart diseases	Males	—	0	0	11	58	169	488	1359	3974	141
Ischaemic heart diseases	Females	—	—	0	2	11	46	206	837	3330	78
Cerebrovascular diseases	Males	—	0	0	2	10	31	127	542	1959	50
Cerebrovascular diseases	Females	—	0	0	2	7	20	92	481	2137	45
Chronic lower respiratory diseases	Males	—	0	1	2	4	26	142	404	863	35
Chronic lower respiratory diseases	Females	—	0	0	1	5	24	92	190	322	19
Transport accidents	Males	—	4	30	18	13	13	17	23	32	16
Transport accidents	Females	—	2	8	5	5	6	6	10	15	5
Diabetes mellitus	Males	—	—	0	2	8	21	66	160	366	17
Diabetes mellitus	Females	—	—	0	1	4	12	38	107	251	10
Intentional self-harm	Males	—	0	20	32	23	19	20	23	32	20
Intentional self-harm	Females	—	0	5	8	8	5	5	5	7	5
Diseases of the nervous system	Males	0	2	3	4	8	17	52	180	554	19
Diseases of the nervous system	Females	0	2	2	3	7	13	42	138	534	16
All causes	Males	6	19	83	135	304	812	2279	5992	16032	681
All causes	Females	5	13	30	65	191	461	1309	3829	12981	430
All causes	Persons	5	16	57	100	248	638	1778	4735	13920	542

(a) Deaths per 100,000 of the estimated mid-year population for each age group used to calculate age-specific death rates other than for age Under 1 year and for Total all ages (b) For age group under 1 year, deaths per 1000 live births used to calculate infant death rates. (c) For total all ages: standardised death rate per 100,000 of the mid-year 1991 population.

Source: ABS special tabulation

Figure 2.3 Australia: Causes of potential years of life lost to age 75, by diagnostic category, 2001

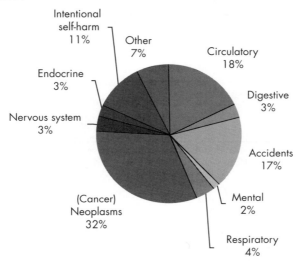

Intentional
self-harm
11%

Other
7%

Circulatory
18%

Endocrine
3%

Digestive
3%

Nervous system
3%

Accidents
17%

(Cancer)
Neoplasms
32%

Mental
2%

Respiratory
4%

Source: Australian Bureau of Statistics, *Causes of Death, Australia*, Cat. No. 3303.0, Canberra: ABS

Table 2.3 also reveals the substantial variation in death rates by age: the death rate for 15- to 24-year-old males is about 10 per cent that for 55- to 64-year-old men. Similar variations occur for women.

One way of combining information on death rates and age at death is to calculate potential years of life lost: the death of a 20-year-old results in more years lost than the death of a 65-year-old. Potential years of life lost (PYLL) is usually calculated as being years lost up to age 75 (PYLL 75). The pattern of causes for potential years of life lost is quite different from causes of mortality (figure 2.3).

Cancer (neoplasms) is the leading contributor to potential years of life lost, accounting for approximately the same proportion of potential years of life lost as deaths. Because deaths from circulatory disorders mostly occur in older age groups, circulatory disorders account for a much lower proportion of potential years of life lost (18 per cent) than of deaths (39 per cent). Conversely accidents and intentional self-harm, with a higher relative incidence in younger age groups, account for a much higher proportion of potential years of life lost (17 and 11 per cent respectively) than of deaths (4 and 2 per cent).

There have been notable changes in cause-specific mortality in the last hundred years (Taylor et al. 1998). One of the great scourges of the nineteenth and early twentieth centuries was infectious diseases, which were then one of the major causes of death. Figure 2.4 shows the trend in the death rate from infectious diseases in Australia from 1921.

It can be seen that there has been a significant reduction in the infectious diseases death rate over the course of the twentieth century, with a steady

Figure 2.4 Australia: Age–sex standardised death rate from infectious diseases, 1921–2001

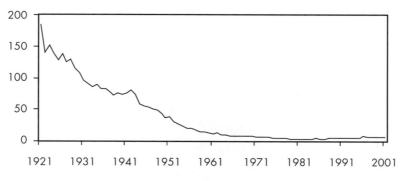

Source: ABS 1997a and later editions

decline from the 1920s to the mid 1970s. The death rate from infectious diseases was stable at around four deaths per 1000 from the early 1980s to the mid 1990s, increasing to about eight deaths per 1000 in 1996, partly due to deaths from HIV. The decline in the infectious diseases death rate in Australia follows the same pattern as in the USA and the United Kingdom (McKinlay and McKinlay 1977), with most of the decline preceding the development of penicillin and most vaccines, highlighting the contribution of other public health measures, particularly sanitary reform.

The most significant other change in mortality has been the emergence and subsequent abatement of the 'epidemic of circulatory disease mortality'. According to Taylor et al. (1998, p. 41): 'This epidemic appears to commence during the mid 1920s and increases rapidly to the mid 1950s ... then flattens until 1970 ... with rapid falls in mortality in both sexes after that date.' There is a similar pattern in trends for cerebrovascular disease (stroke), with mortality rates peaking around 1970 (Dunn et al. 2002). The death rate from lung cancer in males peaked somewhat later, around the mid 1970s, with female death rates still rising (Dunn et al. 2002). This pattern reflects the lagged effect of smoking take up and quitting.

Burden of disease

'Burden of disease' is a measure that brings together cause-specific mortality, in the form of potential years of life lost, and disability attributable to particular conditions (years of life lived with disability). This measure is increasingly being used to aid priority setting. The combination of years of life lost and years of life lived with a disability is called 'Disability Adjusted Life Years' (DALYs). The original studies for burden of disease based the mortality component on (premature) years of life lost to age 75 (Murray and Lopez

1996; see also Paalman et al. 1998 for a critique of the methodology). The Australian burden of disease is based on life expectancy for the cohort alive in 1996 with no upper age limit cut-off; for example, the effect of potential years of life lost for people who die after age 75 is incorporated in DALY calculations based on life expectancy at 75 for that cohort (Mathers et al. 1999).

Several assumptions are involved in measuring the burden of disease, including the extent to which there should be discounting for deaths at very young ages. There is also controversy about whether the burden of disease measure is relevant at all (see Mooney et al. 1997 and Williams 1999a, who argue that the relevant criterion for priority setting is an economic one of the marginal benefit that can be achieved from an intervention relative to marginal cost; see also Butler 1999 for an alternative view).

Figure 2.5 shows Australia's burden of disease for 1996 by major cause, identifying the relative contribution attributable to fatality and that caused by years lived with a (serious) disability. The leading causes of DALYs are cardiovascular disorders and cancer, both accounting for around 20 per cent of all DALYs. Mental disorders account for about one-eighth of DALYs. Mental disorders enter with a significant impact on burden of disease in Australia principally because of their non-fatal impact on people in terms of years lived with a disability. Although overall about half of DALYs are attributable to premature mortality, this fatality ratio varies across disease groups. For cardiovascular disease and cancer, over 80 per cent of the DALYs are attributable to premature

Figure 2.5 Australia: Burden of Disease separated into years of life lost (YLL) and years lived with a disability (YLD), 1996

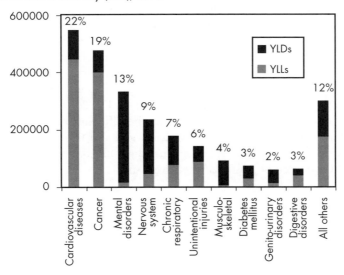

Data Source: Mathers et al 1999

Figure 2.6 Australia: Proportion of total burden of disease attributed to selected risk factors, by gender, 1996

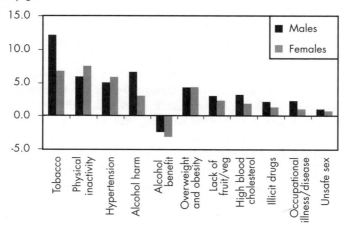

Data Source: Mathers et al 1999

mortality. Not surprisingly, these two conditions also rate highly in terms of the simpler statistics of causes of mortality and premature years of life lost. On the other hand, only 5 per cent of DALYs for mental disorders are attributable to premature mortality. The fatality contribution to total DALYs is 20 per cent for nervous system and sense disorders. Musculoskeletal (8 per cent) and genito-urinary disorders (24 per cent) are other conditions with low fatality contributions. The burden of disease thus presents a very different set of conditions for priority setting relative to the simpler, mortality-focused approaches.

The Australian Burden of Disease study also presents information on the burden of disease attributable to selected risk factors (see figure 2.6).

The mode of presentation in figure 2.6 is based on traditional risk factors rather than what might be underlying causal social or environmental factors. The leading risk factor is tobacco, accounting for about 12.5 per cent of total DALYs in males and about 7 per cent of DALYs for females. The burden of disease presentation also includes the differential effect of alcohol both in terms of its potential to cause harm and also the effect of alcohol consumption in moderation. It is seen that the contribution of illicit drugs to the DALY burden in Australia is relatively small.

Health expectancies

Life expectancy in Australia has been increasing steadily. A critical factor affecting health services and the population is the extent to which this increase in life expectancy is associated with additional years of healthy life or whether the additional years of life gained are associated with disabilities.

Figure 2.7 Australia: Trends in health expectancies by gender, 1981–98

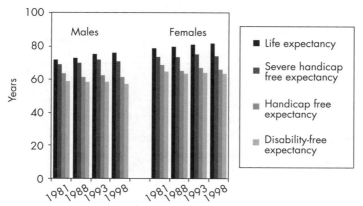

Data Source: Mathers 1999

There is now substantial international literature projecting 'health expectancies', the expectation of healthy life. Major research in this area has been undertaken by Mathers at the Australian Institute of Health and Welfare (for example, Mathers and Robine 1998; Davis et al. 1999; Mathers et al. 2003). Figure 2.7, derived from Mathers 1999, shows the trends in health expectancies at birth over the period 1981 to 1998.

The data points in this graph are the years of the Australian Disability Survey, the most recent of which was in 1998 (ABS 1999b). It can be seen that life expectancy has increased by three years for females and four-and-a-half years for males over the period 1981 to 1998, while disability-free life expectancy has declined for both males and females. About half to two-thirds of the increase in life expectancy entails a period of severe handicap. This trend of increasing severely handicapped expectancy is also apparent in the figures for trends in health expectancy at age 65.

In most OECD (Organization for Economic Cooperation and Development) countries increasing life expectancy has principally been associated with an increase in disability-free expectancy and relatively small increases in severe handicap. The Australian data are thus anomalous and the increase in reported severe expectancy may be artefactual because of changing ways in which questions were asked in the Australian Disability Survey, and changing attitudes to reporting disability rather than a change in the underlying rate of disability (Mathers 1999; Davis et al. 2001). However, if the trend is confirmed in future surveys, this could have a significant impact on demand for health care services (Giles et al. 2003).

Although there have been concerns about the future impact of ageing on health care costs (see National Commission of Audit 1996), more sophisticated studies have shown that ageing accounts for a relatively small proportion of the increased cost in services in recent years (see Richardson and Robertson 1999).

Table 2.4   Australia: Ratio of rate of long-term reported chronic conditions in lowest social status group compared to rate in highest group, 2001

	Asthma	Diabetes mellitus	Malignant neoplasms	Diseases of circulatory system	Arthritis
Household income	1.15	4.23	2.63	2.35	3.35
Index of (geographic) socioeconomic disadvantage	1.08	2.21	1.09	1.43	1.59
Education	1.05	1.29	1.44	1.27	1.44

Data Source: ABS 2002

Equity and ill health

Illness and sickness are unevenly distributed in the population with people in lower socioeconomic status groups experiencing more ill health (McClelland and Scotton 1998; House 2001) and these socioeconomic differences appear to be worsening (Hayes et al. 2002). Walker and Abello (2000) have shown that people on low income report, on average, 40 to 50 per cent more long-term conditions than the rest of the population, while Korda et al. (2002) have shown that, among working adults, professionals had the best self-reported health and blue collar workers, the worst. Table 2.4 shows data from the latest National Health Survey on reported long-term chronic conditions.

It can be seen that for all conditions, people in the lowest social status classification reported higher prevalence, with the household income measure showing particularly strong effects. Mathers (1994) used three measures of class to measure any differences: occupation, education, and income. Moderate (but statistically significant) gradients were found in each case, with the steepest gradients in the sickness (days of reduced activity) rather than the illness measures (recent illness, chronic condition).

In recent Australian studies, Morrell et al. (1998) have shown a strong association between unemployment and ill health, as have Mathers and Schofield (1998). The direction and mechanisms of causation of the socioeconomic effect are complex but in a comprehensive literature review, Jin et al. (1997) have concluded that there is sufficient evidence to say that unemployment causes ill health, a conclusion supported by Mathers and Schofield.

Mortality data show the same gradient as health status, with Lawson and Black (1993) arguing that it is 'by far the most important indicator of premature death for Australian males'. McMichael (1985, p. 220) has noted, for example, that 'Social class has a broad and substantial influence upon health status and risk of disease. The occurrence of congenital malformations, stillbirths, infant mortality, death rates for specific diseases in childhood, and childhood accident and injury rates are all correlated with social class. In adulthood, accidents and injuries, chronic diseases, and total and cause-specific mortality all show strong social class gradients'.

Taylor et al. (1992) have found similar mortality gradients in a study of Sydney local government areas, as have Siskind et al. (1992) in Brisbane, and Burnley (1997) for premature cancer mortality.

In their analysis of occupational mortality, Najman and Congalton (1979) considered whether these differences in mortality rates between occupational groups was better explained by occupation-specific factors or more general factors. First, one could assume that specific work-related events may be associated with specific variation in disease rates. The data do not support this interpretation. As Najman and Congalton point out, 'occupations with high mortality rates tend to have high rates of death from numerous ostensibly different causes'. The alternative interpretation, of 'general susceptibility', was thus favoured. Following this view, they posited that either some occupations involve higher levels of stress (and hence higher mortality for a range of reasons) or 'a combination of more specific hazards or general life style factors characteristic of persons in these occupational groups may explain the mortality variation'.

The mortality variations may be in part due to variations in treatment. Cass et al. (2003), in a study using a geographic measure of disadvantage, found 'marked variations in the proportion of end stage renal disease patients in Australian capital cities who were referred late to nephrologists'. The National Health and Medical Research Council (NH&MRC) has recognised the potential impact of socioeconomic position on each stage of the treatment pathway (susceptibility and prevention, diagnosis, treatment, rehabilitation) by recommending that explicit consideration of social factors be incorporated into guideline development (NH&MRC 2003; this publication also includes reviews of the way in which socioeconomic position impacts on the treatment pathway).

These trends present a challenge to the conventional wisdom of Australia as an egalitarian society: with life chances so dramatically affected by occupation and socioeconomic status, it is hard to argue that all Australians are getting a 'fair go'.

Figure 2.8 Australia: Rate ratio of age-specific death rates, Indigenous versus non-Indigenous population by gender, 1997–99

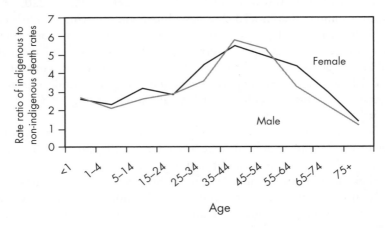

Data Source: ABS 2001

Health of Indigenous Australians

The health of Aboriginal and Torres Strait Islander people is significantly worse than other Australians. Figure 2.8 shows rate ratios of age-specific death rates for the Aboriginal and Torres Strait Islander and non-Indigenous populations.

It can be seen that for most ages, the Indigenous population had an age-standardised death rate at least twice the non-Indigenous population, with a male Indigenous person aged 35 to 44 almost six times more likely to die than a non-Indigenous male of the same age. The same trends are reflected in differences in self-reported health status, recent illnesses, and long-term conditions. Although infant mortality rates per 1000 live births for Aboriginal populations are declining, they are still three times greater than for non-Aboriginal Australians (Mathews 1997). Birth weights for Aboriginal infants are considerably lower than for non-Aboriginal infants.

The causes of the poor Aboriginal health status should not simply be viewed as issues of contemporary lifestyle. Nor are they amenable to a quick-fix change based on improving health services or public health, although these components are a necessary part of any strategy to improve health status. As Mathews (1997) and others (Saggers and Gray 1991; Hunter 1993; Bartlett and Legge 1994) point out, the genesis of problems in Aboriginal health is complex and lies in the dispossession and alienation of the Aboriginal population from their land, caused by colonisation (see figure 2.9).

Colonisation has caused spiritual harm through the loss of traditional lands. However, it has also caused a loss of the traditional hunter-gatherer lifestyle and exposure to the adverse social and health effects of contemporary white society,

Figure 2.9 Historical impacts of white society on Aboriginal culture

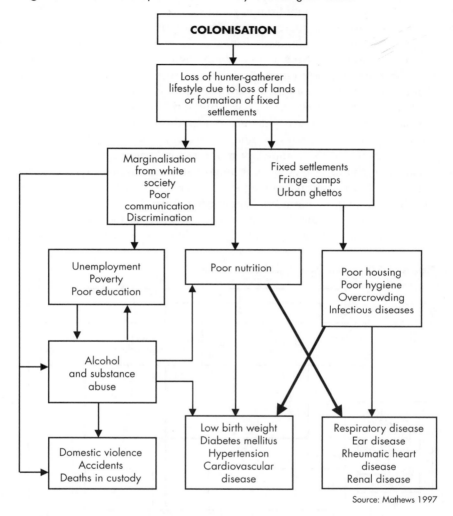

Source: Mathews 1997

resulting in alcoholism, violence, and so on. The loss of the hunter–gatherer lifestyle leads, via a series of intermediate factors, to impacts on health status. Addressing these problems requires working with Aboriginal communities to set priorities for rebuilding Aboriginal and Torres Strait Islander societies.

Health care and health status

Identifying deficiencies in the health status of Australians does not necessarily imply that more health services are required. Indeed, McKinlay and McKinlay

(1977) have argued that medicine and its magic bullets cannot claim the credit for the decline in mortality from infectious diseases in the last century. They demonstrate that it was improved housing, nutrition and so on, as well as other aspects of the social environment, that led to the improvements in health status and reduced mortality. Szreter (1988, 1995) disputes this explanation, arguing that public health interventions, including the work of local authorities, can claim most of the credit for the decline in mortality.

McKinlay et al. (1989) have also advanced the argument that the decline in deaths from the modern epidemics of heart disease and cancer are also not attributable to the successes of modern medicine. Jackson (1985, p. 3) has drawn attention to the complexity of the factors that affect health: 'While behavioural choice or lifestyle is an important factor in determining health status, the choices available to the individual are promoted or constrained by the physical, socioeconomic and family environment'.

Recognition of the interdependence of these factors has important consequences for health planners: it makes little sense to talk about some

Figure 2.10 The creation of health and disease

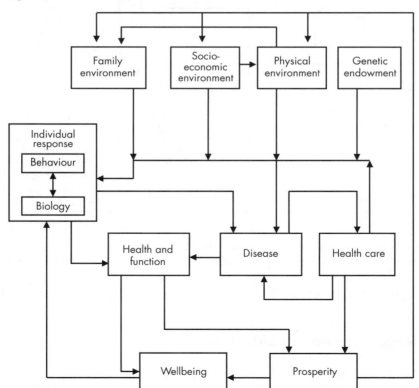

diseases being caused by 'lifestyles' and consequently blame or harass the victim for his or her previous choices (this issue is discussed further in chapter 7).

The interaction of health care and health status is extremely complex, despite the media portrayal, which suggests that all diseases and illnesses can be cured with a magic bullet or a magic scalpel. There are still many conditions for which there is no cure. Further, the media (often citing government or other experts) also presents a relatively simplistic view of how ill health is created. The impression conveyed is that ill health is probably the result of individual 'lifestyle' choices ('individual responsibility') or because of preventable accidents and injuries. However, the factors that affect health and health status are multi-faceted and interactive (see figure 2.10, based on Evans and Stoddart 1990 and modified to take account of the arguments advanced by Jackson 1985).

The top row in the diagram indicates that there are four major factors that impact on health status: family environment, socioeconomic environment, physical environment, and genetic endowment. A person's genetic endowment has an independent and direct effect on an individual. The developments of human genomics (Collins 1999) are increasing our understanding of the impact of genetic factors on health, and genetic factors associated with a range of chronic conditions are now being identified.

All of the four factors in the top row can have an impact on individuals, creating a direct biological response (an illness or disease) or a change in behaviour including health-related actions. For example, the physical environment can have a direct impact on an individual through a lightning strike. However, Jackson (1985) has drawn attention to the limitations of the mono-causal paradigm, highlighting the fact that health is not simply caused by a single factor in the environment or a single behaviour impacting on health. She also argues that conceiving of the creation of ill health as being simply a combination of multiple independent factors such as the environment, behaviour, and hereditary or genetic factors (as postulated in the famous Lalonde (1974) report) is inadequate. Rather, health problems are caused by a complex interaction of factors in the physical, socioeconomic, and family environments, and by individual behaviour. These factors are interdependent, as families and the socioeconomic environment shape behaviour, and the impact of the physical environment is mediated either by the socioeconomic environment or the family (for example, the physical environment may determine food choices but these are generally mediated through culture and family).

A second factor affecting health is the socioeconomic environment. In the Evans and Stoddart (1990) paper this is referred to as the social environment, and includes the work environment (affecting occupationally related conditions), and the school environment (including, for example the effect of peer pressure to smoke). The importance of economic factors in determining health status has been widely recognised. For example, as was shown earlier in this chapter, there are higher rates of illness among lower income households, and in the unemployed compared to the employed. Coburn (2003) has argued that economic globalisation acts to diminish social cohesion and increase income inequalities, which together impact adversely on health and well-being. The political environment is an important component of the socioeconomic environment, not only because political choices might affect systems of health care (Navarro and Shi 2001), but also because of possible direct links between the political environment and health outcomes such as suicide (Page et al. 2002). Finally, the family environment obviously has a critical impact on the health behaviour and health status of an individual. Marriage, for example, has been found to have a protective effect for men but the opposite for women.

The individual's response to factors in his or her environment may lead to diseases and could also have an impact on the health and function of the individual. Functional outcomes are often measured in terms of sickness, such as days of reduced activity, but there can also be positive effects of the environment, for example from participation in social groups in the community, which lead to building up resilience (Antonovsky 1993). The individual's health and function can also have a direct impact on his or her well-being, as well as an indirect effect through their perception of well-being. These both, in turn, affect an individual's prosperity. There is also obviously a link between prosperity and well-being and from well-being to the individual (improved well-being is associated with improved health).

Figure 2.10 also traces the role of health care, which may lead to cure of the disease with a direct impact on an individual, or may lead to a cycle of repeated use of health care services. Improving health care will also impact positively on prosperity, which in turn has an impact on the physical, socioeconomic, and family environment.

Figure 2.10 thus shows the complexity of the interactions involved in the creation of health and disease. Recognition of the complexity of the underlying issues associated with health and disease leads one to question whether measures of the health of the population should simply focus on disease-based measures, or whether we should also be paying more attention to self-perceptions of well-being as incorporated in the SF-36 (short form, 36 questions) National Health Survey, and measures of socioeconomic status, social attachment and cohesion, and the range of non-individual factors that play a role.

Designers of health promotion programs need to take account of the fact that an individual does not function in social isolation but their behaviour and biology are affected by the family environment, socioeconomic environment, and so on. Victim-blaming strategies in health promotion that ignore these factors are bound to have little impact on health status (Crawford 1977). Finally, health care professionals need to recognise that they (and their work) are situated in this broader context, and that health care is but one of the factors that has an impact on disease.

3

Financing Health Care

Health expenditure and health financing policies are rarely off the policy agenda. Health expenditure consumes about 9.3 per cent of Gross Domestic Product (GDP) in Australia, and is a significant proportion of both Commonwealth and state government outlays. With expenditures of this size, health financing is inevitably going to remain a significant policy issue. Understanding the sources and application of expenditure in the health sector facilitates understanding of policy debates and decisions. Australia's health financing system is quite complex, involving provision through public and private sectors. It is further complicated by the involvement of multiple professions and institutions, all of which operate within a federal system.

Critical variables that are often the focus of attention in health policy include the share of health care finance that is met from the public sector and the rate of growth of public or total health expenditure. The desirability (or otherwise) of change in these variables is usually argued on the basis of ideology and self-interest rather than economic analysis. The desirability of a particular rate of growth of health expenditure should only be assessed in terms of the competing use of those funds. For example, if an additional dollar of expenditure in the health sector yields more value to the community than an additional dollar of spending in another sector, then the health expenditure is justified, regardless of the contemporary level of expenditure, its rate of growth, or whether the additional dollar is paid from public or private sources. Additional investment in the health sector may lead to improved economic productivity, which in turn may lead to improved export performance and so on. At the more micro level, employment of additional nurses in the community (at a given cost) may lead to improved immunisation rates, which has a benefit through reduction in disease and suffering in children, but may also lead to improved productivity. It is the ratio of costs to benefits for additional health spending that is the critical variable of policy interest from an economic efficiency perspective. From this perspective, if the ratio of benefits to costs for additional spending in the health sector is better than in other sectors, then the spending is worthwhile.

Similar issues apply when determining the appropriate relative public and private share. Increasing the private share of health expenditure has recently come to be seen as the holy grail of health policy, paraphrasing George Orwell, 'public spending bad, private spending good'. However, there is no intrinsic reason why public spending is worse than private spending; indeed, public financing may be preferred over private financing because of market failure or on equity grounds (Musgrove 1999).

Government performs a number of essential roles in the health system. Davis and Ashton (2001) have suggested six key roles for government that impact on the health sector:

- Establishment of a legal framework for society and the health system including the regulation of private hospitals and public health regulation. This is part of the governance role described in chapter 1.
- Maintenance of law and order and enforcement of regulations including those made by professional regulatory bodies.
- Redistribution of income. A principal instrument here is the use of progressive taxation so that people on higher incomes pay a higher proportion of income for governmental functions than people on lower incomes.
- As a provider of health care services.
- Regulation to ensure consumer protection and promotion of public health; examples include fire regulations, and fair trading controls such as developed by the Australian Consumer and Competition Commission and state fair trading bodies. (This function might also be justified because of market failure.)
- Intervention in the marketplace for reasons of market failure.

The last three roles are all related to 'market failure'. According to economic theory, the market is normally the most efficient way of allocating resources. Under standard market assumptions, consumers have a free choice of purchasing a good or service and their valuation of the good/service is reflected by what they are prepared to pay. Consumers' wishes or demands are thus deemed to be met through the market mechanism. Markets ensure that two of the key criteria for evaluating systems (efficiency and acceptability) are automatically fulfilled. Of course, the market is not usually an equitable way of distributing resources and equity is a third important goal in Australian health policy. However, for markets to work properly certain key underlying assumptions need to be met. Where those assumptions are not met, market failure occurs and governments ought to intervene in the allocation of goods and services, as the market will not be an efficient allocator of resources. The health sector is characterised by a number of examples of market failure and hence government intervention by either regulation or subsidy is appropriate.

There are five key reasons why markets might fail in allocating some health goods and services (see Cohen and Henderson 1988). First, markets assume that the buyers and sellers have perfect information. This is clearly not so, and providers in the health sector, almost by definition, have a greater level of information than consumers because of the providers' training or expertise (see Arrow 1963). This 'information asymmetry' means that consumers most often have to rely on providers to advise them about what health care they 'need'. Some producers may withhold information about the characteristics (such as contents) of their products (ownership interest in a private hospital, for example), so consumers are not able to weigh up the advice they are being given, and thus make a fully informed choice when purchasing the product.

A second assumption of markets that is often violated in the health sector relates to 'externalities'. The operation of markets assumes that the costs and benefits of both production and consumption fall in the same place. This is often not the case: in the absence of government intervention, manu-facturing companies might find it profitable to dispose of wastes into waterways thus polluting the environment; that is, to transfer some of the costs of their production to other producers or consumers. One of the policy responses to this is to develop 'polluter pays' policies or fines to ensure that, if there is pollution, there is a cost to the producer for that. Similarly, policies to reduce the prevalence of passive smoking are designed to ensure that smokers do not cause costs of smoking to fall on other consumers.

A third situation that leads to markets being an inappropriate way of allo-cating health resources is associated with the inherent characteristics of some health care goods. In particular, some aspects of health care (such as prov-ision of medical care) are regarded as a 'merit goods', that is, they are considered to be 'meritorious' so that society benefits by provision over and above the benefit which would be ordinarily provided in the market. Thus members of a society benefit from seeing that other members have adequate access to medical care. Of course, societies may judge various components of the health care system differentially in terms of having characteristics of 'merit goods'. In Australia, there is very strong support for government intervention in ensuring that hospital and medical services are available to all consumers, but there is not such a strong consensus that routine dental care ought to be freely available, and hence one can assume that dentistry is not yet perceived as having the characteristics of a 'merit good'.

Fourth, economics identifies certain goods as being 'public goods'. Markets assume that goods allocated in the market have two characteristics: rivalness and excludability. The assumption of rivalness means that if a consumer consumes a good, it is not available to be consumed by another person. Excludability means that it is possible to exclude consumers from consumption of a particular product. Some aspects of health care, especially public health, do not exhibit these characteristics. The most obvious is the consumption of unpolluted air, as consumption of air by one person does not stop another person consuming it, and similarly, it is almost impossible to exclude anyone from consumption of air. Other examples may be provision of health information on billboards. The absence of excludability or rivalness means that there is no effective mechanism for a market to operate in these areas.

Finally, markets assume that there are many buyers and many sellers and that there are no imperfections on either the supply or the demand side. But competition does not operate perfectly in the health care market. For example, there are barriers to entry to many of the professions in the form of long training requirements. To the extent that free competition among potential suppliers of health care is not operating, the benefit of market allocations will not accrue.

Not every element of the health sector is characterised by these examples of market failure. Government intervention in the health market can be justified for some segments of the health system on the basis of different sources of market failure. Further, as argued earlier, economic efficiency is not the only grounds for government intervention, and pursuit of equity may require government intervention. In Australia, for example, public funding of health care leads to the following redistributive effects:
- from those who have relatively short lives to those who have relatively long lives
- from the affluent to the poorer
- from those without children to those with larger families
- from men to women (Harding et al. 2002).

It is sometimes argued that increasing private spending in order to reduce public spending is inherently a 'good thing' because it allows increased consumer choice and reduced taxes. However, the arguments for this position become quite muddied because advocates of increased private spending are usually from wealthier groups and this advocacy often disguises a redistributive intent from the poor who are more reliant on tax-funded services to the rich, who benefit more from reduced taxation (Evans 1997).

The relative balance of health expenditure between hospital and preventive services is also the subject of policy debates. Again, the issues here are more complex than the fact that prevention only accounts for a small proportion of health expenditure. While there may be strong humanitarian reasons for preventing disease, it is important to stress that from an economic efficiency perspective the optimal expenditure on prevention occurs when an additional dollar spent on preventive activity or community care yields at least the same benefit as a dollar spent on inpatient or other health services.

Despite extensive rhetoric and many policy initiatives aimed at shifting the balance of care between hospitals and the community, the evidence of the value of these initiatives is not strong (Godber et al. 1997). Similarly, many preventive interventions are not as cost-effective as their proponents might claim (Russell 1986, 1987, 1994; Kenkel 2000). This is not to say that community services and preventive expenditures should be avoided, but rather that it is important that these expenditures, as with other proposals for increased expenditure, be evaluated from an economic perspective.

Health expenditure

The main source of information on Australian health expenditure that enables these policy debates to be tracked over time is the annual Health Expenditure Australia series produced by the Australian Institute of Health and Welfare (AIHW). This presents detailed information on the source and objects of health expenditure. The latest edition is usually available on the AIHW web site (www.aihw.gov.au).

Health Expenditure Australia follows the conventions of the National Accounts in terms of presentation. In turn, Australia's National Accounts are based on the United Nations' System of National Accounts that defines what expenditure has to be recognised and how it is to be recognised. Importantly, the National Accounts, and hence Health Expenditure Australia, only recognise expenditure in the traded sector: that is, the National Accounts do not capture any activity that occurs within households, between households where money is not directly exchanged, or by volunteers or unpaid carers.

Provision of neighbourly advice on health care or the value of formal advice by a pharmacist is not captured unless there is a commodity transaction associated with it. So if the pharmacist's advice leads to a sale of a pharmaceutical product, the value of that sale is captured within the National Accounts, but the value of the accompanying advice is deemed to be incorporated within the price of the product. Similarly, the system of National Accounts requires that the value of public sector production, where there is generally no market, be incorporated in the National Accounts at the input costs (what is paid for it). Thus even though health services might contribute more to the economy than the raw input costs, it is only the latter that are incorporated into the health expenditure series (Daniel et al. 1997). This is unlike the situation in the private sector where the price (which might incorporate a large mark-up over the input costs) is fully incorporated into the National Accounts. Finally, the work of volunteers and carers in the health sector, even though they provide a valuable service that may even substitute for a service that might otherwise be paid for, is not currently reflected in health expenditure (Waring 1988, 1999).

Although the UN System of National Accounts obviously has some limitations, it and Health Expenditure Australia are regarded as the definitive frameworks for the presentation and analysis of overall national expenditure including health expenditure. Health Expenditure Australia describes health expenditure according to the National Accounts definition of health. Expenditure in other sectors, although important to health, may not be captured within this framework. The most notable related area not recorded as health expenditure is expenditure on sewage and waste disposal, which is recorded as environmental protection expenditure.

Appendix 1 shows details of Australian health expenditure by area of expenditure and source for 2001/02, extracted from Health Expenditure Australia 2001–02, published in September 2003. This is also the data source used in this chapter.

Overall, Australia spent A$66.6 billion on health services in 2001/02, principally on recurrent expenditure; total capital expenditure (and capital consumption) was less than A$4 billion in that year. Figure 3.1 shows the distribution of expenditure by area of the health system.

It can be seen that over one-third (35 per cent) of recurrent expenditure is spent on hospitals with a further 7 per cent on high level residential care (nursing homes; expenditure on low level residential care or hostels is classified under the System of National Accounts as welfare expenditure). About 18 per cent of all expenditure is spent on medical services with a further 14 per cent on pharmaceuticals.

The objects of health expenditure have changed over time. The hospital share of expenditure has declined from 46 per cent in 1975/76 to 35 per

Figure 3.1 Australia: Distribution of recurrent health expenditure, by area of the health system, 2001/02

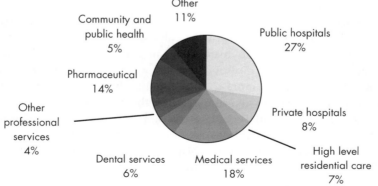

cent in 2001/02. Although the early 1990s could be characterised by tight expenditure controls over hospitals, the 1970s and 1980s involved looser controls. The hospitals' decline is thus probably relative, caused by other expenditure, particularly non-institutional expenditure, having a faster growth rate over this period. Pharmaceuticals expenditure, for example, increased from 11 per cent in 1975/76 to 14 per cent in 2001/02.

Funds flow

All health expenditure is funded by households through taxation, out-of-pocket costs, or health insurance premiums. Providers earn their income from payments from governments or health insurance funds, or from direct payments from consumers. Obviously, health expenditure on providers is also the income for employees of those providers and for private practitioners ('health expenditure = health incomes') and this fact further increases the salience of policy debates about health expenditure.

Figure 3.2 shows a simplified diagram of the flow of funds in the health sector. In fact, the flow of funds in the health care system is substantially more complex than shown in this simple diagram: 'government' incorporates both Commonwealth and state; and providers include public and private hospitals and medical practitioners (see Appendix 2). Figure 3.2 and Appendix 2 are further simplified in that they focus on the domestic flow of funds. The health sector operates in a global market (Barraclough 1997;

Figure 3.2 Simplified flow of health funding in the domestic health sector

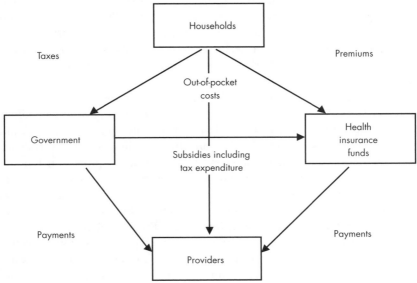

Figure 3.3 Australia: Relative proportions of recurrent health expenditure, 2001/02

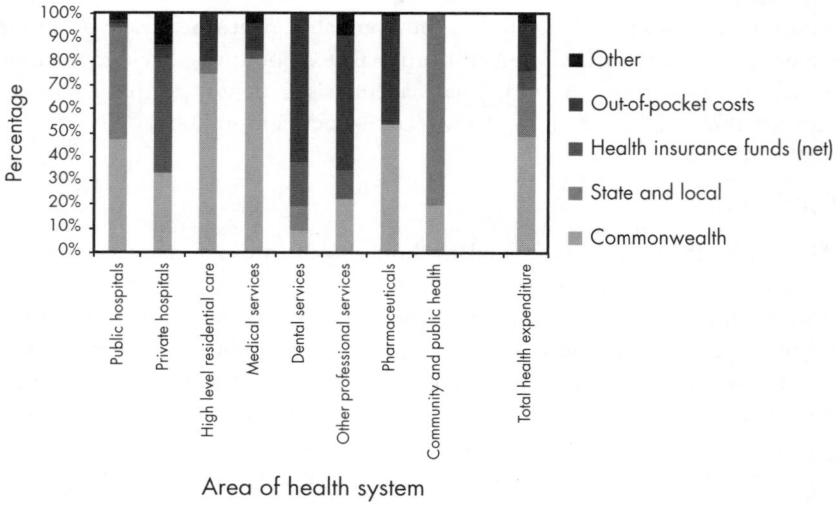

Zarilli and Kinnon 1998; Chanda 2002) and there is an inflow of funds to the Australian health sector from overseas investment and export of health sector goods and services, particularly hospital services (where many Australian hospitals treat international patients). There is also an outflow of funds mostly in investment and to pay for imports of capital equipment.

Because of Australia's universal health insurance system, Medicare, over two-thirds of total health expenditure is from government, with the Commonwealth being responsible for 48 per cent of expenditure and state and local government for 20 per cent. The balance of expenditure comes from out-of-pocket expenses by consumers (20 per cent), with a further 8 per cent being mediated through health insurance funds and 4 per cent from other sources including workers' compensation and motor vehicle third party insurers and donations.

The distribution of sources of funds is quite variable across the health sector; for example most public hospital expenditure is by government, either Commonwealth or state (see figure 3.3). Expenditure on nursing homes and medical services also comes mainly from the Commonwealth government, while private hospital, dental services, and other health profession funding comes from individuals—either via health insurance or as out-of-pocket expenditure. These significantly different shares in funding responsibilities have implications for policy. The Commonwealth government clearly dominates in the area of nursing home care (high level residential care), where it provides 75 per cent of funds, and in medical services (80 per cent). Policy response to issues that arise in these areas is clearly a Commonwealth government responsibility. The same is true in pharmaceuticals where funding is derived from either the Commonwealth government (54 per cent) or consumers (45 per cent). In contrast, public hospital funding responsibility is shared equally between the Commonwealth and state governments; state governments dominate funding for community and public health services (80 per cent). The areas of shared funding responsibilities can cause problems of accountability and 'blame shifting': each level of government is able to blame the other for resource shortfalls. (Commonwealth/state issues are further discussed in chapter 5.)

Health insurance has a particularly important role in funding private hospitals (providing 48 per cent of all funding) and to a lesser extent in dental services (19 per cent) and other professional services (12 per cent).

One of the weaknesses of these shared funding responsibilities is that government (be it Commonwealth or state) may see the health system simply as those parts of the health system that it funds. For example the Commonwealth may equate primary care with primary medical care because of its dominance of funding of medical services and the fact that its expenditure on medical services is significantly greater than its expenditure in community and public health services. This then creates further weaknesses in policy design.

On average, Australian households spent A$32.47 per week on medical care and health expenses according to the most recent household expenditure survey 1998/99 (ABS 2000). This represented about 3.7 per cent of average household income. The distribution of consumer payments (whether through health insurance or as out-of-pocket expenditure) is inequitable, with lower income consumers paying proportionally substantially more (over 10 per cent of income) compared with those on higher incomes (see figure 3.4).

Figure 3.4 Australia: Percentage of household income spent on medical care and health, 1993/94 and 1998/99

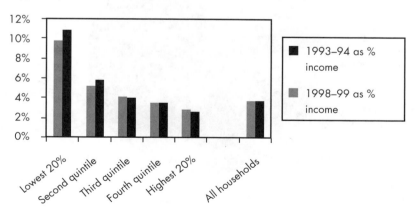

Data Source: ABS 1996c and ABS 2000

Although households in the highest income quintile spent more per week (A\$53) than the poorest 20 per cent of households (A\$17), in percentage terms poorer households spent 10.8 per cent of income compared to the 2.7 per cent of household income for the wealthiest 20 per cent of households. It appears that the distribution of household health spending may be becoming less equitable over time: people in the lowest income percentile having a marginally higher share of household expenditure spent on health services than in the 1998/99 household expenditure survey compared to the 1993/94 survey.

One can also look at expenditure from the perspective of the funder. Public hospitals and community and public health services are the main objects of state and territory expenditure: these two items together account for almost three-quarters of their health expenditure. The main objects of Commonwealth expenditure are medical benefits (30 per cent of its funding), public hospitals (26 per cent), pharmaceutical benefits (16 per cent), and high level residential care (nursing homes, 10 per cent).

The AIHW has embarked on an ambitious project to identify by disease the direct cost to the health system. This will supplement the institutional or sector framework used as a basis for figure 3.1. The direct cost analysis used by the AIHW does not include the costs to the economy of lost productivity, for example, but rather identifies the costs incurred in the health system. Figure 3.5 shows summary results of this analysis.

Figure 3.5 Australia: Costs incurred in the health system, by diagnostic category, 1993/94

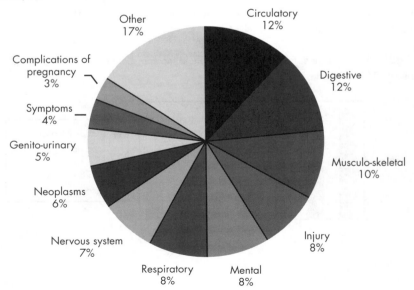

Data Source: Mathers et al 1998

Circulatory and digestive system disorders each account for more than 10 per cent of total direct costs of the health system. The third most expensive disease group, musculoskeletal disorders, accounts for 9.5 per cent of health expenditure. It is interesting to note that cancer (neoplasms), the eighth most expensive disease group, represents about 6 per cent of total direct expenditure but accounted for 27 per cent of all deaths in 1994 (the comparable year) and 28.5 per cent of potential years of life lost, the largest single cause of potential life years lost. In contrast, mental illness was the fifth most expensive disease group (8.2 per cent of all health expenditure) but because it is associated with high levels of disability rather than mortality, it only accounted for 2.1 per cent of potential years of life lost. (For further discussion of burden of disease in Australia, see chapter 2.) These differences highlight the importance of considering a range of different bases when describing the health system.

A further perspective on health expenditure is to consider expenditure on different population groups. About 20 per cent of health expenditure is spent on people over 75 years old with a further 15 per cent of expenditure spent on people aged 65 to 75 years (Mathers et al. 1998; similar results were obtained by Schofield (1997) examining expenditure mediated by health insurance funds). A number of authors have drawn attention to the fact that 'years to death' not 'years from birth' is the better predictor of health expenditure and hence it is not surprising that there is a very high level of expenditure on people, mainly the elderly, in their final years of life (Lubitz and Prihoda 1984; Lubitz et al. 1995; O'Connell 1996; Scitovsky 1988).

Health expenditure trends

As Newhouse (1993) has pointed out, the level of health expenditure is not of great policy relevance. What is important is the extent to which expenditure is changing over time. There are two key indicators that are used for measuring time (or 'secular') trends in expenditure: per capita health expenditure (which standardises for change in the size of the population) and percentage of GDP spent on health (which standardises for change in the size of the economy).

Per capita expenditures particularly need to be adjusted to take account of the effects of inflation and whether prices in the health sector are increasing at a slower or faster rate than prices in the rest of the economy. Over the last decade, health expenditure per head rose from A$1904 in 1991/92 to A$3397 in 2001/02, an average of 6 per cent per annum. Most of this increase is because of inflation in the economy. However, health spending per capita increased faster than the rest of the economy. In real terms, spending rose from $2357 per capita to $3292 (2000/01 dollars), an average

Figure 3.6 Australia: Health expenditure as proportion of GDP, 1975/76 to 2001/02

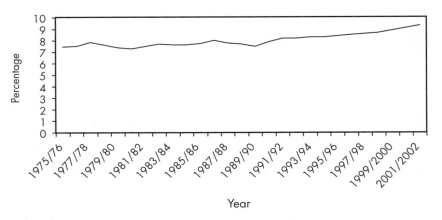

increase of 3.4 per cent per annum. There was a slower real growth rate in the first part of the period (2.8 per cent from 1992/93 to 1997/98) than in the last half of the period (4.1 per cent).

Figure 3.6 shows movement in health expenditure as a percentage of GDP. It can be seen that health spending marginally increased over the period 1975/76 to 1989/90, from 7.5 per cent of GDP to 7.8 per cent. The early 1990s saw the percentage of GDP exceeding 8 per cent for the first time. What distinguished the period 1990–92 was not health sector performance but GDP growth. Average GDP growth in constant prices was 2.4 per cent for the period 1975–90, 0.24 per cent for 1990–92, and 2 per cent from 1992–97. Despite the early 1990s slowdown in the economy, health expenditure continued to rise, and thus the health share of GDP increased. Health spending is considered to be 'sticky downwards': it tends not to show the same oscillation as the rest of the economy, partly reflecting the fact that government expenditure (which accounts for a large percentage of health expenditure) is less responsive to movements in the general economy.

Health expenditure share of the economy continued to rise to the mid 1990s at around 0.1 per cent per annum. A new trend emerged in the late 1990s with faster health spending growth: since 1998/99 health spending as a share of GDP has been increasing at around 0.2 per cent per annum. This faster increase is in part due to growth in pharmaceuticals expenditure (which has been growing at more than 10 per cent per annum over this period) and partly to growth in expenditure on 'other health professionals' (other than medical and dental practitioners) that has exhibited similar rates of growth, partly underwritten by private health insurance.

Another important trend in health expenditure has been in terms of the role of government, particularly the Commonwealth government. Figure

Figure 3.7 Australia: Relative share of total health expenditure, 1970/71 to 2001/02

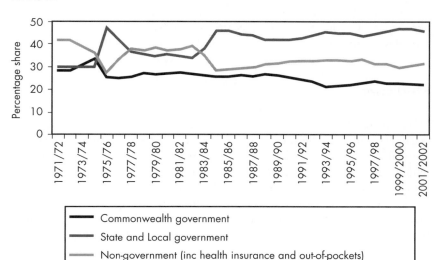

3.7 shows the relative shares of total health expenditure over the last 30 years. A significant feature is the instability revealed in funding shares between Commonwealth and state governments over the period 1975 to 1985. This period covered the introduction of Medibank in 1975 (when the Commonwealth's role and funding increased significantly and the state share concomitantly decreased). This policy initiative was slowly dismantled under the Fraser government and the Commonwealth share decreased and the states' share increased. With the reintroduction of Medicare in 1984 the Commonwealth and state roles again reversed. The state share has marginally declined from the early 1990s level of around 25 per cent to 22 per cent in 2001/02 with a marginal increase in the Commonwealth share over the same period from 42 per cent to 46 per cent. The distribution of Commonwealth funding to the states is discussed further in chapters 5 and 6.

The Commonwealth share of expenditure is also affected by 'tax expenditures', that is, tax forgone by government (in Australia usually the Commonwealth government) in the form of rebates or subsidies to households (Butler and Smith 1992). Until 1997/98, the most important of these was the income tax rebate for medical expenditure over a threshold of A$1250 per individual. As few taxpayers claimed this rebate, the effect of this rebate is relatively small, around A$160 million in 2001/02. In 1996/97, the Commonwealth government introduced a new tax measure, effective 1 July 1997, which provided a means-tested rebate (or subsidy) for purchase of health insurance, estimated to cost about A$420 million in a full financial year. This scheme was subsequently replaced (1 January 1999) with a rebate of 30 per cent against the cost of hospital and ancillary insurance. In 2001/02 the premium rebate was estimated at A\$1950 million or about 6 per cent of Commonwealth government health expenditure. Appendix 3 provides a summary of the changes in health insurance policy since 1975.

Medicare

Medicare is an important part of the health policy landscape in Australia because it provides the mechanism for financing two key provider groups: hospitals and doctors. The principal objective of Medicare is to remove (or reduce) financial barriers to access to health care for all Australian residents. (Medicare also provides benefits for residents of certain countries with whom Australia has signed a Reciprocal Health Care Agreement, currently Denmark, Finland, Ireland, Italy, Malta, Netherlands, New Zealand, Norway, Sweden, and the United Kingdom (see also Barraclough 1997).)

Medicare arrangements for hospital services

Historically, hospitals developed as a state responsibility and the Common-wealth's hospital Medicare policies are thus implemented via the states. The Commonwealth government has entered into agreements with each state that provide for the Commonwealth to fund the states for hospital services. In return for this funding the states agree to abide by a number of conditions including:
• to provide a network of hospital services
• to allow all consumers to be able to access inpatient services in these hospitals as 'public patients' free of any cost.

The agreements provide that states are responsible for the full marginal cost of any increase in hospital budgets during the term of the agreement. Conversely, states accrue the full benefit of any reduction in hospital budgets over this period. Commonwealth Medicare funding is formula-driven during the course of an agreement with the formula being un-related to actual hospital budgets, adjusting only for exogenous factors such as population growth and ageing. This places strong incentives on states to achieve efficiency improvements, or reduce hospital budgets through other strategies. The formulae enshrined in the agreements have changed over time.

The first Medicare hospital agreements (1984–88) were designed to compensate states for specific additional costs incurred as a result of the introduction of Medicare and, because of this focus, were known as Medicare Compensation Agreements. Compensation was provided for revenue losses associated with reduction in inpatient revenue (both price and volume) and for other revenue forgone (for example, lower numbers of private patients reduce the revenue stream for public pathology services). Compensation for cost increases was based on the number of 'shift bed days', which was based on the proportionate change in the public:private bed day ratio, assuming no increase in volume (Duckett 1988 describes both the 1984–88 and 1988–93 agreements). Funding under the 1984–88 agreement supplemented the ongoing Commonwealth funding known as the 'Identified Health Grant'.

The two subsequent Medicare Agreements (1988–93 and 1993–98) and the first Australian Health Care Agreements (1998–2003) have attempted to address perverse incentives in Australia's health care system and to achieve specific Commonwealth policy objectives; the second Australian Health Care Agreement (2003–08) was designed by the Commonwealth to improve transparency of funding and to force states to at least match Commonwealth funding growth (see table 3.1).

Table 3.1 Key elements of Commonwealth–state hospital funding agreements

Agreement	Political objective	Key principals
1984—88 ('Medicare Compensation Agreement')	• Introduction of Medicare	• Compensation for cost increases and revenue losses • Transparency • Accountability • Dynamic
1988—93 ('Medicare Agreement')	• Consolidating Medicare • Growth and reform of public provision	• Incentives for system reform • Penalties for lower public:private bed day shares and excess private medical service use
1993—98 ('Medicare Agreement')	• Entrenching Medicare • Expansion of public provision	• Reward for relatively higher levels of public provision and for increasing public provision relative to other states
1998—2003 ('Australian Health Care Agreement')	• Continuing with Medicare • Increased Commonwealth funding with increased accountability for States	• Post 1996, accountability for negotiated outcomes • Increased accountability on states for activity level changes
2003—08 ('Australian Health Care Agreement')	• Continuing with Medicare • Increased accountability of states • Reduced growth in outlays	• Increased clarity of Commonwealth responsibility if health insurance levels change • Improved reporting, especially of state spending • Requirement on states to at least match Commonwealth funding increases

The first Medicare agreements focused on facilitating the implementation of Medicare; the 1988–93 agreements reflected a move to a more institutionalised status for Medicare, incorporating a series of components relating to system reform rather than determining appropriate compensation. In particular, the agreements incorporated incentives for states to increase either the proportion or the number of patients treated as public patients to attempt to ensure that states maintained their level of provision and responded to the emerging political problem of waiting lists.

The 1988–93 agreements replaced the Identified Health Grant and the Compensation Grant with a single grant, thus increasing the amount of money formally paid via the agreement. This change was mainly symbolic as the bulk of the agreement funding (the Base Grant) was, like the Identified Health Grant, subject to Grants Commission equalisation (see chapter 5).

The 1993–98 agreements were negotiated in the run-up to the 1993 election; indeed the agreements were signed on the day the writs for the election were issued (see Butler 1993 and Pearse 1994 for detailed discussion). From the Commonwealth government's perspective, the agreements were meant to ensure Medicare's continuance, even if Labor lost the election: the agreements were enshrined in legislation and major changes to the agreements had to be approved by the Senate.

Following the signing of the 1988–93 agreements it became clear that although states had acceded to the key obligations of Medicare, both politically and in the form of the signed Medicare agreements, states and/or their hospitals had attempted to circumvent their obligations through cost shifting and other stratagems. The 1993–98 Medicare agreements were therefore revised mid-term to incorporate more directly objectives related to the expected negotiated levels of throughput and performance in other key policy areas, such as waiting lists and emergency department waiting times.

An important dynamic element of the 1993–98 agreements was a requirement to 'review' Commonwealth funding if health insurance declined by more than 2 per cent. Although these reviews did take place, the states were dissatisfied with the outcome as the Commonwealth did not provide any additional funding in the face of the states' arguments that there was increased demand on state hospital systems because of the decline in insurance.

The 1998–2003 Australian Health Care Agreement built on the frameworks of the earlier Medicare agreements. It had three main funding streams:

- an admitted patient component, which included a specification of the target public patient admission rate in each state, which increases by 2.1 per cent per annum over the course of the agreement because of 'utilisation drift' caused, for example, by technological change
- a non-admitted patient component

- funding for mental health and palliative care (carried over from the previous Medicare agreement), together with new components for quality enhancement and system restructuring (Bigg et al. 1998).

Like previous agreements, the 1998–2003 agreement provided for funding increases for change in the size or age–gender composition of the population. However, unlike the predecessor agreements it had several important dynamic elements:

- an explicit funding adjustment if health insurance declined (or increased) beyond a threshold
- recognition of the costs of 'demand growth' or utilisation drift of 2.1 per cent per annum
- commitment to rationalise funding of hospital pharmaceutical services.

The first Australian Health Care Agreement also included provision for external review in the event of disagreement between the Commonwealth and the states. This provision was exercised in 1999 when the Commonwealth failed to adhere to a provision relating to development of a new cost index for use in the agreement. The independent reviewer proposed a modified cost index but the Commonwealth rejected this proposal

The second Australian Health Care Agreement (2003–08) was presented as a *fait accompli* to the states with strong financial incentives on states to sign, which they did on the deadline. The most significant elements of the new funding arrangements are:

- a base grant, which is increased for weighted population increases, a further 1.7 per cent increase for utilisation drift, and indexation for wage movements
- a withheld amount of 4 per cent of the grant paid on compliance with reporting schedules and funding growth matching requirements
- a capital funding scheme to facilitate improvements in services involved in the transition from hospital to home ('Pathways Home Program')
- funding for palliative care, mental health, and safety and quality initiatives.

The second Health Care Agreement commits the Commonwealth and states to work towards reform in a number of areas including the interface between hospitals, primary care, and aged care; continuity of care particularly in cancer care and mental health services; and continued work on pharmaceuticals reform. Whether these aspirations will be achieved, given the acrimonious exchanges prior to signature of the agreement, is a moot point. The second agreement also strengthened reporting requirements on the states, with penalty provisions for noncompliance. These stronger reporting frameworks built on the trend from the previous agreements and responded to a critical Auditor-General's report (Auditor-General 2002), which concluded that the Commonwealth did not have all the performance information required to administer the Commonwealth funding allocated under the agreement.

Medicare arrangements for medical services

The Commonwealth plays a more direct role with respect to medical services, with medical funding being directly administered by a Commonwealth agency, the Health Insurance Commission (HIC). Medicare provides for rebates against the costs of medical care at the rate of 85 per cent of a scheduled fee for out-of-hospital services with a maximum per item gap between the rebate and the schedule fee of A$57.10 (November 2002 levels). There is also a safety net: Medicare pays 100 per cent of the rebate when total gap payments exceed A$319.70 per family in a calendar year. The fee schedule and gap limits are updated by the Commonwealth on a regular basis. Medicare also pays a rebate of 75 per cent of the scheduled fee for medical services provided to private inpatients (with no maximum gap).

Doctors can send their bill to the Commonwealth (Health Insurance Commission) through a process known as 'bulk' or 'direct' billing, in which case the medical practitioner must accept the rebate in full settlement of the account. Alternatively, doctors can bill patients and there is then no limit on fees that may be charged; patients then obtain a rebate from the Commonwealth (Health Insurance Commission) for the relevant percentage of the government schedule fee. Further information on the prevalence of bulk-billing and observance of the fee schedule is provided in chapter 8; Deeble (1999) provides a good review of trends in Medicare services and expenditure.

Health insurance funds are generally not allowed to cover any charges by medical practitioners above the schedule fee. This policy was designed to place financial pressure on doctors to influence their fee charging behaviour. However, since 1996, insurers may make contractual arrangements (known as Medical Purchaser Provider Agreements) with doctors providing services to (private) hospital inpatients to pay rebates above the schedule fee.

Medicare is funded from general taxation. However, Australia's income tax laws provide for a 'Medicare levy', currently 1.5 per cent of taxable income (see Appendix 3 for changes in levy rates over time). Differential low income thresholds (below which no levy is payable) are set for individuals, single parents, and couples. Couples and families with a combined income over A$100,000 who do not have health insurance which provides cover for hospital care are liable to a levy surcharge of a further 1 per cent of taxable income. (The single person cut-off is A$50,000.)

The Medicare levy is not intended to cover the full cost of Commonwealth health expenditure (or indeed total expenditure on health) but rather was introduced as a financing measure to raise additional revenue to pay for the introduction of Medicare in 1984. The levy is not a 'hypothecated' tax; that is, Medicare levy collections are not specifically allocated to the health portfolio, although the need to increase health spending is often used as a political justification for increasing the levy. The levy is thus simply another tax which flows into the pool of funds from which Commonwealth expenditure derives. In 1999/2000 total revenue from the Medicare levy was A\$4.2 billion, representing about 16 per cent of total Commonwealth health expenditure.

Health insurance

Patterns of private health insurance largely reflect changes in government and national health policy. Prior to the introduction of Medicare in 1984, health insurance accounted for about 20 per cent of all health expenditure. Immediately following the introduction of Medicare (1984/85), the health insurance share of expenditure declined precipitately to 8.8 per cent of health expenditure, with a slight increase in the intervening period to its current (2001/02) level of 8 per cent of expenditure. The proportion of the population with health insurance declined up to the late 1990s, despite the introduction of significant tax rebate incentives to take out private health insurance (Hall et al. 1999). The introduction of 'Life Time Cover' led to an increase in health insurance in 1999.

As figure 3.8 shows, the proportion of the population with private health insurance has been declining since the 1970s, with a steeper decline associated with the introduction of universal health insurance in 1984. There has been a differential rate of decline in the prevalence of insurance across different population groups, leading to a change in the composition of the insured population. Middle income families were more likely to drop insurance relative to high income and lower income families, and younger families were more likely to drop insurance relative to older families (Schofield et al. 1997).

Figure 3.8 Australia: Percentage of population with private health insurance, 1970–2002

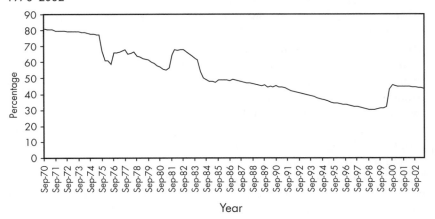

Data Source: Private Health Insurance Administration Council 2003 and prior years

For much of the 1970s, health funding policy was in a state of flux with frequent gyrations of policy, as the then Fraser Government used health policy as an instrument of economic policy and repeated attempts to induce greater take-up of private health insurance (Duckett 1979, 1980, 1984; Scotton 1980; Gray 1996). Appendix 3 summarises the variations of policy since that period in terms of medical rebates, hospital access, and changes to the Medicare levy and private health insurance.

The Labor government from 1984 to 1996 provided some stability to health policy and pursued a passive policy of allowing health insurance to continue to decline (Duckett 2003). The major changes introduced in the Labor period were to remove most implicit subsidies to health insurance (in the early years of the Labor government) and towards the end of its term, to allow health insurers to negotiate with doctors and hospitals to ensure there were no out-of-pocket costs for patients following private inpatient treatment. An implicit subsidy remains as bed day charges for private patients in public hospitals are significantly below average cost.

The return of a Liberal government in 1996 marked a resurgence of policy interest in the level of private health insurance, ostensibly because increased private insurance might reduce demand on public hospitals (Duckett and Jackson 2000; Vaithianathan 2002). Although the new government introduced a rebate/subsidy for health insurance in its first budget, this did nothing to reverse the decline in the proportion of the population with insurance, and was followed by a more generous rebate/subsidy scheme introduced in 1999. Partly in response to the higher drop-out rate in younger families, and the consequent risk of a deteriorating age profile of the insured population, in 1999 the government changed the regulatory controls on funds to allow them to offer health insurance products with premiums varying with age of entry in the insurance market. People who first take out health insurance over the age of 30 face a 2 per cent per annum cumulative increase in premiums (capped at 65); thus a person who first takes out insurance at 35 faces a 10 per cent higher premium than would have applied if they had taken out insurance at age 30. This latter policy (known as Life Time Cover) led to an increase in health insurance to around 45 per cent of the population (Butler 2002), but since that peak, insurance has declined to stand at around 43 per cent in June 2003 and recent health insurance data shows that the risk profile of health insurance is again worsening with younger people dropping out of health insurance (Butler 2002; see also www.phiac.gov.au).

A number of studies have shown that health insurance is unevenly distributed in the population: those with health insurance are wealthier, better educated, and older than the uninsured (Cameron et al. 1988; Cameron and Trivedi 1991; Willcox 1991; Burrows et al. 1993; ABS 1994; Cameron and

McCallum 1996; Hopkins and Kidd 1996; Schofield 1997). Evidence about the risk profile of the insured population is mixed. The Productivity Commission (1997, pp. 196, 244–6) suggested that 'adverse selection', that is, disproportionate recruitment and retention of contributors with health problems that make them more likely to claim benefits, accounted for 17 per cent of the increase in health insurance premiums between 1990 and 1995. On the other hand, the same report from the Productivity Commission also noted that the probability of holding health insurance was higher with better self-assessed health status (p. 195) and that the insured population used fewer hospital bed days per capita than the uninsured (p. 187). Because of the greater take-up of health insurance among the wealthy, rebates/subsidies to health insurance are inherently inequitable: the wealthy benefit more from the subsidy (Smith 2001).

Regulation of health insurance

The private health insurance industry is subject to regulation by two industry-specific bodies established by the Commonwealth government: the Private Health Insurance Administration Council (PHIAC) and the Private Health Insurance Ombudsman. In addition, the health insurance industry is subject to normal trade practice laws and is thus monitored by the Australian Competition and Consumer Commission (ACCC) in common with other industries. The ACCC has taken action against a number of health insurance funds to protect consumers or private hospitals against inappropriate pressure from funds. The Senate has also requested the ACCC to produce a six-monthly report on anticompetitive practices by health insurance funds that describes some of these actions (see www.accc.gov.au/pubs/catalog.htm).

The Private Health Insurance Administration Council

PHIAC is an independent body established under the National Health Act responsible to the Commonwealth Minister for Health and Aged Care. It is the main regulatory body supervising health insurance organisations. PHIAC consists of five members appointed by the minister. The key functions of PHIAC include:

- providing comparative data to the health insurance industry and the public
- monitoring solvency and capital adequacy of health insurance funds
- administering the Health Benefits Re-Insurance Trust Fund.

To achieve these ends, it has broad general powers to receive reports, to appoint investigators, and, where necessary, to appoint administrators of health insurance funds. PHIAC has published standards for monitoring solvency and capital adequacy. It is also responsible for collecting health insurance coverage and expenditure data from funds and publishing these on a quarterly basis.

The Private Health Insurance Ombudsman

The Private Health Insurance Ombudsman, in contrast to PHIAC, does not have regulatory power but functions more as a mediator. The Private Health Insurance Ombudsman, who is appointed by the Commonwealth Minister for Health, receives and investigates complaints (from consumers, hospitals, medical practitioners, or health insurance organisations) about health insurance. The Ombudsman's powers are to investigate, mediate, and make recommendations to the health insurance fund the Commonwealth Minister for Health, and the ACCC.

About one-fifth of the complaints received in 2002/03 were about costs, with differential rates of complaints across funds probably related to the size of increases in premiums and the way premium increases were notified.

International comparisons of health expenditure

Cross-national studies of health expenditure attempt to explain variations in health expenditure associated with different types of health systems. An important finding from these studies is that wealthier countries tend to spend more on health as a proportion of GDP. Figure 3.9 shows the relationship between per capita GDP and health expenditure for a number of OECD countries including Australia and the USA.

Figure 3.9 Health expenditure and GDP per capita, OECD countries, 2000

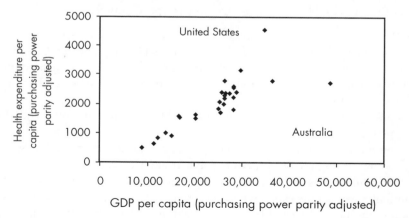

Data Source: OECD 2003

Health expenditure and GDP per capita are highly correlated and Australia's expenditure on health is almost exactly on any prediction equation: its health expenditure being as expected based on its GDP per capita. The USA, on the other hand, is a significant outlier and spends a higher proportion of its GDP on health than would be predicted based on its GDP.

Other conclusions from the literature on cross-national studies of health expenditure are:

- health expenditure tends to increase faster than GDP (Pfaff 1990; Gerdtham et al. 1992; see also McGuire et al. 1993, who summarised 10 previous studies)
- a higher public proportion of health spending is not associated with higher health spending overall (Pfaff 1990) and may be associated with lower spending (Gerdtham et al. 1992; Jönsson and Eckerlund 2003)
- higher consumer co-payments or higher cost-sharing does not lead to lower health expenditure, either per capita or as a share of GDP (Pfaff 1990)
- health care expenditure is greater in countries where fee-for-service is the dominant way of remunerating medical practitioners (Gerdtham et al. 1992).

There does not appear to be a relationship between health expenditure and health status (McGuire et al. 1993; but see Mathers et al. 2003 for a contrary view) possibly because of the number of intervening variables, for example whether provided services are effective (Filmer and Pritchett 1999).

The existence of primary care-gatekeeping for access to secondary and tertiary care does not appear to affect total health expenditure (Barros 1998; Delnoij et al. 2000; Jönsson and Eckerlund 2003; but see Starfield and Shi 2002 for a contrary view).

The relationship between public expenditure and total expenditure is an interesting one. Evans (1995) has argued that public expenditure lowers total GDP share because the stronger the role of a public funder, the greater the likelihood of the use of methods to control provider incomes (especially through capping hospital expenditure and moderating medical fees). Limiting the number of funding sources for health providers reduces providers' ability to play one off against the other and enhances the potential for the funder/purchaser to use monopsony power in the health care marketplace.

The relationship between total health spending and the proportion of the population aged over 65 is unclear. Some studies have found no relationship (Pfaff 1990; Gerdtham 1992; O'Connell 1996; Zweifel et al. 1999; Moïse and Jacobzone 2003), others that increased ageing is associated with increased expenditure (Gerdtham et al. 1992). The O'Connell study helps to explain the different conclusions. She examined ageing effects in different countries over time and found that in about one-third of OECD countries there was a positive relationship between the proportion of population over 65 and health expenditure; in one-third (including Australia) the relationship was negative, and in one-third the relationship was not statistically significant. The age relationship is therefore sensitive to the countries included in the analysis (Jönsson and Eckerlund 2003). A further explanation is that there may be different relationships between expenditure and costs at different ages (Seshamani and Gray 2003). A number of studies have found that health expenditures are concentrated in the last few months of life (Lubitz and Prihoda 1984; Lubitz et al. 1995; O'Connell 1996; Scitovsky 1988; Zweifel et al. 1999; Moïse and Jacobzone 2003), suggesting that health expenditure is better predicted by years till death rather than years from birth. Propper (2003) concludes that the impact of ageing will thus be to push the high levels of health care expenditure to later in individuals' lives rather than to increase per capita expenditure.

These findings about the ambiguous relationship between health expenditure and age have important policy consequences. As was shown in the previous chapter, older people have higher use of services and in most countries, including Australia, health expenditure increases with age (Moïse and Jacobzone 2003). This has led to scaremongering about the implications of an ageing Australian population (Clare and Tulpulé 1994) with the assumption that the ageing population will bankrupt Australia unless draconian action is taken. Schulz (1998) has referred to the basis of this argument as 'voodoo demographics', as it rarely takes into account the effects of economic growth, and in the Australian case, may be based on invalid assumptions (Kinnear 2001). Further, the Australian elderly make up a smaller proportion of the population than in many European countries that provide levels of social support similar to those in Australia, and those

Figure 3.10 Per cent of GDP spent on health by source of funding, selected countries, 2000

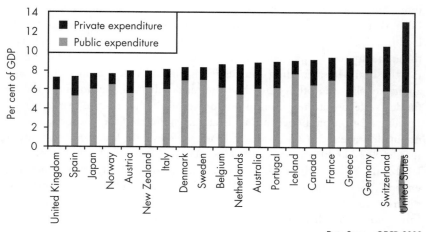

Data Source: OECD 2003

countries have coped well with this higher proportion of the elderly (Gibson 1998; Richardson and Robertson 1999). Moïse and Jacobzone (2003) have also discounted the doomsday scenarios by pointing out that older people tend to be treated less aggressively than younger people, a finding confirmed in Australia (Duckett and Jackson 2003).

The USA, the main outlier in any analysis of health care expenditure, is the only OECD country where private expenditure accounts for more than half of the total expenditure on health care. A relatively high proportion of Australian health expenditure (28 per cent) is also from private sources, principally out-of-pocket costs (20 per cent). For most OECD countries, public expenditure on health services in 2000 was around 6.3 per cent of GDP (see figure 3.10). Private expenditure appears much more variable around the mean of about 2.6 per cent of GDP (mean of 2.3 per cent excluding the USA), ranging from 1.3 per cent in Sweden and 1.4 per cent in the United Kingdom to 7.3 per cent in the USA. The variation in the health share of GDP is principally explained by variations in the private share: it appears that private spending does not substitute for public spending but is additive. Differential private shares may thus reflect different perceptions of the potential contribution of medical care to improving health status. Different countries may be situated at different points on a 'production possibility frontier' that describes this relationship (Cutler 2003).

Because private expenditure is not proportional to income (health insurance, for example, being typically a fixed sum regardless of income), health financing arrangements in countries that have a relatively large private sector share are less equitable than in countries that have a smaller private sector share (Wagstaff et al. 1999).

Finally, it is important to stress that the level of health expenditure in a given country is a matter of political and individual choice: politics may make a difference! Navarro and Shi (2001), for example, have examined social welfare spending in OECD countries categorised in terms of their predominant political complexion over the period 1945–80. They demonstrate significant differences in public expenditure on health, and public medical care coverage between 'social democratic', 'Christian democratic', 'Liberal Anglo-Saxon', and 'Former fascist dictatorships'. Their findings were not confirmed by Harrinvirta and Mattila (2001) who concluded that left-wing governments are not associated with higher public spending.

How should health expenditure be controlled?

One of the key concerns of policy makers in Australia over recent decades has been with control or reduction in health expenditure. Restructure of health insurance in the Fraser years was often claimed to be based on controlling health expenditure, and health care reform at state level is also associated with policies for controlling or reducing health expenditure (for example, the introduction of casemix funding in Victoria and South Australia). However, as indicated earlier in this chapter, Australia's total health expenditure is not proportionately high when compared with other countries with a similar GDP per capita. Further, economists argue that control of health expenditure is an unusual and inappropriate objective from an efficiency perspective: what should be of concern is the extent to which marginal increases in health expenditure lead to marginal improvements in health outcomes.

The focus on control of expenditures derives in part from a perception by policy makers, and occasionally policy analysts, that current levels of health spending are not appropriate. The evidence base for this assumption is not clear. However, there is an extensive rhetoric that the health care production function is characterised by diminishing marginal returns and that additional investments in health care are unwarranted (or, a stronger conclusion, that reallocation of health spending to other sectors will lead to improvements in total well-being). This rhetoric is often based on assumptions that much of health care is unevaluated (see, for example, Evans 1990a, p. 106: 'so much of what is done in health care is ineffective, questionable, or simply unevaluated...'). The lack of relationship between health care utilisation rates and health status (in the light of wide variation in utilisation) is also used as evidence of the lack of benefit of additional health expenditure and addressing 'overuse' is regularly postulated as a cost-saving initiative (Wennberg et al. 2002).

Certainly, it would appear that policy makers and formulators of Commonwealth and state budgets have adopted a modus operandi with an implicit assumption that the opportunity costs of increasing health expenditure are high, and/or that current levels of health expenditure are inappropriate.

There are a number of ways of attempting to 'control' expenditure. However, it is important to recognise that health care is a labour-intensive industry: what is seen as health care expenditure by a payer is seen as health care income by providers. Although payers have an interest in controlling or reducing health expenditure, providers have an interest in increasing health expenditure (or at the very least, changing the distribution of health expenditure from other providers to themselves). As Evans (1990b) has pointed out, these opposing forces in health care financing debates lead to opposing strategies, termed tension and compression. These forces of tension and compression can also lead to 'shear'—strategies to transfer costs from one group to another. In Australia this latter strategy is exemplified by cost shifting (for example, state-funded agencies attempting to shift costs to the Commonwealth) and arguments for patient co-payments (shifting costs on to consumers). Consumer co-payments, of course, significantly reduce equity, as well as being a relatively inefficient way of controlling total costs.

Table 3.2   Targets of health care cost control

	Demand side	Supply side
Price	• Consumer co-payments	• Design/structure of fee schedule (e.g. casemix funding)
Volume	• Assessment processes for eligibility	• Regulating capacity • Utilisation review

A number of authors have reviewed the instruments, strategies, or targets of health cost control (the language used varies; see White (1999) for the development of a coherent framework). In broad general terms, cost control strategies can attempt to influence the behaviour of suppliers or providers (such as hospitals and medical practitioners) on the supply side, or consumers on the demand side (Rice 2002; Carrin and Hanvoravongchai 2003). Given that health care expenditure is determined by the multiplication of price of services by the volume provided, strategies can also be categorised into these two broad targets: control of price or control of volume.

Table 3.2 (based on Scotton 1977) portrays these choices in a 2 x 2 table, with an example of policy instruments in each cell.

The relative emphasis that is placed on demand side versus supply side and price versus volume strategies varies across the health sector. For example, a key component of Medicare is that there are no consumer co-payments for access to public hospital care. On the other hand, consumer co-payments have been incorporated into the design of the funding arrangements for pharmaceutical benefits.

The relative emphasis on the use of strategies in any of the cells of the table needs to take into account their impact on other cells in the table (for example, squeezing providers on price may result in providers increasing their volume to achieve a target income). Also, instruments and policies focusing on one area need to take account of the interaction with, and consequences for, substitutes. For example, very high co-payments in general practice may result in consumers increasing their use of hospital emergency services where co-payments are either nonexistent or not as high.

Interests in the health sector are differentially affected by the policies shown in table 3.2. For example, providers are generally opposed to supply-side strategies focused on price, which are designed to reduce provider income. Providers thus can typically be expected to attempt to focus on strategies in the other cells in table 3.2, in particular, cost shifting or attempting to focus policy attention on the demand side (Evans 1997). Cost-control strategies have rarely been evaluated and arguments for change are thus rarely evidence-based. This is particularly the case with consumer co-payments where the evidence for the effectiveness of consumer co-payments in re-ducing demand is very slight indeed (Carrin and Hanvoravongchai 2003), to the extent that this focus of attention has been described as being akin to a walking zombie (Barer et al. 1993; Evans 1995).

Finally, it is important to recognise the interaction of health care cost control strategies, which focus on the efficiency attributes of the health system, with the other key elements of system design, namely equity, qual-ity, and acceptability. For example, the introduction of extensive consumer co-payments will have a differential impact on the poor and hence affect equity. Some strategies to affect volume, by restricting consumer choice, may also have an adverse impact on consumer and provider acceptability (Flynn and Smith 2002). Further discussion of contemporary policy initia-tives with respect to cost control will be undertaken in subsequent chapters.

4

The Health Workforce

The knowledge, skills, and attitudes of the health workforce are critical to the quality of care received by a patient or consumer; the structure and functioning of that health workforce is critical to the structure and functioning of the health system overall. To a very large extent, diagnosis and treatment decisions call on the training and experience of the health professional. Health professionals' attitudes to updating their knowledge, using contemporary evidence in treatment and learning from mistakes, impact on a patient's quality of care. The interpersonal and technical skills of health professionals determine the quality of the interaction with patients or consumers. In a sense, health workers are important in defining the very nature of health care services. The significance of the health workforce is further highlighted by the fact that, as is typical of most service industries, labour costs account for a large proportion of health costs (around 70 to 80 per cent).

There are two ways of looking at the health workforce. First, in terms of the health professions, that is, groups that have specific training related to diagnosis and treatment of patients or consumers, and/or the organisation of health care delivery. The second way of looking at the health workforce is in terms of those people who work in the health industry, be they health professionals or people from a different background. Table 4.1 shows information on the place of the health workforce (using both approaches) in terms of the Australian labour market.

The health industry accounts for 6.72 per cent of the employed workforce, smaller than the health share of GDP. Health professionals account for 43 per cent of employment in the health industry (other groups include managers, cleaners, social welfare professionals, people in trades, and so on). Nurses comprise the single largest health profession, accounting for just over one-quarter of all health industry employment.

Many industry sectors have a role in promoting or protecting health, for example local government, water supply authorities, and so on.

Table 4.1 Australia: Number of persons in health occupations in health and other industries, 2001

Industry	Medical practitioners	Nursing professionals	Other health professionals	Total health professionals	Other occupations	Total
Hospitals and nursing homes	12,725	111,359	11,370	135,454	145,955	281,409
Medical and dental services	28,711	9242	10,974	48,927	69,850	118,777
Other health services	3994	27,597	25,395	56,986	100,490	157,476
Total health industry	45,430	148,198	47,739	241,367	316,295	557,662
All other industries	2781	23,409	24,047	50,237	7,690,707	7,740,944
Total	48,211	171,607	71,786	291,604	8,007,002	8,298,606
	16.53%	58.85%	24.62%	4.0		

Source: ABS unpublished
Census cross-tabulations

However, over 90 per cent of medical practitioners and over 85 per cent of nurses are employed in the health industry, with the remainder being employed across a range of industries including tertiary education and the government sector. About two-thirds (65 per cent) of nurses are employed in hospitals and nursing homes.

The number and distribution of health professionals

Table 4.2 provides more detailed data on the number of persons in health occupations in Australia.

Note that the variation in numbers between tables 4.1 and 4.2 is partly the result of a different data source (2001 Census for the occupations for table 4.1, the quarterly Labour Force Surveys for table 4.2), and also table 4.2 is for a later time period (August 2002) compared with the table 4.1 (2001 Census data).

Table 4.2   Australia: Persons employed in health occupations, 2002

Occupation	Males ('000)	Females ('000)	Persons ('000)	Mean weekly earnings in main job ($)
Generalist medical practitioners	15.8	11.2	27.0	1492
Specialist medical practitioners	10.6	*2.9	13.5	2517
Registered nurses	13.4	152.3	165.8	713
Other nursing professionals	*3.5	18.8	22.3	870
Dental practitioners			*2.5	*1519
Pharmacists	4.6	5.2	9.8	899
Occupational therapists			*3.5	*722
Optometrists	*2.8	*1.5	*4.3	*833
Physiotherapists	*2.7	6.6	9.2	704
Speech pathologists	*0.0	*3.3	*3.3	*648
Chiropractors and osteopaths	*1.0	*0.0	*1.0	*1909
Medical imaging professionals	*3.8	6.5	10.3	867
Other health professionals	*3.6	9.0	12.5	793
Total employed in health occupations	64.5	220.6	285.1	898
Other occupations	4202.6	3439.3	7641.9	692

An asterisk (*) indicates that the estimate has a Relative Standard Error (RSE) of greater than 25 per cent and care should therefore be exercised in using it.

Source: ABS, Employee Earnings, Benefits and Trade Union Membership Survey (ABS data available on request)

Nurses represent two-thirds of the health professional workforce with medical practitioners being the second largest group (14 per cent of the health workforce). The next major health professional groups are radiographers ('medical imaging technologists'), pharmacists, physiotherapists, and dentists, together accounting for a further one-ninth (11.7 per cent) of the health workforce.

The health workforce is predominantly female (77.4 per cent) although the higher income professions tend to be male dominated (79 per cent of specialist medical practitioners are male; males make up 59 per cent of generalist medical practitioners, compared with 8 per cent of registered nurses and 18 per cent of physiotherapists). Specialist medical practitioners earn substantially more than other professionals. The overall pattern is that groups with a larger proportion of women tend to have lower earnings. Health professionals generally have higher earnings than people in other occupations.

The health workforce has grown substantially over the last 40 years. The 1961 Census, for example, recorded a total 72,598 health professionals (that is, people with health professional qualifications, whether employed or not), 56 per cent of whom were registered nurses, 16 per cent were medical practitioners, and the remaining 28 per cent all other health professionals. By 2001, the health workforce had quadrupled to 291,604 with nurses now accounting for 59 per cent, medical practitioners 17 per cent, and others 24 per cent. The number of health professionals per head of population increased from 6.9 per 1000 population in 1961 to 15.4 per 1000 population in 2001. (The proportion of nurses reported here probably exaggerates the growth in this profession as the 1961 figures do not include an additional 20,000 student nurses employed, but not counted in the professional workforce.)

The health workforce is now characterised by a large number of separate professions, each with a different course of preparation, a different emphasis in practice and, to some extent, a different ideological foundation in terms of the way in which the profession interacts with other professions and with patients or consumers. The workforce has changed dramatically over the last 20 years with increasing specialisation in the workforce, both within professions (for example, additional specialisations in medicine and nursing) and also by the creation of new professions. To some extent, this specialisation has led to increased quality of care as individual professionals have been able to develop in-depth skills across a narrower range of areas. However, in the late 1990s there was a recognition that this increasing specialisation may have a downside in increased coordination costs, leading to inefficiency and problems of continuity of care.

The change in the composition of the health workforce has also been accompanied by the feminisation of many of the professions. This makes the older workforce planning terminology of 'manpower planning' particularly inappropriate. Figure 4.1 shows trends in the proportion of women in health professions over the Census years 1961 to 2001.

The male:female ratio in most of the health professions is converging to

Figure 4.1 Australia: Trends in proportion of women in health occupations, 1961–2001

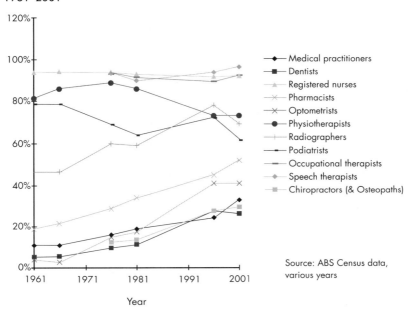

Source: ABS Census data, various years

the population ratio. There has been a significant increase in the proportion of women in a number of health professions including medicine, radiography, and pharmacy. On the other hand, the proportion of males in physiotherapy and podiatry has declined over this period. The nursing profession, however, stands out as remaining a predominantly female profession. The reasons for the changes in most of the health professions are multifactorial. In part, they reflect societal changes in the perceptions of the appropriateness of women studying for and becoming members of these professions. This in turn is part of a wider change relating to the place of women in the workforce. In the late 1950s and early 1960s, for example, many women were implicitly discouraged from studying sciences at school which meant they were unable to meet prerequisites for some of the university-based health professions at that time (Reid 1978). There have been few studies of the reasons for school leavers choosing to study the different health professions in Australia.

Registration and regulation

Most of the health professions are subject to regulation through state or territory professional registration boards. Despite several attempts, especially in the late 1980s and early 1990s, to establish a set of common national principles for regulating health professions, decisions to register and regulate each profession are made by states and territories independently and, as a consequence, there is variation in which professions are regulated in each state and territory.

There is some commonality, with older health professions registered in all states and territories (for example, medical practitioners and nurses). Increasingly, laws establishing registration boards specify that the board exists to protect the public interest rather than to protect the interest of members of the profession. The professions where interventions can carry a high degree of risk, and hence where protection of the public interest is greatest, are registered in all states. Of course, many health professionals, whether in registrable professions or not, may be involved in activities that are potentially harmful to patients, and hence the variety of decisions about registration. Professions that are not regulated by state and territory registration boards are typically subject to self-regulation by professional associations. However, because membership of a professional association is voluntary, the professional associations cannot debar a person from practice and can mostly only exercise moral authority over their members. Access to rebates from private health insurance funds is usually restricted to professionals who are registered with state/territory registration boards or who are members of certain designated professional associations.

The registration boards specify the criteria for registration (for example, the nature of the required educational preparation), and decide on who can describe themselves as being a member of that particular profession. The boards also regulate the practice of (registered) members of the profession. Breen et al. (1997) describe how the medical profession is regulated, but regulation in other professions is similar. Depending on the profession, the registration boards may also regulate particular techniques or practices, whether or not they are carried out by registered practitioners (for example, certain interventions may only be able to be legally performed by registered practitioners). Because registration is effected at state level, there are differences in approach to registration across Australia including differences in composition of registration boards, procedures, and definitions of misconduct (Brodie and Barclay 2001; Bryant 2001). Rights of professionals to prescribe medication is regulated by state and territory Drugs and Poisons Acts.

The work of health (and other) professionals, whether or not they are registered, is also governed by the general legal framework including, for example, commercial law.

Members of the professions are required to exercise an appropriate level of skill in their dealings with consumers, and specialists are expected to exercise a higher level of skill (Zipser 1999). Health professionals are also expected to take account of the circumstances of the patients or consumers they are treating and ensure that they provide them with adequate information. In a key High Court judgment on this issue (Rogers v Whitaker

(1992) 175 CLR 479) it was stated that the professional's obligation is to regard the 'paramount consideration [to be] that a person is entitled to make his [sic] own decisions about his [sic] life' (at 487).

The practices of individual health professionals and health professional associations are also regulated by the (Commonwealth) Trade Practices Act 1974 (and equivalent state Acts), which prohibit anticompetitive practices such as collusion, price fixing, and misleading advertising. The ACCC is the independent statutory authority that, among other functions, is responsible for compliance with and enforcement of the Trade Practices Act.

Preparation of health professionals

Education of most health professionals takes place within the general framework of tertiary education. Since the mid 1980s there have been two broad streams of post-secondary education: a university sector and a vocational education and training sector, the latter principally providing non-degree programs. Most health professionals now receive their initial educational preparation in universities with course length varying from three to six years (for example, three years in the case of nursing and health information management; four years for pharmacy, physiotherapy, occupational therapy, speech pathology, and podiatry; five years for dentistry and some medical programs; and six years for other medical schools).

University-based preparation for the health professional is a relatively recent phenomenon. Until the 1960s, most health professionals received education in hospital-based programs or in state- or profession-run, professional-specific colleges. University education in most states was confined to preparation of medical and dental practitioners. The transformation of the tertiary education sector that took place in the late 1960s and early 1970s, following the creation of Colleges of Advanced Education, provided a new framework for non-medical health professional education.

In New South Wales and Victoria, two Colleges of Advanced Education specialising in the education of health professionals were established (New South Wales College of Paramedical Studies, subsequently Cumberland College of Health Sciences; in Victoria, the Lincoln Institute of Health Sciences). In other states, health professional education was transferred to generalist colleges. The major profession that remained outside of the general tertiary education system at this time was nursing, which retained its hospital-based focus. There was considerable controversy as to whether it was appropriate for nursing to transfer to colleges, the fear being that nurses would lose their 'practical' orientation. However, the leadership of the nursing profession was steadfast in its support for college-based education. Prior to its election in 1983, the Labor Party promised to support the

Figure 4.2 Australia: Trend in higher education course completions for health professionals, 1984—2000

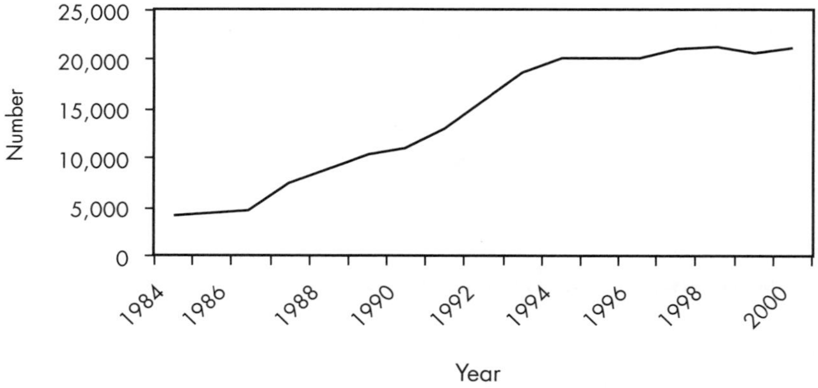

Data Source: Department of Education, Training and Youth Affairs, *Selected Higher Education Statistics: Higher Education Students Time Series Tables 2000,* Pub. No. 6714HERCO1A, DETYA, 2001

transfer of nurse education into the tertiary education sector and this was effected over the ensuing five years.

There was a further restructuring of the tertiary education sector in the late 1980s with the discontinuation of the 'binary' system (universities and the more vocationally oriented colleges), the merger of Colleges of Advanced Education with universities, and the establishment of new universities out of former colleges. The New South Wales and Victorian health sciences colleges merged with the University of Sydney and La Trobe University respectively. As a result of these changes there has been a significant increase in health sciences graduates from universities. Figure 4.2 shows the growth in health sciences graduations from universities over this period.

The vocational education and training sector provides shorter educational preparation leading to non-degree qualifications for occupations, most notably in the area of nursing (for associate professionals, variously termed 'enrolled nurses', 'division 2 registered nurses': nursing personnel who have not received educational preparation allowing them to practice independently as registered nurses). Although all health professionals receive on-the-job clinical education as part of their initial education, there tends to be a higher proportion of clinical placements as part of a program in the vocational education and training sector compared to universities.

Most professions have developed common national standards for defining the necessary educational preparation for entry to the profession, typically in terms of the competencies to be expected of a new graduate. The state registration boards have in many cases effectively delegated their powers to approve educational programs to national bodies (for example, the Australian

Medical Council in the case of approving medical courses; the Australian Council of Physiotherapy Registration Authorities for physiotherapy courses). The national bodies are designed to ensure consistency across Australia in standards for entry into the professions. The national bodies often are also able to ensure common decision-making standards in terms of recognition of which educational qualifications obtained internationally should be recognised as being equivalent to an Australian qualification for registration purposes.

Since the late 1980s there has been agreement on the need for harmonisation of the registration requirements for all professions, including health professions, to facilitate labour market flexibility across state boundaries. This process, known as mutual recognition, now ensures that a professional registered in one state or territory would automatically be able to meet registration requirements in every other state or territory. This process is obviously facilitated by the development of the national competency criteria for the professions and national processes for approving educational programs. The mutual recognition process also applies to New Zealand and, except for medical practitioners, professionals on a register in New Zealand are normally entitled to register in all Australian states and territories.

The 1990s saw a number of changes to the initial preparation for health professionals including the development of shortened, graduate entry programs. In these programs, rather than only selecting students following secondary school, selection is made after completion of a first degree. The prerequisite study requirements vary across programs. Graduate entry programs are now available in medicine, nursing, and most of the other health disciplines.

The initial educational preparation of a health professional generally needs to be consolidated by structured experience immediately post-graduation. In some cases (for example, medicine) there is a compulsory 'intern' year that provides supervised experience to consolidate the university-based preparation, and must be undertaken before the new graduate can practise outside the supervised environment of a hospital. In other professions (for example, nursing), structured experience immediately post-graduation is encouraged but is not compulsory.

In many of the health professions there is a tendency towards specialisation post-graduation. In some cases, specialist training is provided in universities and in others by professional colleges.

The structure for postgraduate education of health professions in universities follows that for other aspects of tertiary education, with a hierarchy of graduate certificates (the equivalent of one semester of full-time study), postgraduate diplomas (the equivalent of two semesters of full-time study), and Masters degree by coursework. Research degrees (master and doctoral) are also available. A number of universities also offer 'professional doctorates' which incorporate a mix of coursework and a research thesis, with the balance between the two areas varying between universities. (The Australian Qualifications Framework, introduced in 1995, specifies nomenclature for qualification levels, titles, and so on, for both universities and the vocational education and training sector.)

In medicine, clinical specialisation post-graduation is primarily the province of the Royal Clinical Colleges (for example, the Royal Australasian College of Physicians, and the Royal Australasian College of Surgeons), which supervise structured programs leading to recognition as a specialist in those clinical areas, such as Fellowship of the Royal Australasian College of Physicians (FRACP). Generally, medical specialty training takes about five to seven years and involves written and clinical examinations together with a range of clinical experiences in generalist or sub-specialty areas. Specialty training may take account of different locations of future practice, particularly the difference between rural and urban practice (Hays et al. 1997).

A number of universities also provide postgraduate qualifications in medicine in research (for example, doctoral degrees) and in coursework programs (such as in epidemiology, women's health, geriatrics). Postgraduate specialist education in a number of other health professions is also beginning to emulate the medical 'clinical college' model (for example, physiotherapy specialties, and podiatric surgery).

The nursing workforce is also increasingly specialised into areas such as midwifery, acute and critical care, and community health. Education for these specialties is now principally undertaken in universities, often linked to hospitals or health centres for clinical experience.

Postgraduate coursework opportunities are also provided by universities for other health professions such as physiotherapy (manipulative and sports physiotherapy). Universities also offer research training through doctoral degrees and Masters by research, and multidisciplinary postgraduate programs in areas such as occupational health, epidemiology, health promotion, and public health.

Continuing education is available from professional associations and colleges, universities, and independent organisations. A number of professions have requirements for a minimum level of participation in continuing education to maintain membership or to attain higher status within the association or college.

Models of provider payment

One of the most contentious aspects of health workforce policy relates to the way in which providers are paid for health care (Robinson 2001). Figure 4.3 shows a number of different models of provider payment.

The simplest model (A) is based on a consumer–provider dyad. Under this model consumers pay providers directly for services received. This is the most common method for many health providers operating in a simple professional environment without any form of insurance. From a provider's

Figure 4.3 Models of provider payment

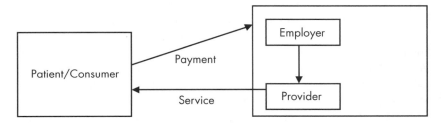

Model A: Simple 'commercial contract' model of payment

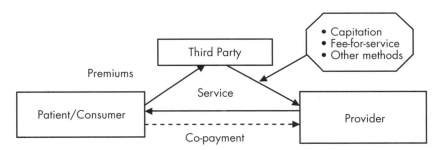

Model B: Employment contract model of payment

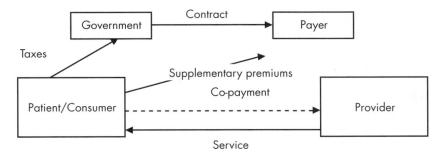

Model C: Third party payer model of payment

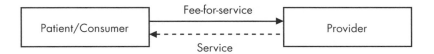

Model D: Government—payer split model of payment

perspective it involves a direct relationship with the consumer, with no interference from any other payer and so maximises professional autonomy. Of course, the interaction between the consumer and the provider is still regulated by professional registration board requirements in terms of advertising and the nature of services that may be delivered, and by the standard principles of commercial contract and other aspects of the commercial environment (such as truth in advertising, and fair dealing). From a consumer's perspective, this model maximises the likely responsiveness of the provider to the wishes and demands of the consumer. The simple, 'commercial contract' model of payment operates for professional work in many other parts of the economy (for example, legal services).

As described in chapter 3, the health care market is not typical of other markets and that leads to deficiencies in the commercial contract model. Arrow (1963), in a seminal paper, outlined a number of aspects of market failure in health care, most notably problems relating to information asymmetry: that the provider necessarily has different information from the consumer. An important consequence of information asymmetry is that consumers find it difficult to judge between the knowledge and skills of competing providers and hence cannot make a fully informed choice of providers. Further, they are not well placed to evaluate the services their provider might recommend. The simple commercial contract model also has no mechanism for addressing equity issues, as the full cost of services falls on the individual consumer.

The second simple model of payment (B), the employment contract model, represents the situation where professional services are provided by a health professional employed by a larger organisation. It reflects the situation of services provided to consumers by hospitals, community health centres, and local government (in maternal and child health provision). In this arrangement, the employer provides a salary (including part-time or sessional payments) to a provider in exchange for the health professional working within the organisation. A component (which may be the entire component) of the health professional's work will be providing service to the consumer. The consumer may be required to make a payment directly to the organisation which may or may not cover the direct costs of the service that the consumer received (that is, there may be some cross-subsidies within the organisation). Although the interaction between the health professional and the consumer is still regulated by the professional registration board (if any) which covers the professional, the direct relationship with the consumer is weakened in that the provider's accountability is in part to the consumer, but in part to their employer. The provider may thus be constrained to work within certain guidelines as to the amount of time available to the consumer or the services that can be provided. This in turn may cause some ethical issues about the provider's relationship to the consumer. There is a developing body of literature, mainly from the USA, related to ethical problems associated with the professional's complex balancing of accountability to consumer and the employer (Rodwin 1995, 1996).

The most common application of the employment contract model in Australia involves public hospitals and community health centres and is associated with government subsidies paid to the employing organisation. This substantially improves access for consumers, which to some extent offsets the potential negatives of the model.

Another way of subsidising consumers' use of health care (thus increasing equity and access) is used in most developed countries. This entails the creation of third party payers to equalise risk over time for individual consumers by providing cross-subsidies between consumers (model C). Private health insurance arrangements and Medicare are both variants of this model; with Medicare there are no premiums and the payer is funded by taxation. The third party may pay the provider in a number of ways: fee-for-service, salary, or capitation (a fixed amount per person per annum, with the provider assuming all responsibility for the care to that individual or family). The consumer may be required to make some co-payment to the provider for any services received. Consumers also may be able to make supplementary premium payments to ensure differential entitlement for services.

If the insurance system is compulsory and a broad risk pool across the whole population is thus insured, this model addresses many of the equity issues that beset the simple commercial contract model. Depending on the nature of consumer choice in any system and the ability of consumers to exercise choice among providers, this model can also address some of the weaknesses of the employment contract model. Providers, however, may have less autonomy than afforded by the simple commercial contract model because third party payers may exercise some constraint over the provider in a way similar to the employment contract model.

The most complex model (D) is a more recent policy approach that distinguishes between government's funder and payer roles. In this model the government contracts on behalf of consumers with a payer, which in turn contracts with providers. Advocates of this model argue that specialist payers (especially private payers) are able to develop more sophisticated contracts with providers that provide for enhanced accountability of the provider to the payer. To some extent, the model involves an inherent and planned confusion of government accountability: government can claim that it does not specify the nature of contracts between the payer and the provider (or between the consumer and the payer). In this model, payers are not normally government organisations so there is also a loss of democratic accountability.

The contract between the government and the payer organisation is a critical feature of this model as it needs to specify the scope of services to be covered and how payers will be funded by government. There is now an extensive literature on the ways in which government can set a 'risk adjusted' premium to payers designed to ensure an appropriate payment for necessary care. Despite the advances in risk adjustment (Iezzoni 1994), the payment rates may be such that the paying organisation has an incentive to 'cream skim' (that is, attempt to recruit consumers who are healthier than average) so as to increase profits or margins. This more elaborated government–payer split model is now increasingly used in the USA as part of government health sector payment arrangements (so-called 'managed care').

Different payment models have different policy consequences. Models involving third parties (C and D) obviously allow treatment choices of providers to be influenced by those payers. In Australia, third party payers have, by and large, not attempted to influence treatment choices of consumers. This is not the situation in the USA where many forms of 'managed care' have involved restrictions on consumers in terms of their choice of the providers from whom they can seek treatment, and restrictions on providers in terms of the need to get clearance from the third party payer prior to payment approval (most widespread is the need to seek 'pre-admission certification' prior to hospitalisation). There are a variety of forms of managed care in the USA with wide variations in the kinds and levels of restrictions (Hacker and Marmor 1999).

The different models of provider payment provide different opportunities for controlling expenditure (the more provider or consumer choices are limited, the more opportunities there are for a third party payer to exercise control over treatment choices) and provide different incentives for expansion of services, different patient experiences, and may lead to differences in quality of care (Gosden et al. 2001). Payment models that link income to activity or are based on provider costs also have different incentive effects (Jegers et al. 2002). For these reasons, third party payers often seek to change payment arrangements in ways that generate political heat. Some analysts, for example Scotton (1999), argue that the government should transfer the risk of growth in health expenditure to other third party payers by moving from the current Medicare model (C) to one in which 'independent' third party payers assume those risks (D). One of the main ways expenditure growth risk can be managed in this model is through change in consumer behaviour, and thus consumers are likely to see little benefit in moving away from the contemporary system where they have a high degree of choice. Third party payers also need to be paid for assuming risks so this model may be inherently more expensive than its alternative.

As was indicated in chapter 3, health care costs as a proportion of GDP are close to what would be predicted based on the size of Australia's economy. While this does not prescribe the ideal level of spending for a society, it does not provide support for a dramatic change in the nature of payment arrangements in Australia.

Issues in health workforce supply and demand

An important and regularly recurring policy issue relating to the health workforce is the adequacy of supply to meet demand: do we have enough doctors, are we facing a nursing shortage crisis? Increasingly, governments are concerned to ensure that there is an adequate supply of skilled labour in all areas of the economy, usually implemented through education and training policy. In Australia, government has historically been active in health workforce issues, particularly relating to the medical workforce, because of the government's role as both a funder and provider in the health sector. Health workforce policy has usually been driven by health (rather than education and training) portfolios and policy levers applied to influence the supply and distribution of the health workforce have been a mix of 'health' and 'education' instruments (see table 4.4).

There are three main committees that have been established to co-ordinate health workforce planning in Australia:

- The Australian Health Workforce Officials Committee (AHWOC), which consists of senior staff from each of the state health authorities, and from the Commonwealth education and health departments. This committee aims to provide national oversight and coordination across all health workforce planning activities.
- The Australian Medical Workforce Advisory Committee (AMWAC) has membership drawn from medical associations and colleges, representatives of universities and consumers, experts (for example in health economics), and nominees from state and Commonwealth departments and agencies.
- The Australian Health Workforce Advisory Committee (AHWAC) is responsible for providing advice on the non-medical workforce: nursing, midwifery, and allied health. Its membership includes representatives of the professions, universities, and bureaucratic agencies.

All three committees report to the meeting of heads of health authorities/departments (Australian Health Ministers' Advisory Council, AHMAC) and all are serviced by a secretariat based in Sydney.

Health workforce policy attention is directed to whether the workforce is in balance at a state or national level as well as whether segments of the market (specialty, location) are in balance. Ensuring a balance of supply and demand in the health workforce is difficult for a number of reasons:

- low mobility of health professionals means that there can be oversupply in some areas and undersupply in others, thus reducing the likely success of training additional professionals as a means of redressing imbalances
- long lead times for education and training of health professionals, especially specialists

Table 4.3   Costs of workforce imbalance

Costs of undersupply	Costs of oversupply
Poor access, unmet need, potentially poorer outcomes	Unnecessary costs incurred in education sector in training workforce
Overworked and stressed workforce (which may make the profession/area unattractive and further reduce supply)	Unnecessary services provided where workforce can create own demand
Increased costs of alternative provision (e.g. travel costs)	Workforce may not maintain skills because of insufficient consultation rate

Source: AMWAC and AIHW 1998

- long-term predictions must also take account of changes in technology in the health industry (and hence demand) and yet technological change is quite rapid, possibly invalidating even recent predictions.

Health workforce policy is further confounded by the existence of real costs associated with an imbalance, both in terms of undersupply and oversupply (see table 4.3).

Typically, health workforce policy attempts to influence supply, viewing demand as exogenous. This is not the case, however, as changes in broad policy settings or the labour force may in turn affect demand for consultations with health professionals. There can also be policies to affect demand for health consultations; for example, providing additional information to consumers may increase their ability to self-manage a particular condition.

Figure 4.4 summarises the key flows that affect the size of the health workforce.

The key inflows are new graduates, internationally trained health professionals, and people returning to the workforce. Major outflows are retirement and death, and other exits including emigration. A key focus of policy attention is the flow of new graduates into the health workforce. Here, there are three major factors:

- the number of entrants into educational programs, that is, the size of the intakes into university and other training programs
- the proportion of intakes who graduate (flow A) and who then enter the workforce. The dropout rate from universities in the higher status health professions (such as medicine or physiotherapy) is quite low but there is significant dropout from other professions, such as nursing
- the number of graduates who eventually enter the workforce.

Most graduates of health professional programs enter the workforce immediately after graduation (around 90 per cent of 1996 graduates (Johnson 1997)). However, there is a significant number who do not immediately enter the workforce because of an interest in further training (in postgraduate programs, including research programs), who defer entry into the Australian

Figure 4.4 Factors affecting health workforce supply

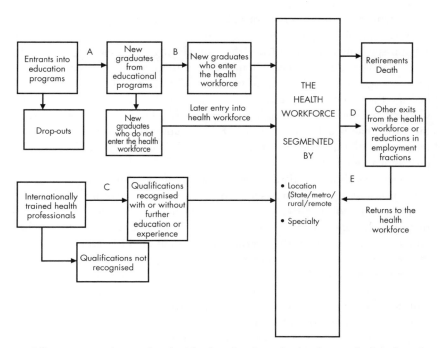

workforce to travel, or who decide that, having obtained a professional qual-ification, they do not propose to enter that profession.

A second major flow relates to the number of internationally trained health professionals who enter the workforce. Given the long lead times involved in adjusting workforce supply by increasing student intakes, the flow of internationally trained workers is critical to workforce planning (Walker and Maynard 2003). Australia is a relatively attractive country for internationally trained health professionals and a significant number of pro-fessionals seek to migrate to this country. Australian immigration rules tend to discourage migration from professional groups seen to be in oversupply through allocation of priorities for migration work permits. A further bar-rier to immigration comes from the processes for recognition of education or experience. Obviously, if a profession is not regulated in a given state then there is no barrier to practise. But in those states or territories where a pro-fession is regulated, there are usually three hurdles prior to registration:

- a test of communication skills, most commonly operationalised as the 'Occupational English Test' which assesses reading, writing, and listening skills in English
- a written examination on professional knowledge (often undertaken as a multiple choice test)

- an examination of clinical skills (normally, this examination is available only in Australia).

In some professions, certain qualifications from overseas programs are automatically eligible for professional registration. Typically, these are programs in English-speaking countries such as the United Kingdom, Ireland, and Canada. The professions differ markedly in this respect. In medicine, for example, automatic recognition is only given to graduates of New Zealand medical schools, because the schools have been individually assessed by the Australian Medical Council, the body that assesses Australian medical schools. In physiotherapy, on the other hand, a broad range of overseas universities have been granted recognition. In other circumstances, internationally obtained qualifications give professionals the right to sit written exams or the clinical examination.

Decisions about standards of entry into the professions are controversial. The health professions themselves often have an economic incentive to reduce competition in the marketplace, and hence may place tight restrictions on the entry of overseas graduates. This situation has also applied where the Commonwealth government has attempted to reduce the supply of overseas medical graduates in order to reduce pressure on its expenditure under the Medicare Benefits Scheme. The flow of internationally trained professionals into the workforce can be a significant reason for growth in workforce supply. The economic incentive to reduce competition is often argued on the grounds of the need to maintain 'standards'.

The effect on overseas-trained health professionals who cannot obtain registration to practise in Australia can be quite traumatic (Kunz 1975; Kidd and Braun 1992). In some professions, internationally trained professionals may be restricted to practise in rural and remote areas in order to address the perceived shortages of professionals in those areas.

The health workforce is obviously reduced by retirements and deaths. Although there is no requirement for persons to retire at a particular age, there is a tendency for most health professionals to retire between 60 and 65 years of age, with some reducing their practice involvement on a graduated basis starting some years earlier. This is especially the case for those professionals whose work requires a high level of physical activity or manual dexterity.

Professionals might also leave the health workforce (either temporarily or permanently) for a host of other reasons including overseas travel, child rearing, pursuing other opportunities, and so on (flow D in figure 4.4). This flow is particularly influenced by the broader economic situation, including the relative attractiveness of working in the health professions (relative wages and conditions). Those health professions that have a higher proportion of females are particularly affected by temporary and permanent exits from the workforce associated with family formation.

Depending on the length of time absent from the workforce, the professional may need to undergo retraining prior to re-entry. Again, the flow back into the health workforce (flow E) of those who temporarily exit is affected by opportunities within the workforce for retraining, support arrangements such as child care and flexible work arrangements that make return to employment easier. It is also affected by the general economic situation, including relative wages and employment prospects in the health sector versus other sectors, by employment opportunities for spouses, and by broad societal trends such as attitudes to women's employment.

The health workforce for any profession is highly segmented in terms of both location at state level (persons who trained in one state tend to work in that state) and also within the state in terms of metropolitan, rural, and remote practice. There are different market conditions applying in metropolitan and rural areas, both in terms of the nature of the profession and also the remuneration.

As indicated earlier, many of the professions now involve specialisation in a particular skill area and this further segments the workforce. The effect of this segmentation is that workforce planning normally needs to be undertaken at a specialty level (for the example of specialist physicians, see Dent and Goulston 1999).

Identifying whether there are shortages or surpluses of a particular profession requires analysis of both workforce supply and demand. As indicated above, there can be interactions between supply and demand; for example if

Table 4.4 Options for addressing workforce imbalances (shortage)

	Demand Side	Supply side
Price	Increase/introduce consumer co-payments	Increase relative wages/fees for health professionals
		Increase/introduce recruitment/retention bonuses (flows D and E)
		Introduce retraining incentives to reskill professionals to skill area of short supply
		Introduce mobility incentives to encourage relocation of professionals to geographic area of short supply
Volume	Encourage use of substitute professionals	Increase educational intakes (flow A)
		Reduce program dropouts
	Encourage self-management of care needs through information provision or other strategies	Increase flow of internationally trained professionals into the workforce (flow C)
	Support informal carers	Facilitate re-entry (flow E) through retraining programs, job redesign
	Reduce demand through changing consumer expectations	Increase use of technology to expand available provision (e.g. e-health)

there is a severe workforce shortage, this may create queues and waiting lists, which in turn may reduce demand. Table 4.4 shows several options for addressing an imbalance between workforce supply and demand.

For ease of presentation table 4.4 has been structured in terms of addressing a workforce shortage; addressing a workforce oversupply involves symmetrical strategies. Each of the strategies in the table needs to be assessed in terms of the general criteria for assessing health systems: efficiency, equity, quality, and acceptability. In terms of equity, the co-payment strategies, for example, will have an adverse effect on equity; other strategies may have adverse effects on acceptability (for example, encourage self-management of care needs) or efficiency. The strategies also need to be assessed in terms of their cost-effectiveness and whether they will establish precedents that would result in increased expenditure for professions or specialisations that are not subject to a workforce imbalance.

The nursing workforce

In 2001 there were 268,873 nurses in Australia, 80 per cent of whom were registered nurses. Nursing represents the largest component of the health professional workforce. The most recent source of nursing workforce data (AIHW 2003f) provides a range of data on nurses and most of the data in this

Figure 4.5 Australia: Trends in nurses per 100,000 population, by state or territory, 1993–99

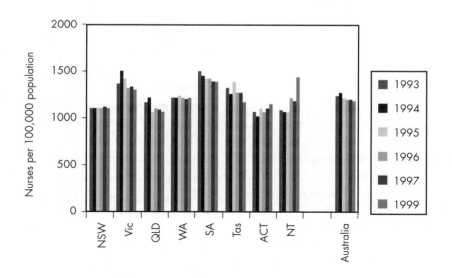

section are taken from that publication. Updates of nursing labour force data are available on the AIHW web site (www.aihw.gov.au).

Figure 4.5 shows that in Australia in 1999, there was an average of around 1200 nurses per 100,000 population. There is about a 15 per cent variation in the number of nurses per 100,000 population between the highest provision state (Victoria, 1297; the AIHW views the Northern Territory data as being less reliable than the other states and territories) and the lowest provision state (New South Wales, 1093). Despite increased demand for hospital and other health care services, the number of nurses per capita has declined about 4 per cent over the period 1993 to 1999, with larger declines in some states (e.g. Tasmania, 12 per cent).

There is currently (2003) a shortage of nurses nationally and in most states: most categories of nurses are listed on the Department of Employment and Workplace Relations' National and State Skills Shortage List (www.workplace.gov.au/WP/Content/Files/WP/EmploymentPublications/NSSFeb2003.pdf) and on the Department of Immigration and Multicultural and Indigenous Affairs' Migration Occupations in Demand List (MODL; www.immi.gov.au/migration/skilled/modl.htm). One way of assessing shortages is to monitor advertising of job vacancies. The Department of Employment and Workplace Relations publishes a data series based on a count of advertisements in major daily newspapers on the first Saturday of each month (see figure 4.6).

Figure 4.6 Australia: Trends in nurse vacancies as advertised in metropolitan daily newspapers, 1981–2003

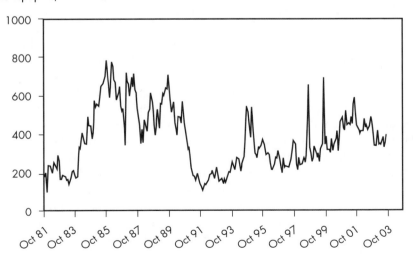

Data Source: DEWR special tabulation

Figure 4.7 Australia: Ratio of employed registered nurses to employed enrolled nurses, by state or territory, 1989–2001

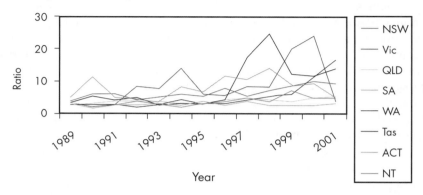

Job advertisements' series are affected by contraction or expansion in the industry and consequential impacts on job creation/contraction, industry practices about advertising in newspapers, and by recruitment difficulties (the same job being advertised more than once). The pattern revealed in figure 4.6 is of a severe shortage of nurses in the mid 1980s, which appeared to be resolved in the early 1990s (probably because of budget cuts at that time and contraction of the industry). Job shortages re-emerged in the mid 1990s.

There are significant differences in the nursing workforce skill mix (the ratio of registered to enrolled nurses) between the states (see figure 4.7).

In 2001 registered nurses comprised 94 per cent of the employed nursing workforce in Victoria and 78 per cent of the South Australian workforce. It can also be seen that in every year there are more employed registered nurses per enrolled nurse in Victoria than in New South Wales, reflecting the higher proportion of enrolled nurses in Victoria. This probably reflects a tendency for there to be a relatively higher skill mix, especially in nursing homes in Victoria, with enrolled nurses replacing non-nursing staff. In Victoria, 52 per cent of enrolled nurses work in aged care, compared with an Australian average of 33 per cent (New South Wales, 24 per cent; Queensland, 23 per cent). There has also been a substantial increase in the ratio of registered to enrolled nurses over the last five years. This shift has been most notable in Victoria where the ratio has increased from 3.5 to 16.8 over the period 1996 to 2001.

Figure 4.8 shows the significant variation in employment patterns of nurses by location, with provision in remote centres being at lower levels than in capital cities and other metropolitan areas.

Interestingly, unlike the situation with respect to medical practice, large rural centres have very high levels of supply of nurses. The availability of nurses in large rural centres may in part reflect the more widespread availability of nursing education. Many large regional centres have nursing schools on

Figure 4.8 Australia: Trend in employed nurses per 100,000 population, by region, 1993–99

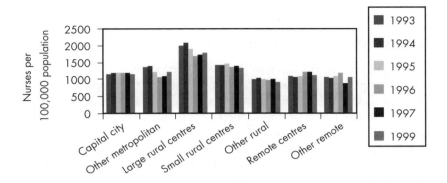

the campus of the local university. This is unlike the situation for medical training where most of the medical schools are located in capital cities.

One reason for the volatility in the nursing workforce may be associated with volatility in enrolments in nursing education at universities. Figure 4.9 shows the number of nursing course commencements over the period 1989 to 2001.

New nursing students increased from 6747 in 1989 to a peak of 9325 in 1991 before declining to around 7000 from the mid 1990s. The number of entrants is in part a reflection of choice by students about whether they wish

Figure 4.9 Australia: Commencements in basic nursing courses by Australian citizens and permanent residents, 1989–2001

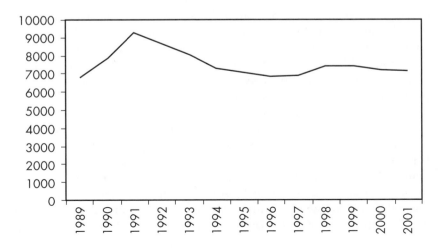

to enrol in nursing as a course and in part choices by institutions about how many places they will make available. A number of universities have reduced the places available to nursing students in the late 1990s as part of a strategy to increase the tertiary entry score required for entry to the profession.

Contemporary issues in the nursing workforce

A review of nursing education in Australian universities in 1994 (Commonwealth Department of Human Services and Health 1994) identified a range of policy issues affecting the nursing workforce, including issues of labour force planning, career pathways, and educational preparation. In its report, the review made a large number of recommendations for change and development that received little policy attention. National policy interest in nursing was reawakened in 2001 with two inquiries being established, one by the Senate (Senate Community Affairs References Committee 2002) and one by the Commonwealth government (National Review of Nursing Education 2002). In addition there had been a number of state-based reviews of nursing (see listing in Senate Community Affairs References Committee 2002, p. 3). Both national reviews recognised there were significant problems in workforce planning for the nursing profession. The 2002 National Review, for example, highlighted:

- the lack of long-term planning for the health workforce and nursing specifically
- the fragmentation of the responsibilities for different aspects of nursing and nursing education combined with the different contexts in which nurses work (p. 107).

Fragmentation of responsibility means that there are four parties who need to be involved in addressing issues relating to the nursing workforce: universities that make decisions about intakes and curriculum design and development (which affect retention in courses); health agencies that have responsibility for employment practices (which affect retention); states and territories that make decisions about award pay and conditions; and the Commonwealth government, which funds universities and regulates migration intakes. Unfortunately there are no structures that bring these parties together to ensure a coherent and combined response to nursing workforce issues.

Both recent reviews of nursing identified critical shortages of nurses (see pp. 14–17 and 48–52 of the Senate report and pp. 188–9 of the 2002 National Review). The extent of the shortage of general nurses has been estimated at 40,000 by 2010 (see National Review 2002, p. 188). Shortages of nurses are also reported in the USA (for example see Coile 2002; Sochalski 2002) and in other countries. Given the international migration of nurses, recruitment of Australian nurses to work overseas might exacerbate the forecast shortage. Although the response to a shortage of the magnitude forecast must include provision of additional nursing places in universities, restructure of the workplace and changing demand patterns for nurses must also be considered.

A major issue for nursing workforce policy in the medium term therefore relates to the role of the professional (registered) nurse. Without clarification of the role of the nurse, there cannot be clarity about how many nurses are needed in the workforce, and educational institutions will find it difficult to make coordinated decisions about design of curricula and appropriate number of nurses that ought to be enrolled in nursing education programs.

The competency standards for the nursing profession published by the Australian Nursing Council Incorporated (www.anci.org.au/competency-standards.htm) are broad and aspirational. The Australian Nursing Council has also published a statement on the role of the nurse that is also phrased in broad generalities. There is good reason for this, as an alternative approach focusing on particular tasks may make the competency standards and role statements out of date relatively quickly.

The role of the nurse is the subject of a number of pressures, posing both threats and opportunities to the profession. In the first instance, the educational preparation of all nurses is improving, associated with the move to university-based education and the continuing refinement of university curricula. This broader educational preparation of nurses provides a foundation for nurses to undertake more complex roles and tasks. Failure to provide challenges in the workplace may lead to dissatisfaction among nurses with contemporary levels of educational preparation and affect retention. Further, as the postgraduate preparation of nurses is also now largely university-based, this provides further opportunities for developing highly skilled nurses. There is now a developing literature about the potential for nurses to undertake roles that were previously the sole preserve of doctors (Richardson and Maynard 1995; Sakr et al. 1999; see also Sergison et al. 1999 for a comprehensive bibliography on skill mix in primary care). Some studies have suggested that up to 30 per cent of the work of doctors could be undertaken by nurses. Whether this substitution is cost-effective depends not only on the relative pay rates of nurses and doctors but also the relative time taken to complete the tasks.

New South Wales was the first state to consider the potential for nurses taking broader roles through a series of pilot programs under the general rubric of 'nurse practitioner'. This is an unfortunate term as it is poorly defined. The New South Wales nurse practitioner pilot programs initially focused on practice in rural and remote areas where there is said to be a shortage of medical practitioners. Developing the nurse practitioner model in the other states has not been limited to rural and remote practice (Offredy 2000).

Nurses can substitute for general practitioners in many primary care tasks, for residents in intensive care units, and can undertake high level triage functions in hospital emergency departments. Midwives also play a significant role in maternity care. In Australia, most experience in substitution has occurred in areas that are relatively unattractive to medical practitioners (for example rural areas, aged care, services for Aboriginal people and Torres Strait Islanders) and hence substitution strategies have not caused conflict with the medical profession.

The basis for independent nursing practice is a sound educational base to make diagnosis and treatment judgments. Opportunities for substitution would be substantially greater if nurses had independent prescribing rights (for either a limited range of drugs, or according to specific protocols). The extent to which nurses should have independent prescribing and practice rights is thus a critical issue for determining the future role of the nurse. It is also likely to be a contentious one, attracting opposition from the medical profession, as did the transfer of nursing education to universities in the 1980s (Hazelton 1990).

Discussion of the development of expanded nursing roles (including prescribing) is confused by a focus on the payment arrangements; for example, an automatic assumption that the development of a 'nurse practitioner' means a change of payment arrangements from the employment contract model (B in figure 4.3) to either an independent commercial contract model (A) or a third party payment model (C). There is no reason why the development of a nurse practitioner model needs to involve independent fee-for-service practice.

The economic viability of substitution and enhanced nursing roles must also take account of the effects on treatment thresholds. If nurses become the first point of contact with the health care system, this may change the perception of consumers about whether or not they should initiate a health consultation. Conditions that might have previously been self-managed may, in the new environment, lead to a professional consultation, with consequent increases in the volume of consultations and total costs.

Policies on substitution should also involve consideration of whether all the tasks currently undertaken by professional nurses should continue to be undertaken by those nurses, or whether they can be delegated to other personnel, either associate professionals (enrolled nurses) or persons with shorter, more generic training.

Change in roles, including greater substitution, needs to be carefully planned and accompanied by appropriate legal protection (Dowling et al. 1995, 1996). As was noted earlier, there are considerable differences in the relative proportions of professionals and associate professionals in the nursing workforce, partly reflecting decisions in different states about which tasks can be undertaken by enrolled nurses and which can be undertaken by other personnel. This is particularly important with respect to employment in nursing homes. If professional nurses are to undertake an expanded role, some tasks currently undertaken by nurses will need to be delegated to other personnel. Given constraints on health funding and available places in universities, a significant expansion of the nursing workforce is relatively unlikely.

Finally, resolution of legal, economic, and organisational issues relating to broader nursing roles will not necessarily mean that implementation of the new roles is easy. Opposition to broader roles may well derive from ideological/value differences or opposition to a perceived market competitor. Broader roles for nurses may eventually lead to increased power for nurses in policy debates, to the detriment of those, especially the medical profession, who occupy that policy space at present.

Issues relating to substitution in the health workforce lead to consideration of what is the appropriate model for nursing workforce development. At present there are three major levels of entry into the nursing workforce: a registered nurse who graduates from a three-year university program, a 12- to 18-month trained enrolled nurse, and a nursing assistant with very short training in the vocational education and training sector. An alternative model would be a structure involving an initial preparation of four years for registered nurses, and two years for enrolled nurses, with the nursing assistant level unchanged. An enrolled nurse with two years training could undertake a much broader range of tasks and should be able to provide the predominant staffing in most hospital settings.

A model of this design, which increases the average length of training, would be substantially more expensive if current roles were to continue. However, in order to be cost-effective the model would need to be accompanied by a major change in roles and a significant reduction in the demand for four-year trained registered nurses. In this model, the registered nurse would be employed in professional and consultative roles as well as having prescription rights and would function in a way analogous to the autonomy exercised by other health professionals. In turn, this model would require a review of the current ratios of registered to enrolled nurses. Such a model could only be implemented in a phased way given the large number of existing nurses who would need some additional educational preparation.

The nursing workforce is increasingly segmented into specialties, for example midwifery, intensive/critical care nursing, emergency nursing, and so on. These specialties generally parallel medical specialties, many of which could not function without appropriate specialist nursing support (AMWAC 1998b). The education pathway for each of these nursing specialties is different and thus the workforce needs for each must be planned separately. AHWAC has undertaken workforce studies of midwifery (AHWAC 2002a) and of critical care nurses (AHWAC 2002b). The differences in the areas mean that drivers of demand are quite different (for example, fertility versus intensive care bed requirements), and training patterns also differ. However both areas reported substantial contemporary shortages and needs for increases in supply.

As mentioned earlier in this chapter, responsibility for initial preparation of nurses rests with the universities, loosely coordinated by the Commonwealth government. Each university makes an independent decision about course design, number of entering students, postgraduate course offerings, and so on. University decisions have critical consequences for the health and community service sectors in terms of the numbers of entering registered nurses, and yet there are no mechanisms at the national level and few mechanisms at the state level to ensure that these decisions have a positive impact on future workforce requirements. The need for national co-ordination in this area is self-evident but sadly lacking.

Unless issues of the appropriate role and composition of the nursing workforce can be resolved, nurse workforce planning cannot be undertaken in any meaningful way.

The medical workforce

The medical workforce accounts for about 13 per cent of the entire health workforce. The most recent source of data on the medical workforce is for 2000 (AIHW 2003d; note this is a summary publication, full data are only available for 1999, AIHW 2003c; data in this chapter are drawn from those sources). Figure 4.10 summarises the overall medical workforce situation.

There are approximately 50,000 individual medical practitioners working in Australia. There are approximately 62,000 medical practitioners on state and territory registers, but this includes multiple state registrations as well as medical practitioners currently working overseas. Of the individual practitioners registered, 94 per cent are in the medical workforce, most of these being clinicians (90 per cent).

The clinical workforce is divided into primary care practitioners (about 45 per cent of the medical workforce), hospital-based non-specialists (11 per cent), specialists (34 per cent), and specialists in training (11 per cent). The proportion of women in each of these areas differs remarkably, with 32 per cent of primary care practitioners being female compared with 14 per cent of specialists. It is interesting to note that there is a larger proportion of female specialists in training relative to the female specialist workforce, which may suggest that, over time, the proportion of women in the specialist workforce will increase to that in the primary care practitioner workforce, subject to similar attrition patterns.

The female proportion of medical graduates increased from 40 per cent in 1988 to 47 per cent in 1994 and has stabilised since then. Females therefore comprise a significantly higher proportion of entrants into the medical workforce as a whole. As figure 4.11 shows, females have a different work pattern from males, with a lower proportion of the female workforce

Figure 4.10 The Australian medical workforce, 2000

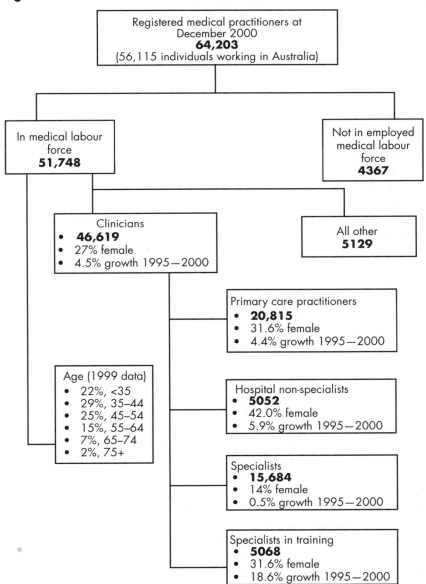

Figure 4.11 Australia: Employed medical workforce by hours worked per week, 1995 and 1999

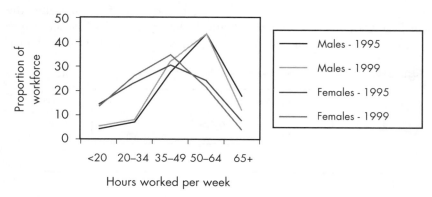

working full-time. Comparing 1995 to 1999, fewer males and females are working longer hours, possibly reflecting the realisation that long working hours could impact adversely on patient safety.

'Feminisation' of the medical workforce results in fewer effective full-time medical practitioners being available. Although the proportion of female medical practitioners working full-time may increase as family-friendly workplace policies are introduced, the relative proportion of female practitioners in the workforce will remain a significant variable to be taken into account in workforce planning (for comprehensive reviews of this issue see AMWAC and AIHW 1996 and 1998 AMWAC, Reports 1996.7 and 1998.4).

The clinician workforce has grown by about 4.5 per cent over the period 1995–2000, but with almost no growth occurring in the specialist workforce. It is interesting to note that the number of specialists in training is growing rapidly. This suggests that, as the trainees graduate, the specialist growth rate will begin to increase. The rapid growth in specialists in training may be driven by government policy to limit access to Medicare provider numbers to specialists and FRACGPs (or equivalent).

The hospital non-specialist workforce is growing faster than clinicians as a whole. This growth is also a result of specific policies at both Commonwealth and state level, in this case to change the composition of the workforce in hospitals by using career medical officers to undertake work previously undertaken by specialists in training or junior doctors (Mason et al. 1993; van Konkelenberg and McAlindon 1993). Use of career medical officers reduces the overtime hours of trainees and also provides experienced personnel in a range of specialty areas, albeit without specialist qualifications.

As figure 4.12 shows, there is considerable variation in the number of employed medical practitioners (full-time equivalent clinicians) per 100,000 population around the Australian average (326.6).

Figure 4.12 Australia: Employed medical practitioners (clinicians) per 100,000 population, 1999

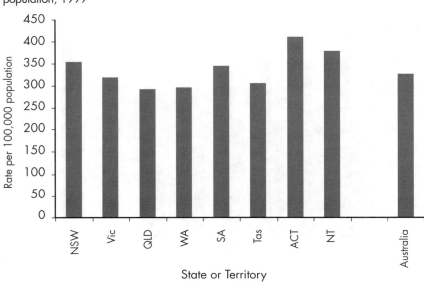

The highest ratio of employed medical practitioners, in the Australian Capital Territory (413), is 40 per cent above the ratio in the lowest state (Queensland, 290). The Australian Capital Territory ratio may be inflated in that Canberra serves as a referral centre for the rural areas in New South Wales that surround it. The population that it serves is thus greater than the recorded Australian Capital Territory population. The New South Wales ratio (354), which would not be affected by referral patterns, is 22 per cent above the Queensland ratio.

Figure 4.13 shows trends in general practitioner:population ratios in urban and rural areas in Australia. Over the 15-year period 1984/5 to 2000, there has been a 66 per cent increase in the number of general practitioners per capita. Rates of growth were fairly evenly distributed across all geographic classifications, although there were particularly high rates of growth in remote areas where the provision doubled on a per capita basis. The pattern of lower provision in smaller rural communities relative to larger rural centres is consistent with a previous study (Richardson et al. 1991), which found that the likelihood of general practitioner presence increased with town size and a threshold effect for presence of other medical specialists. Brasure et al. (1999), in a US study, found a similar threshold effect, and noted that the population increment needed to attract a second medical practitioner was less than required to attract the first. There has been a significant increase in general practitioner provision in both metropolitan

Figure 4.13 Australia: General practitioners per 100,000 population, 1984/85 to 2000

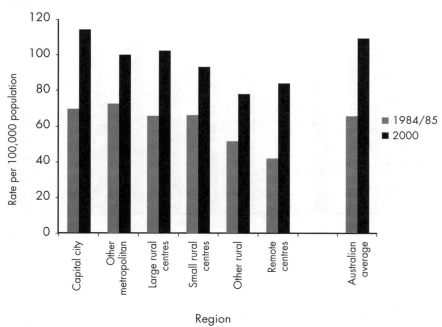

and rural areas, with a higher ratio in capital cities relative to rural and remote areas. What is remarkable about this is that, although there is a perception of underprovision of general practitioners in rural areas, and a significant focus of policy attention on access in rural and remote areas (Humphreys et al. 1997) and factors affecting medical practitioners' choosing rural practice (Laven et al. 2003), the contemporary level of rural access is above the metropolitan level in 1984/85. As figure 4.13 shows, the general practitioner:population ratio has increased over the period 1984/85 to 2000. However, regular reports of high levels of dissatisfaction and disillusionment among general practitioners (for example, Douglas and Saltman 1991) prompted government and the profession to develop organisational strategies to reduce general practitioner isolation and provide a framework for general practitioner involvement in local health services development (Pegram et al. 1995). Divisions of General Practitioners were created covering designated regions as voluntary associations of general practitioners. Infrastructure funding from the Commonwealth to the divisions enables these divisions to employ staff and undertake projects. Funding is also provided to facilitate achievement of negotiated objectives, such as increased immunisation rates in the region covered by the division. The emphasis of Commonwealth funding in the 1990s was through these divisions for a wide range of medically led projects (such as health promotion projects—see Commonwealth Department of Human Services and Health 1995) in contrast to the community-led approaches that characterised Commonwealth funding in the 1970s.

As figure 4.4 shows, the size of the medical workforce is affected by the flow of internationally trained practitioners. There are three main pathways for internationally trained medical practitioners to enter the Australian medical workforce. Two pathways lead to a permanent stay and on-going registration as a medical practitioner. Of these, the most common is the pathway for general registration. In the period 1997–2000 an average of 746 candidates presented to the Australian Medical Council for the multiple choice questionnaire component of its examination each year. An average of 303 candidates passed the examination each year (41 per cent pass rate), with an average of 197 per annum passing the clinical examination and being eligible for registration. An alternative pathway for those seeking permanent residency is through specialist recognition, assessed by the relevant specialist college. On average 51 people achieved specialist recognition per annum in the period 1997–2000.

In contrast to the 250 or so medical practitioners who gain registration through the paths outlined above, there are almost 10 times this number of medical practitioners who come to Australia on a temporary basis. There are two main classes of visas for medical practitioners who wish to work in Australia on a temporary basis, one relating to 'areas of need' and one for occupational trainees. Over the period 1998–2000, an average of 763 doctors migrated to Australia for a short stay (less than one year) and a further 1535 migrated temporarily for a long stay. Almost 60 per cent were doctors trained in the United Kingdom or Ireland, with a further 10 per cent trained in the USA and Canada, and 10 per cent in New Zealand. Doctors from these countries are often able to achieve temporary registration to fill positions in areas of designated workforce shortage, especially rural areas, without any further examination. They are obviously an extremely important component of the medical workforce in Australia. AMWAC has estimated the contribution of Temporary Registered Doctors (TRDs) to the medical workforce during 1997, about 50 per cent more TRDs contributed to the medical workforce than had arrived in that year (AMWAC 1999). Further, as at December of that year, there was approximately the same number of TRDs working as had arrived in that year. Assuming the same pattern holds for later years, in 2000 there were about 2400 TRDs employed in Australia.

TRDs comprise a larger proportion of the workforce in rural areas (6.3 per cent of the workforce in 1997) than in metropolitan areas (3.1 per cent), and in hospitals compared to other areas (TRDs comprised 13 per cent of the metropolitan and 33.7 per cent of the rural hospital non-specialist workforce in 1997).

Figure 4.14 Specialist and general practitioner workforce per 1000 population, selected countries, 1999

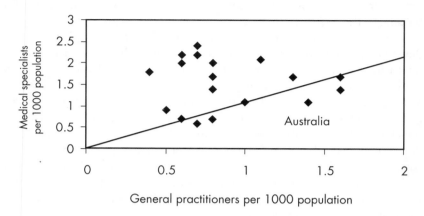

General practitioners per 1000 population

Data source: OECD 2003

There is considerable international variation in per capita provision of medical practitioners, in the relative proportion of general practitioners to specialists (see figure 4.14) and in the ratio of medical practitioners to other workers (Gupta et al. 2003). Australia is one of the few countries that have relatively more general practitioners than specialists (the countries below the diagonal line in figure 4.14). This reflects the strength of primary medical care in Australia relative to other countries. The USA, for example, has a ratio of 0.8 general practitioners and 1.4 specialists per 1000 population. Many of the countries with more specialists than general practitioners are in Eastern Europe.

Workforce planning for the specialist medical workforce involves the same considerations as for the general practitioner workforce. However, because the number of personnel involved is obviously a subset of the total workforce, planning involves finer detail in decisions in terms of increasing or reducing supply. In a provocative paper, Paterson (1994) suggested that there was considerable imbalance in the specialist workforce, principally based on the differential earning power of the different specialties. In the context of the debate about Paterson's thesis it was suggested that a number of specialty associations were restricting entry into the specialty in order to maximise income. As indicated earlier, restriction on supply is often justified on the basis of the need to maintain quality.

A major review of the surgical specialist workforce in 1994 (Baume 1994) argued that there were shortages in a number of surgical specialties and recommended improved processes to address surgical supply. Since then, medical workforce planning has improved with the creation of AMWAC. A recent review suggested that further improvements in its methodological

Table 4.5 Population catchment requirements for a viable resident service as defined by specialist medical colleges, 1998

10,000—20,000	20,000—60,000	50,000—80,000	80,000 or more
General surgery	General physician/ cardiology	ENT Surgery	Urology
Anaesthesia	Obstetrics and gynaecology	Dermatology	Diagnostic Radiology
	Paediatric medicine	Rehabilitation medicine	Cardiology
	Psychiatry	Neurology	Intensive care
	Orthopaedic surgery	Thoracic medicine	Nephrology
	Geriatric medicine		Medical oncology
	Pathology		Radiation oncology

Source: AMWAC 1998b

approach and transparency could be made (Brooks et al. 2003). AMWAC has responded, in part, by publishing a guide to its planning process and advice to specialty workforce planning committees (AMWAC 2003). AMWAC has produced a number of reports on a range of specialties, the recommendations of which often include increasing the number of trainee positions. These recommendations are often adopted by states that fund and regulate hospital training positions. AMWAC reports on progress on implementing its recommendations in its annual report.

AMWAC has elicited from the specialist colleges and associations what these bodies perceive as the population base necessary to support a viable specialist service in rural areas. As shown in table 4.3, there are costs of both an oversupply and undersupply, and it is important that there be an appropriate range of work to ensure that a specialist does not lose his or her skills. Table 4.5 shows the specialists' views on viable population size.

These results need to be interpreted carefully, as they may be aspirational in terms of ensuring a desirable target income for the specialty. However, the existing level of provision across Australia is by and large in line with the ranges proposed by the colleges.

Contemporary issues in medical workforce planning

Policy on the development and management of the medical workforce has changed dramatically since the 1970s. There have been four major policy reviews of the medical workforce in this period with significantly different recommendations (see table 4.6). There has been a complete reversal of policy over this period.

Table 4.6   Medical workforce policy recommendations

Report Year	Direction	Key recommendations
Karmel 1973	Expansion	Increase graduates by about 300 per annum New medical schools at: University of Newcastle James Cook University in north Queensland
Doherty 1988	Stable	No need for reduction in medical school intakes but review in five years New graduates expected to be around 1160 in early 1990s and this is adequate
Commonwealth Government Budget 1995	Contraction	Aim to reduce medical school intakes from around 1200 to around 1000 per annum
Commonwealth Government Budget 2000	Expansion	Funded expansion of medical school intakes of 100 per annum, targeted at rural students
Commonwealth Government Budget 2003	Expansion	An additional 234 medical school places, to be filled by students 'bonded' to work in rural areas New medical schools at: Notre Dame University in Western Australia Griffith University on the Gold Coast in Queensland Australian National University (announced March 2001)

Development of policies on the medical workforce is confounded by two conflicting objectives of government. On the one hand, government, through Medicare, is the major funder of medical services in Australia. Viewed from that perspective, government objectives are associated with minimising growth in medical expenditure. On the other hand, government also has objectives about ensuring adequate access to medical services as part of its health policies. During the mid to late 1990s, government pursued two strategies with respect to restraining expenditure. The first, implemented by the Labor Government in 1995, was an attempt to reduce the number of medical graduates produced in the country by limiting intakes into medical schools (flow A in figure 4.4). Although some temporary reductions were achieved and there was some redistribution of intakes from South Australia to the Northern Territory, this strategy failed to effect any long-term reduction in medical school intakes. The second strategy, implemented by the 1996 Liberal Government, separated medical registration from entitlement to bill Medicare for medical services. The government introduced a policy of restricting new Medicare provider numbers to people who had achieved specialist, including College of General Practitioners, recognition. Simultaneously, the government also introduced steps to address the perceived relative shortage of services for medical services in rural Australia.

A critical issue in medical workforce planning relates to the future role and place of the medical profession. There can be considerable overlap in the role of nursing and medical practitioners in primary care and in major hospitals (see also Dowling et al. 1995). Nurses, especially if granted limited prescribing rights, can undertake many of the contemporary functions of medical practitioners in primary care without any reduction in quality of care (Sergison et al. 1999). Given the difficulty of attracting medical practitioners to rural areas, a nurse-led strategy would seem to form a key part of addressing rural medical workforce shortages. Similar strategies could also be applied in metropolitan areas.

There are also potential overlaps in some areas of the specialist workforce. For example, in the USA, nurse anaesthetists play a significant role in the provision of anaesthetic services, complementing and substituting for medically qualified anaesthetists. In the USA and the United Kingdom, podiatric surgeons undertake some orthopaedic surgery which in Australia tends to be the preserve of orthopaedic surgeons. These issues of substitution and role clarification are going to become increasingly important as the cost of educating nurses, podiatrists, and others is substantially less than educating general practitioners, and the average earnings of these groups are lower than for the general practitioners or specialists for which they substitute. It would appear cost-effective for there to be wider use of alternative personnel in provision of health care, subject to ensuring that the time taken to perform similar tasks is around the same and that the quality of care is not affected. In the long run, however, wage creep might change the salary relativities. Identifying what is the unique role of medical practitioners then becomes an important issue for policy.

Workforce supply is determined by multiplying two variables: the number of professionals and the hours each professional works. The increase in feminisation of the medical workforce will impact on the average hours worked of medical personnel and hence will reduce the effective supply. The extent to which a given level of workforce supply can meet demand is affected by a further variable: the consultation rate per professional per hour. This latter variable is particularly amenable to short-term change through financial incentives to change the average length of consultation, and by improving efficiency through better organisation of a practice. For example, increased productivity in medical practice could be achieved by consolidating medical practices into larger practice groups and using auxiliary personnel. This may also have benefits in terms of increasing quality by improving patient access to practitioners with a different set of skills in the health team (such as nurses or physiotherapists).

Policy change on length of consultation time is quite complex, as very short consultation times are often perceived to be associated with poorer quality care. Workforce policy thus needs to be clear with respect to the trade-offs it is trying to achieve.

As already discussed, the medical workforce is segmented both by a series of specialties and by location. Medical workforce policy needs to be quite sophisticated to ensure that relative shortages in labour market segments are addressed without creating excess supply in other segments of the market. This suggests that financial incentives, when used, need to be carefully targeted. Workforce segmentation also highlights the importance of training (and retraining) programs.

Globalisation of the international economy will also have an impact on the medical workforce, with pathology and radiology services probably the first to be affected with the dissemination of technology for the digital transmission of views of specimens and medical images. This will mean that a specialist pathologist or radiologist, located remotely from the patient, will be able to provide a report on the examination. Internationalisation of the ownership structure of pathology and radiology practices is already occurring.

Policy on 'e-health' has typically focused on the potential to improve services in remote Australia by telecommunication connection to metropolitan areas. However, there is no technological reason why the communication cannot be to a pathologist or radiologist in another country. The extent to which this occurs will in part depend on financial incentives (Medicare may not pay for these services), and legal constraints (Is the pathologist or radiologist providing a medical service in Australia? Are they registered? Do they need to be registered for this purpose? Can another doctor rely on a pathology or radiology reported by a practitioner who may not be registered in Australia? Who is legally liable for negligence and how is that enforced?). Nevertheless, inevitably there will be increased emphasis on e-health that will have an impact on labour force requirements.

The development of the European Union has also meant that there is free movement of labour between European Union countries. A medical practitioner who is trained in Germany is able to work in any other European Union country, despite the different approaches to medical education and medical practice across member countries. A similar economic zone in the Asian area (which might emerge from Asia–Pacific economic cooperation) would also have profound implications for the medical workforce.

Chapter 8 includes further discussion on remuneration of the medical workforce, on the role of the medical professional, and on provision of medical services in the community.

Other health professionals

About one-fifth of the health professional workforce consists of people trained in a wide variety of professions including pharmacists, dentists, chiropractors, therapists (for example, physiotherapists, occupational therapists, speech pathologists), and non-medical professionals trained to assist in diagnostic techniques (for example, medical imaging technologists). Some of these groups are able to diagnose and treat patients independently (dentists, podiatrists, chiropractors). Others may not have direct interactions with patients (for example, health information managers and those supporting diagnostic modalities). These health professionals are involved in a range of employment locations. Unlike nursing staff, the vast majority of whom are employed in hospitals, only a minority of these other health professionals (around 20 per cent) are employed in institutional locations with the majority employed in non-institutional settings, including private practice.

The AIHW collects and publishes data on a number of the allied health professions including physiotherapists (AIHW 2001b), podiatrists (AIHW 2002d), optometrists (AIHW 2000a), pharmacists (AIHW 2003g), and, for selected states, occupational therapists (AIHW 2001a). Its Dental Statistics and Research Unit publishes data on dentists (Brennan and Spencer 2002a, b). Figure 4.15 shows the number of allied health personnel per 100,000 population derived from these publications.

Obviously, the professions are not of equal size: there are about 11,000 physiotherapists in employment in Australia (60 per 100,000 population), compared with only 2800 optometrists (15 per 100,000) and 2000 podiatrists (11 per 100,000). There is also significant variation in provision across states in all professions, with close to twofold variations occurring in provision in occupational therapy (Western Australia at 43 per 100,000 versus Queensland at 22.2), podiatry (South Australia at 16.4 versus Queensland at 7.0), and dentistry (Tasmania at 25.2 versus South Australia at 49.7). This variation cannot be explained by demographic characteristics and 'need' for services (for example, differences in the age profile of the population). The variation

Figure 4.15 Australia: Allied health workforce per 100,000 population, 1998–99

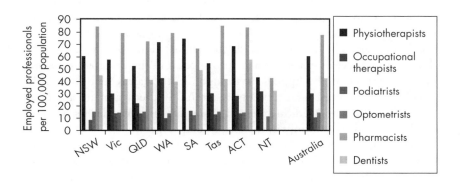

can in part be explained by availability of education programs (for example, there is no dental school in Tasmania). Most of these professions are growing rapidly. For example, 128 students completed podiatry programs in Australia in 1999, a ratio of about one for every 16 employed podiatrists. In contrast, in medicine the graduating to employed ratio is 1:40.

Unlike the situation with respect to 'private' medical practice, which is underpinned by public health insurance through Medicare, no similar direct public support for independent private practice is available for most of these professions. The major exception relates to optometry, which is encompassed within the Medicare arrangements. As part of the negotiations for inclusion of optometrists within the Medicare Benefits Schedule, the optometrical profession agreed that MBS benefits would only be paid to optometrists who committed to charging all patients at or below the schedule fee and direct (bulk) billing all pensioners (Scotton and Macdonald 1993). This 'participating optometrist' scheme is unique in Medicare and has led to continuing high levels of direct billing (around 95 per cent of all optometrical services). About one-sixth of income for optometrists in private practice comes from direct billing, with 80 per cent of income being from sales of glasses, frames, and contact lenses (ABS 1999f).

Pharmacy also attracts public support as the Pharmaceutical Benefits Scheme (PBS) provides important underpinning for private community pharmacy through the mark-ups paid by the Commonwealth for medication dispensed under the PBS (discussed in Chapter 9).

Although the Medicare schedule is principally focused on rebates for the work of medical practitioners, it includes a number of items that do not require the direct personal provision by the medical practitioner. These items can be rendered 'on behalf of' a medical practitioner where another professional, either employed by the medical practitioner or 'acting under the supervision of the medical practitioner', renders the service. In either case the service must be billed in the name of the medical practitioner who accepts full responsibility for the service. Typically, where the other health professional is not directly employed by the medical practitioner, there would need to be quality assurance processes for data acquisition and the medical practitioner would sign off on the report, presumably after analysing the data reported by the other health professional. The most widespread use of billing for services not 'personally provided' is in the provision of pathology services but it also applies in a range of other areas such as radiation oncology where imaging technologists administer the treatment, audiology, and orthoptics. The Medicare Benefits Schedule also provides for a subsidy for dental services, but only in the area of oral surgery.

The major sources of funds for professional services are shown in figure 4.16. This figure does not include expenditure in the category 'community and public health' which would also encompass expenditure on health

Figure 4.16 Australia: Expenditure on dental and other health professionals, A$million, by source of funds, 2001/02

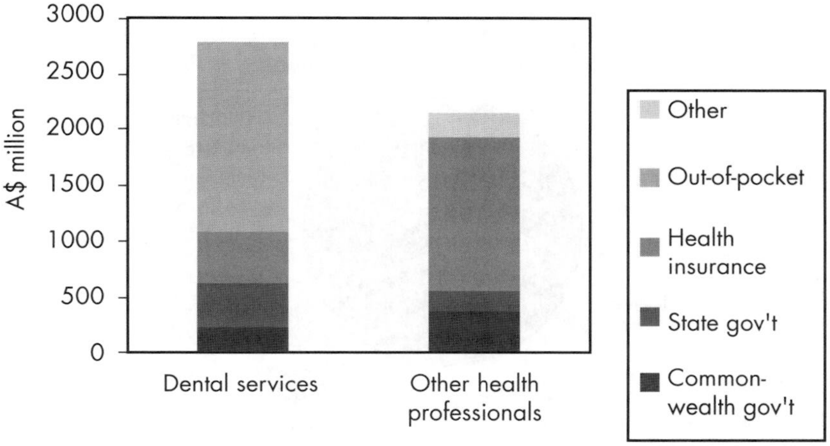

Data source: AIHW (2003) Australian Health Expenditure 2001–02

professionals such as physiotherapists. Over A$2 billion was spent in this category, and is principally sourced from government, the majority being from state government. This category is not further subdivided in the published data and also includes expenditure on nursing, medical, and other services. The AIHW category 'other health professionals' thus primarily relates to health professionals in private practice. Information on pharmaceuticals is also not included in figure 4.16.

For both dentists and other health professionals, over 60 per cent of funding comes from patients themselves as out-of-pocket costs. The Commonwealth government rebate of 30 per cent of the cost of health insurance also provides a significant indirect subsidy to fees for these services. About 9 per cent of funding for dental services is from the Commonwealth, and about 6 per cent overall is Commonwealth expenditure via the rebate. State dental schemes account for about one-eighth of dental expenditure. Commonwealth expenditure for other professionals is a higher proportion of expenditure (17 per cent) but a relatively smaller proportion (3 per cent of all expenditure) is via the rebate. The Commonwealth has a number of programs to support allied health and other professionals, especially in rural areas. 'Other' sources, such as third party and workers' compensation insurance arrangements, account for about 10 per cent of the funding for other professionals.

Private health insurance provides 17 per cent of the funding for dental services and 9 per cent of funding for other professionals. Almost half the payments from ancillary insurance tables is for dental services with optical services accounting for almost one-sixth of expenditure (although optometry is covered by Medicare, the cost of glasses is not covered by Medicare).

Figure 4.17 Australia: Distribution of benefits paid from ancillary insurance, June quarter, 2003

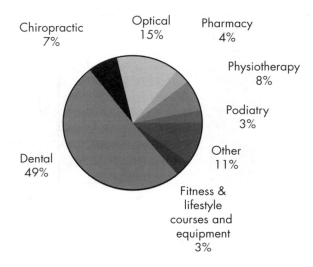

Chiropractic 7%

Optical 15%

Pharmacy 4%

Physiotherapy 8%

Podiatry 3%

Other 11%

Dental 49%

Fitness & lifestyle courses and equipment 3%

Other significant expenditures from ancillary tables are for physiotherapy and chiropractic services (see figure 4.17).

Like insurance for hospital care, ancillary insurance is more common among people with higher incomes. Given the significant proportion of funding raised from insurance, it is not surprising that higher income groups have better access to services such as dental, physiotherapy, and chiropractic (Schofield 1999).

Challenges facing health professionals

The working environment for other health professionals in the public sector has been significantly affected by the financial squeeze in that area (Ferguson 1998). The non-medical, non-nursing health professionals have been trad-itionally relatively weak in hospital power structures as they do not have the status and role in attracting and treating patients directly that medical practitioners do, nor the numerical dominance of nurses. As a result, these health professionals have felt excluded from the decision-making processes of hospitals. The strategy of the mid to late 1980s to counteract this was the creation of 'allied health divisions', to parallel similar structures for the medical profession, and the creation of senior allied health leadership pos-itions in hospitals to head the division. However, these leadership positions were often removed with the funding reductions of the mid to late 1990s.

The increased use of casemix funding in hospitals has called into question the contribution of the health professions to the treatment process.

The evidence about the extent to which therapy services contribute to improved outcomes or improved efficiency is somewhat mixed (Liang et al. 1987; Haas 1993; Cherkin et al. 1998). This may in part be due to the fact that most of these professions were relative latecomers to university education and so do not have a long tradition of research to determine their effectiveness. This is changing, and for the last decade all of these professions have been educated in university settings and there has been a parallel development of research into these areas.

Although many of the professions are educated in faculties with multidisciplinary focuses, only a small proportion of the undergraduate curriculum is designed to foster the teamwork necessary in these professions postgraduation. As a result there is some disjunction between the expectations of therapists on graduation and the nature of the work that is undertaken. This means that, as with medicine, people graduating in other health professions require consolidation of their professional training through a formal (or informal) internship arrangement. Unfortunately, the funding reductions in the hospital sector have tended to reduce these learning opportunities.

The increased use of multidisciplinary care plans (Tallis and Balla 1995; Wang et al. 1997) which systematised the treatment and care processes in hospitals has provided increased opportunities for the various health professions to articulate and demonstrate the contributions they can make to improving outcomes or increasing efficiency in hospitals. Although care plans cover a minority of the care provided in hospitals, they at least provide a framework for ensuring that the roles of all the health professions are clearly recognised.

As relative latecomers to university-based education, the non-medical professions do not have as strong a research base as the medical profession, nor do the university-based health professional schools have the generous funding that medical schools have been able to garner. However, university-based education and the development of clinical academics in the non-medical professions means that the scientific base of these professions is increasing, as is their visibility in the workplace and in policy formation. In the long term, these changes may begin to address some of the power imbalances in the health sector and provide a sounder basis for more equitable teamwork in health care. This will be to the long-term benefit of patients and other consumers.

Conclusion

The health sector is at a critical juncture, requiring a major rethink of the way its workforce is organised. Significant shortages are foreshadowed in nursing, the largest of the health professions. Changes in the organisation of medical work in hospitals, and the reduction in average hours worked by medical practitioners, also presage further workforce change. The health workforce is an input into provision of health services and therefore health workforce planning should not simply be concerned with planning the numbers required in each profession but rather should focus on planning the provision of professionals with the mix of skills necessary to ensure adequate provision of services. Further, expanding intakes into health professional courses will not be sufficient to meet the emerging needs. New roles and new patterns of working will be required. At present the health sector does not have the right structures to facilitate a rethink of workforce roles, let alone implement them.

Workforce redesign is complex. It can involve four types of changes:

- moving a task up or down a traditional uni-disciplinary ladder (for example, senior medical staff doing work previously done by junior staff)
- expanding the breadth of a job (for example, rehabilitation practitioner working across traditionally determined boundaries)
- increasing the depth of a job (for example, nurse practitioners)
- creating new roles formed by combining tasks in a new way (NHS Modernisation Agency 2003).

Workforce substitution may involve conflict between the health professions. The interests of the professions are not coincident because substitution affects the professions differentially. Nursing staff may substitute for medical staff in rural communities; similarly, substitution can also occur in major teaching hospitals where nursing staff could appropriately substitute for some medical staff in intensive care units, cancer treatment, emergency departments, and patient admissions. In some states, hospital funding design militates against such substitution, for example by providing a significant subsidy for employing hospital-based registrars. There are similar possibilities for substitution of allied health for nursing staff (and vice versa) and other non-medical disciplines for medical practitioners (Brooks 2003).

Workforce substitution will initially be facilitated by specifying protocols for performance of the new roles outside traditional professional boundaries. Protocol-based care might improve the quality of care by ensuring a sounder evidence base for provision.

The health professions themselves are also facing a range of problems. Some of the problems being faced by the professions are similar: during the 1990s all hospital-based staff have been subject to reduced funding and organisational restructuring. The reduced funding has often been associated with increased accountability through casemix funding and calls for a greater emphasis on evidence-based practice.

The political environment in the institutional sector means that the professions have not been equally affected by these changes. Medical staff have traditionally had greater power in the sector and, although they have not escaped unscathed, their power has ensured that the medical profession has not been challenged to the same extent as the two other main groups of professionals—nurses and 'allied health staff'. The impact on these two other groups has principally come through reduction in the number of staff and increased intensity of the workplace (reduced staffing per patient and increased acuity or complexity of patients). These changes are often short-sighted because of the role of professions, such as occupational therapy and social work, in facilitating discharge. Indeed, expansion of these services may be a cost-effective use of institutional funds.

Workforce policies, as in other areas of health policy, should be informed by research and evidence. However, the track record of health workforce planning studies in getting projections 'right' is not good (Walker and Maynard 2003). Although there have been methodological improvements in workforce studies in recent years (Antonazzo et al. 2003), workforce planning in Australia and many other countries is still weak. Bloor and Maynard (2003) present this damning indictment: 'The basis of current physician workforce planning is incomplete and mechanistic, using fixed ratio relationships that have no empirical validity'. They argued this situation has continued because of a 'combination of the ignorance of policy makers … and the failure of economists and other researchers to convince policy makers that different methods may be productive'.

As argued in this chapter, there is an urgent need to address workforce issues. Creative policy development, underpinned by sound evidence and research, is clearly long overdue. Although health professionals take between four and six years to enter the workforce, change to employment patterns and roles could occur rapidly. Hopefully, the health workforce of 2020 might thus be quite different from that which new graduates entered a decade earlier.

5

Departmental and Intergovernmental Structures

Government plays a critical role in the health sector as funder, regulator, and provider. As seen in chapter 3, government provides about 70 per cent of health sector finance, all of which is mediated through government departments and much of which involves both the Commonwealth and state governments.

Government departments

The structure and functioning of government departments clearly have an important influence on the operation of the health system. The scope of a department influences the extent to which 'boundary' issues, such as co-ordination of health and disability services, require liaison across organisational boundaries (and budgets) or are the subject of intra-organisational coordination strategies. Similarly, internal structures of departments can affect the design of programs and often the perspectives of departmental managers.

The influence of management and operational styles of a department extends beyond the department and affects the agencies that it funds. Some departments adopt a laissez-faire approach allowing a high degree of autonomy in the way funded agencies operate, with accountability focused on outcomes and performance against articulated goals. Other departments are more interventionist and specify the ways in which funded agencies are to operate. These require a high degree of consultation with (or approval from) the department on a range of matters. Different parts of a department may adopt different operating styles and departments may change styles with a change of minister or bureaucratic head. (The bureaucratic head is variously styled secretary, director general, commissioner, or chief executive.)

The extent of interchange of staff between funded agencies and the department also affects the way in which a department operates.

Government departments function within a bureaucratic frame: they are mostly staffed by career public servants, many of whom have had careers outside the health portfolio in other government departments and see their career progressing through other government departments. The public service at both Commonwealth and state levels is organised into various grades of staff. The extent to which positions are advertised outside the public service, thus facilitating career interchange between funded agencies and the department, varies between states and also with the level of the position. Most senior management positions are now routinely advertised outside the public service to broaden the applicant pool.

Departmental scope

Boulding (1967) observed that '"social policy" is a vague term, the boundaries of which are ill defined…' (p. 3). The same is true of 'health policy' and it is thus not surprising that the scope (or jurisdiction) of health departments changes over time. Aspects of health policy have an impact on a number of government departments and thus require a close interrelationship with other spheres of policy. It is a matter of bureaucratic and political choice whether a particular area of policy is principally the responsibility of the health portfolio in liaison with another portfolio or vice versa.

Two examples of these boundary areas that have changed portfolio focus are occupational health and safety (which has interrelationships with industrial relations) and policies with respect to air and water quality ('environmental health' which has interrelationships with general environmental policy). Until the 1960s, health departments in most states had principal responsibility for both these areas. Since the early 1970s, these functions are more commonly vested in other portfolios (industrial relations and environment respectively) and health's role is to provide the requisite technical or professional advice, with the shape and emphasis of policy being vested in the non-health portfolio. There may be significant policy consequences of changing bureaucratic alignments. Allison and Zelikow (1999) have pointed out the importance of organisational politics in the decision-making process. A shift of a policy area out of a health portfolio almost inevitably leads to a de-emphasis on technical health issues, while increasing the emphasis given to the dominant field of the new bureaucratic location.

Typically, the key policy areas of health and community care include: acute health and hospitals; mental health services; community health services; public health; aged care; disability services; environmental health; and occupational health. Other functions are sometimes added to create a 'super department', for example incorporating responsibility for family services, youth welfare and/or housing.

Prior to the early 1970s, many of these core health functions were split between separate departments, commissions, and 'authorities' in a single state. New South Wales, for example, had a Hospitals Commission and a Health Department; Victoria had a Hospitals and Charities Commission, a Mental Health Authority, and a Health Department. Mergers of these separate bodies occurred in the 1970s creating integrated 'Health Commissions'. In the early 1980s there was a tendency to separate 'health' and 'community care' functions, the latter typically involving disability, into distinct departments. In some cases this created unworkable anomalies: Victoria separated residential aged care from community services for the aged at a time when Commonwealth policy was emphasising the interdependence of the two. The late 1980s and early 1990s saw some rationalisation of these splits.

At the Commonwealth level and in a number of states, boundary issues have been addressed by creating large departments ('super departments') thus internalising many bureaucratic coordination problems (Halligan 1987; Halligan et al. 1992; Nethercote 2000). These large departments incorporate most aspects of health and community services into a single bureaucratic organisation, in some instances reporting to more than one minister. Internalising coordination issues does not automatically improve coordination; purposive action needs to be taken lest the separate divisions within the organisation operate autonomously with relative disregard for interrelationships with other parts of the same department. However, use of internalisation strategies does mean that the bureaucratic or ministerial head of the department can deal with many coordination issues, and budget allocations are not 'frozen' into separate departments or ministerial portfolios.

The defining feature of health departments is responsibility for acute health, public health, community services, and mental health services. Beyond these core areas, there is some variability across Australia in terms of scope of departmental responsibility, although the trend at state level is towards super departments covering all aspects of health and community care. The Commonwealth, which pioneered multi-ministerial super departments, reduced the scope of its 'health' portfolio in 1998 by transferring disability and child care services to the Department of Family and Community Services.

Departmental structures

The structures adopted by health departments reflect choices about three key issues: the organisational structures to support policy and program direction; structures to support advocacy and equity; and organisational arrangements for line management and relationships with funded agencies. There is no 'right answer' to the question of organisational design, and each structure has relative strengths and weaknesses. The choices made reflect organisational history, contemporary organisational priorities, the organisation style of the minister or departmental head, and the scope of departmental responsibility; the reasons behind those choices reflecting interplays of power, context, and personalities (Ranson et al. 1980).

Policy and program direction

There are two broad choices for structures to support policy development and program direction. First, the department can be organised along programmatic lines. Contemporary approaches to government financing adopt a 'program budget structure' that identifies the key objects of government expenditure and allocates funding to these key programs. Program budget structures typically identify separate programs for acute health, public health, community health or primary care, mental health, and aged care. Other programs, such as dental health, may be separately identified or may be part of community health. The Commonwealth Department of Health and Ageing and a number of states are structured along programmatic lines.

The alternative design is to emphasise common functions such as planning and strategic direction, finance, and so on. Osborne and Gaebler (1992) proposed distinguishing the functions of owner, funder, purchaser, and provider, and a number of health authorities have experimented with organisational structures that identify and separate these functions (or, at least, the latter two: purchasing and provision). The New South Wales Department of Health is an example of a health authority that has adopted a primarily functional approach (Baldwin and Walker 1995).

There is no ideal way of structuring a department and both types of structures have strengths and weaknesses. The 'programmatic' approach provides for unambiguous program direction, with clear accountability for success or failure of policy in the relevant area. The 'functional' structure, on the other hand, emphasises integration of functions across a range of areas, thus facilitating priority setting across policy areas and coordination of the interrelated parts of the portfolio. The tension between the benefits of the 'programmatic' and 'functional' structures is one reason why organisational structures of health departments are regularly reviewed.

The need to balance the various tensions in organisational design has led to a number of states elevating geographic considerations to a second tier split in the departmental structure. This approach was first adopted in the South Australian Department of Human Services. The second tier split in that department is partly on geographic and partly on programmatic lines. All rural services are grouped into a single division, recognising the strong interrelationship between functions that occur in rural towns; but metropolitan services are split into separate divisions along programmatic lines. Metropolitan health services are also organised in a separate division. Victoria and Western Australia have adopted a similar approach, an example of what DiMaggio and Powell (1991) call 'institutional isomorphism', that is, the tendency for organisations in similar areas to evolve so that they look more alike in their organisational forms.

Organisational arrangements need to be made for input or support services for the operation of the department. Typically, the key inputs involve finance, personnel (often coupled with industrial relations), information services, and capital planning. These areas have a higher prominence in the 'functional' rather than 'programmatic' approach to organisational design, as programmatically structured departments typically organise these functions into a single 'resources' division whereas in functionally organised departments, finance and personnel often have separate status as major organisational units.

Advocacy and equity

Since the 1970s a number of government departments have been created based on 'social identity': women, youth, aged, etc (Fells 2003). These portfolios promote the interests of the groups that they represent. They provide policy advice on relevant issues, and aim to influence policy development and budget decision making to ensure that the concerns of the groups are considered and addressed. In addition, they implement policy and program responses to promote equity and provide support services to assist these groups (Fells 2003, p. 105). These portfolio-level structural changes have often been replicated within departments.

Most government departments now recognise a responsibility to address the needs of social identity groups whose health and community care needs require specific planning and attention. The population groups recognised as warranting specific policy consideration vary from jurisdiction to jurisdiction and over time, reflecting political pressures, ideological factors, the size of the relevant groups and objective 'need' factors. Typically, population groups identified for organisational recognition include women, persons of non-English speaking background, Aboriginal and Torres Strait Islander peoples, people in rural and remote areas, and people with disabilities. In some organisations a specific unit is established with funding and policy responsibility for each relevant population group. The effectiveness of this approach depends in part on the level of the unit within the organisation. In other departments, the needs of all special population groups are dealt with in a single 'policy' group within the organisation.

A third approach requires all organisational subunits to address the needs of special population groups. This 'mainstreaming' approach can lead to integration of the concerns of the various population groups with those of the rest of the population, although a risk associated with this strategy is that specific needs may not be identified and addressed. High level coordination committees (either bureaucratic or ministerial) might also be used to ensure that the needs of special groups receive appropriate attention.

Line management and relationships with funded agencies

The third key structural choice for organisation design relates to the arrangements for line management. Since the early 1970s, most health authorities have adopted some form of 'regionalisation': establishing 'regional offices' or 'area administrations' to facilitate line management of direct service delivery and relationships with local funded agencies. The extent of autonomy allowed to regions varies between jurisdictions and within jurisdictions over time.

Schon (1971) has argued that tensions between central parts of an organisation and its periphery are inevitable. Regions are in part created to respond to regional diversity, but the more autonomous and flexible regions become in responding to local needs, the more the organisation as a whole suffers from the effects of centrifugal force and loses its unified character. Thus, there tends to be a continuous process of rebalancing regional autonomy and central direction.

Another source of tension arises if policy development becomes divorced from implementation, or if the key members of the executive group of an organisation have little experience in, or contemporary knowledge of, issues related to regional operations. This tension occurs particularly in structures where regions report through a 'Director of Regional Services' or 'Director of Operations', and/or where there are a significant number of peers with policy responsibilities in specific areas, but no formal responsibility for implementation of policies they develop. An innovative response to this problem has been structures that assign the line management role for one or more regions to each program director. This increases peer accountability among the senior executives, as each can legitimately comment on proposals that may impinge on their own policy area, or which might be implemented in regions for which they are responsible.

The effect of these tensions and other organisational choices (see Bolman and Deal 1991, especially pp. 80–5) is that health authority structures are changed frequently. Table 5.1 summarises key aspects of department organisation design at 2003.

Most departmental structures involve a mix of programmatic and functional approaches, so the table shows the main structural frame. Most jurisdictions have adopted a programmatic approach, with services integrated into the structure. The 'regional' structures in New South Wales are known as area health services and are separately incorporated with their own boards.

Table 5.1   Departmental structural approaches, 2003

	Primary Organisation Frame	Regional Reporting Arrangements
Commonwealth	Programmatic	To Secretary (effectively through Deputy Secretary)
New South Wales	Functional	To Deputy Director-General (Operations)
Victorian	Programmatic/ regional	Metropolitan health services to Executive Director, Metropolitan Health and Aged Care; rural services, via Regions, to Executive Director, Rural Health and Aged Care
Queensland	Functional	To General Manager (Health Services)
South Australia	Programmatic/ regional	Metropolitan to Executive Director, Metropolitan Health Division; country services to Executive Director, Social Justice and Country Division
Western Australia	Functional/regional	Metropolitan services to Director General; rural services to Executive Director, Country Services
Tasmania	Programmatic	Hospitals report to Director, Hospital and Ambulance Division
Australian Capital Territory	Programmatic	Services report to Deputy Chief Executive
Northern Territory	Programmatic	Hospital services report to Assistant Secretary, Acute Care

Associated agencies

Most health portfolios have a number of associated agencies: independent statutory bodies with boards usually appointed by the minister (or by the Governor-General/Governor on the advice of the minister), charged with specific functions of an administrative or regulatory nature. At the Commonwealth level, the largest of these is the Health Insurance Commission, responsible for paying benefits under Medicare, the Pharmaceutical Benefits Scheme, and child care payments. At the state level, typical associated agencies include professional registration boards and hospital or area health boards. Most of these bodies employ their own staff, have separate parliamentary appropriations and report separately to Parliament in terms of an Annual Report. Ministerial control over these agencies is generally not as clear as for the departments of state; ministerial direction may be limited by statute and directions may have to be tabled in Parliament.

Commonwealth Department of Health and Ageing

Figure 5.1 shows the central office structure for the Commonwealth Department of Health and Ageing in 2004 (updates of the structure are usually available on the departmental web site at www.health.gov.au).

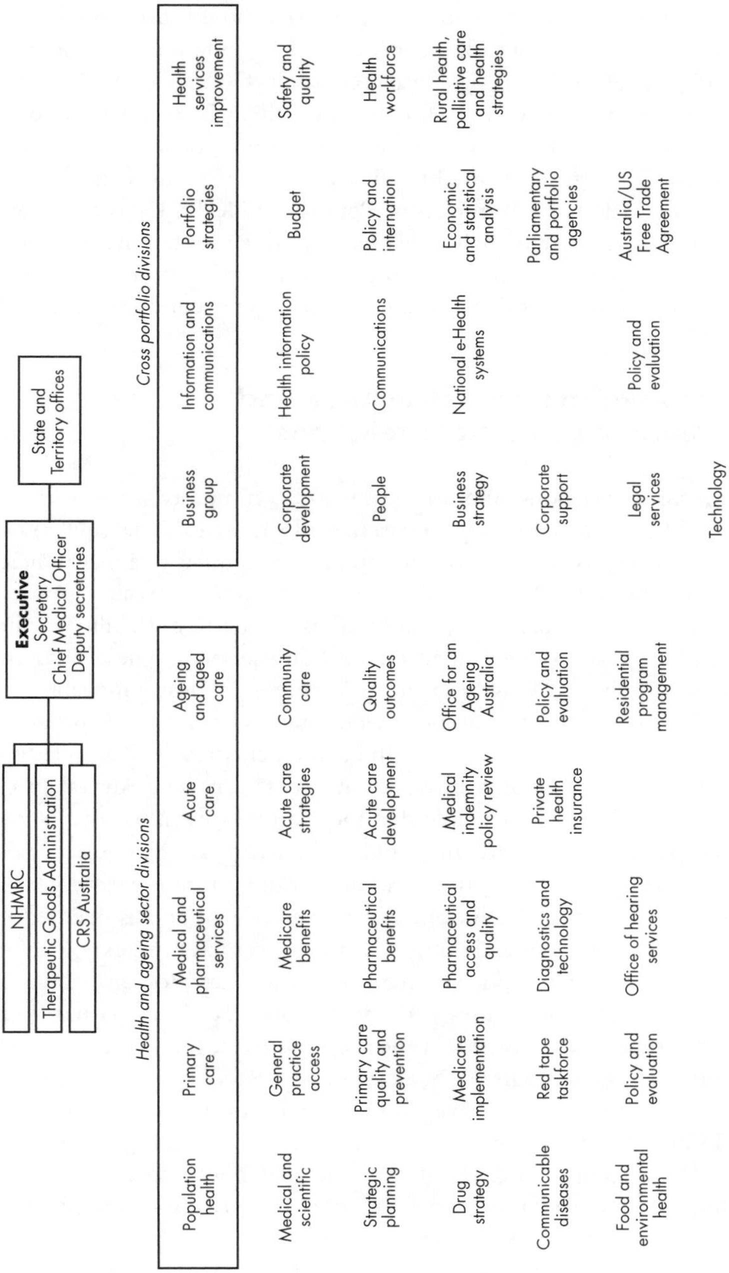

Figure 5.1 Organisational structure, Commonwealth Department of Health and Ageing, 2004

Executive
Secretary
Chief Medical Officer
Deputy secretaries

- NHMRC
- Therapeutic Goods Administration
- CRS Australia

State and Territory offices

Health and ageing sector divisions

Population health	Primary care	Medical and pharmaceutical services	Acute care	Ageing and aged care
Medical and scientific	General practice access	Medicare benefits	Acute care strategies	Community care
Strategic planning	Primary care quality and prevention	Pharmaceutical benefits	Acute care development	Quality outcomes
Drug strategy	Medicare implementation	Pharmaceutical access and quality	Medical indemnity policy review	Office for an Ageing Australia
Communicable diseases	Red tape taskforce	Diagnostics and technology	Private health insurance	Policy and evaluation
Food and environmental health	Policy and evaluation	Office of hearing services		Residential program management

Cross portfolio divisions

Business group	Information and communications	Portfolio strategies	Health services improvement
Corporate development	Health information policy	Budget	Safety and quality
People	Communications	Policy and internation	Health workforce
Business strategy	National e-Health systems	Economic and statistical analysis	Rural health, palliative care and health strategies
Corporate support		Parliamentary and portfolio agencies	
Legal services	Policy and evaluation	Australia/US Free Trade Agreement	
Technology group			

The Commonwealth department is organised into five programmatic divisions, five 'cross-portfolio' divisions (mostly functionally organised), and five distinct management units reporting centrally for governance reasons (audit and fraud control) or because they function quasi-autonomously (National Health and Medical Research Council). As is typical of a programmatic structure, the link between the principal funding programs of the Commonwealth department and its organisational structure are clear and explicit. The structure within divisions also maintains this programmatic structure and so, for example, the Population Health Division incorporates a number of separate branches that have specific programmatic responsibilities and budgets. The structures adopted in other jurisdictions are normally published in the relevant department's Annual Report and/or on its web site.

Intergovernmental structures and Commonwealth–state relations

Government responsibility for health and community services in Australia is shared between the Commonwealth and the states. This split responsibility means that it is difficult to develop comprehensive national policies. States have responsibility for hospital services, the Commonwealth assumes responsibility for medical services, and both take some responsibility for home and community care projects, and for disability services. These divisions render coherent policy making, even at the state level, almost impossible.

The problems of Commonwealth–state relations stem in part from the nature of the Constitution and the agreements reached on relative roles of the states and the Commonwealth at Federation. The Australian Constitution is based on the principle that the Commonwealth Parliament does not have power to legislate in a policy area unless that area is specifically mentioned in the Constitution as an area of Commonwealth power. In the absence of a specific mention, governance of that area is deemed to be the responsibility of a state. Commonwealth power has been extended, however, by use of its explicit power over corporations and foreign affairs including matters covered by treaties and conventions that Australia has signed. The High Court has accepted that the Commonwealth can make laws to implement treaties it has signed (for example, to protect the environment), even in areas where it does not have explicit constitutional power (Commonwealth v Tasmania (1983), 158 CLR 1). The Commonwealth government also has power over corporations and has used that power to regulate the way in which these corporations act in a variety of areas (for example, to prohibit advertising of tobacco products).

Where the Commonwealth does have constitutional power it is pre-eminent, that is, its laws override those of a state or territory. The Constitution provides in section 109 that 'when a law of a state is inconsistent with a law of the Commonwealth, the latter shall prevail and the former shall, to the extent of the inconsistency, be invalid'. The landmark Engineers' Case determined that the pre-existing doctrine of implied immunities, which emphasised the independent and sovereign role of the state and the Commonwealth governments in their respective spheres, was not a proper interpretation of the Constitution (Amalgamated Society of Engineers v The Adelaide Steamship Co Ltd (1920) 28 CLR 129). When the Federal Parliament could make laws in relevant areas they overrode those of the state, and thus state instrumentalities, for example, were subject to those federal laws (see Zines 1989 for a discussion of the evolution of Commonwealth power).

The Constitution, as originally proclaimed, limited the role of the Commonwealth in health services to matters relating to quarantine (section 51 (ix)). Even in this area, the Commonwealth role was limited and states often imposed their own quarantine restrictions. A series of outbreaks of infectious diseases from 1918 onwards showed the farcical nature of existing quarantine coordination arrangements (for a catalogue of these events, see Cumpston 1953). The failure of state activity was generally recognised, and a Commonwealth Department of Health was established in 1921, initially through transfer of the quarantine division of the Department of Trade and Customs. However, more formal coordinating and leadership roles were soon recognised as necessary, and following a report of the Royal Commission on Health in 1926, a Federal Health Council was established consisting of the Commonwealth Director General of Health and the professional heads of the state Health Departments (see Abbott and Goldsmith 1952). In 1937, the Federal Health Council was expanded and renamed the National Health and Medical Research Council (NH&MRC) with additional membership including medical representation from the Colleges of Physicians and Surgeons, medical schools of the universities, and the British Medical Association, as well as two non-medical members.

The states have had somewhat of a 'renaissance' in the last decade (Parkin 2003). A benefit of a federal system is supposed to be that states can act as 'laboratories', experimenting with policy ideas. In the USA this is more a potential than a reality (Holahan et al. 2003), and there is a similar lack of experimentation with policy design in Australia. Victoria's adoption of casemix funding for its hospitals is perhaps the most notable exception.

Central governments in federal systems have increased their relative roles since their foundation (Wheare 1963, p. 237). Oates goes so far as to suggest that these centripetal tendencies are inevitable and that central power will continue to increase (Oates 1972, pp. 223–5). This is certainly the case in Australia. The Commonwealth government now dominates health policy in Australia. When states require extra money for their hospital systems, their first port of call is the Commonwealth. Health insurance policy is set by the

Commonwealth government which in turn means that the Commonwealth exerts a major influence over the demand for public hospital care. Medical fees policy is also the preserve of the Commonwealth government.

The growth of Commonwealth constitutional power

A major part of the Curtin–Chifley scheme of postwar reconstruction was the development of a pharmaceutical benefits scheme. The Pharmaceutical Benefits Act 1944 provided for the establishment of a Commonwealth pharmaceutical formulary which listed approved medicines that were obtainable from approved chemists on a doctor's prescription free of charge. The medical profession was strongly critical of the Pharmaceutical Benefits Scheme, saw it as the first step to nationalised medicine (Kewley 1973, p. 344), and favoured health policies that limited the role of the Commonwealth government and relied relatively more heavily on payment by individuals.

In a landmark decision in 1944, the High Court ruled that the Curtin–Chifley legislation was invalid, a decision that also called into question the validity of other benefit packages which had widespread community support (Attorney-General for Victoria (ex. rel. Dale and others) v Commonwealth (1945), 71 CLR 237). The government proposed a new clause in the Constitution which was approved at a referendum and gave the Commonwealth power to make laws with respect to: 'The provision of maternity allowances, widows pensions, child endowment, unemployment, pharmaceutical, sickness and hospital benefits, medical and dental services (but not so as to authorise any form of civil conscription), benefits to students and family allowances' (section 51 (xxiiia)).

This amendment gave the Commonwealth clear powers to provide hospital and other benefits and there was for the first time a conjunction of political will with constitutional power to legislate in this area. However, the Pharmaceutical Benefits legislation was again challenged in the High Court and was declared invalid on the basis of a relatively restrictive definition of civil conscription (British Medical Association v Commonwealth (1962) 79 CLR 201). Subsequent cases have led to a weakening of this original restrictive interpretation (General Practitioners Society of Australia v Commonwealth and others (1980) 145 CLR 532), and the Commonwealth now appears to have the power to impose reasonable conditions on medical practitioners as part of its management of the Medicare benefits arrangements.

The other major head of Commonwealth power in health comes from its power to make grants to states: section 96 of the Constitution provides this power and the ability to set conditions on these grants. In addition to these key heads of power, health policies can be based on several of the other constitutional provisions, such as insurance (see McMillan 1992 and also Reynolds 1995 for a review of constitutional issues relative to public health).

The need for coordination

Despite the widening of Commonwealth power provided by section 51 (xxiiia) and the ability to make grants under section 96, governments of both political persuasions have emphasised state government roles in health, especially hospital services. Apart from a brief flirtation with the possibility of establishing Commonwealth public hospitals in the Whitlam era (1973–75), Commonwealth governments have recognised the need to work with states in implementing national policies.

As Reagan (1972) points out with regard to similar currents in the USA: 'Federalism is [now] a political and pragmatic concept stressing the actual interdependence and sharing of functions between Washington and the states and focusing on the mutual leverage that each level is able to exert on the other' (p. 3).

Substituting Canberra for Washington, this situation also describes the Australian context. Sharman (1991) suggests that: 'The operation of state and national governments involves such a degree of interpenetration that it is hard to find either an area of Commonwealth activity that does not impinge on state policies, or state administration that does not entail some Commonwealth involvement' (p. 23).

Reagan also argues (p. 145) that federalism should be recast in terms of this interdependence (or interpenetration as Sharman calls it) rather than the more traditional conceptions of federalism implying that the jurisdictions are independent (for the traditional approach, see Wheare 1963). In Reagan's terms, federalism in the USA is: 'Now best described as that states ... have won the right to be heard in the design of programs and a right to share in the implementation of programs' (p. 159).

This essentially describes the nature of Commonwealth–state financial relations in Australia today, especially in health. This compromise in turn means that formal and informal coordinating mechanisms need to be established to allow opportunities for states to be 'heard in the design of programs'. Commonwealth–state negotiations are now less determined by the precise phrasing of the Constitution and more influenced by political and electoral politics. As May (1971) points out: 'The way in which a Federation develops is determined largely by bargaining between governments, in response to outside pressures and the demands of electors. The Constitution provides an important element in this bargaining process, stating some of the rules of the game but it does not pre-determine the outcome' (p. xi).

Informal bargaining processes

The relative power and roles of parties in the informal bargaining processes of Commonwealth–state relations vary over time and with the issue under negotiation. French and Raven (1959, 1968) outlined five key bases of power: resource, referent, expert (including information), coercion, and legitimate authority. Each of these is relevant in Commonwealth–state negotiations.

A key basis for Commonwealth influence is its resource power. The High Court in a series of cases has effectively increased the Commonwealth government's taxing powers and, concomitantly, reduced the scope of state taxation. The Commonwealth government now controls the key growth taxes (such as income tax), and thus often has more ability than the states to develop new policy initiatives that involve additional spending. Negotiations surrounding the introduction of a Goods and Services Tax (GST) from 1 July 2000 ensured that the states collectively accrue all the revenue of the GST. The GST is seen to be a growth tax and its introduction may equalise the resource bases of the Commonwealth and the states.

The Commonwealth often attempts to use legitimate authority, not in the hierarchical sense originally contemplated by French and Raven (1959, 1968), but through reliance on an assumed national leadership role. Although this role is not recognised in the Constitution and is not always accepted by states, the Prime Minister is generally seen by the public as being 'senior' to and more important than state Premiers. Depending on the status of an individual Commonwealth Health Minister, he or she is also often able to rely on this Commonwealth pre-eminence to achieve support for policy initiatives.

The relative power of the various states is affected by a version of 'legitimate authority' based on their populations. The two largest states, New South Wales and Victoria, generally have more influence in negotiations than the smaller states and territories. (The seating arrangements at formal meetings reflect this population hierarchy with the Commonwealth and the two largest states sitting nearest the Chair, with other states arranged further from the Chair in line with population.) However, the fact remains that in most Commonwealth–state forums each jurisdiction has one vote, which provides equal formal power between all states and territories.

Referent power is also used in informal negotiations at both bureaucratic and ministerial levels. Many Commonwealth and state health officials have worked with each other over many years and friendships develop across the negotiation table. At ministerial level, party bonds are also used to influence the outcome of negotiations.

Any participant in Commonwealth–state negotiations can exercise expert power. Some state officials, even from quite small states or territories, have recognised expertise in particular areas and can exercise national leadership or influence the course of negotiations.

Lukes (1974) has criticised the approach to power adopted by French and Raven and others, arguing that the exercise of power is multidimensional. In Lukes's view, power is seen not only in overt conflict, but in 'latent' conflict, where the powerful influence, shape, or determine the wants of the less powerful (p. 23).

The combination of the bases of power identified by French and Raven (1959, 1968), especially the effects of the resource and legitimate authority bases, means that the Commonwealth has the potential to exercise national leadership on many issues, taking an 'agenda shaping' role in Commonwealth–state relations (Lukes 1974). Although states may add matters to the formal agendas of Commonwealth–state forums, those matters rarely progress if the Commonwealth exhibits no interest or does not pick up the idea or proposal. Commonwealth leadership thus can be exercised alone but also can be used to shape a national consensus, essentially as *primus inter pares*. The Commonwealth may also play a negative, blocking role by refusing to commit resources to a program.

Commonwealth–state negotiations are generally conducted harmoniously, with little involvement of the media or the public. Occasionally one or other side of the negotiation uses the media to attempt to influence the outcome and to change relative power in the bargaining process. Negotiation processes usually conclude with a formalised agreement specifying the agreed bargain.

Formal coordinating mechanisms

Important components of Commonwealth–state relations are the formal coordinating councils, termed 'executive federalism' (Sharman 1991). All government portfolios (and the health portfolio is no exception) have formal mechanisms for Commonwealth–state discussion and decision making, including meetings of ministers (ministerial councils) and meetings of the chief executive officers of the relevant portfolios (Hede 1993). The ministerial councils in health and community services are the Australian Health Ministers' Conference, the Community Services Ministers' Conference and the Health and Community Services Ministerial Council. These include ministers from the Commonwealth, the states and territories, and New Zealand and Papua New Guinea, the latter two countries either as full members or observers. Commonwealth representation normally includes one or more ministers from the health and community services portfolio (however named), depending on the assignment of responsibility at Commonwealth level.

Ministerial councils meet annually with the chair of the ministerial council being the host state health minister. In general, ministerial councils work on a consensus basis, although votes can be taken. Decisions of the ministerial councils are not legally binding on members (who are accountable to their own parliaments). Ministerial council meetings are highly political and decisions can be an important part of political negotiations and positioning. Ministerial council meetings are attended not only by ministers but also by advisers from their personal offices, and senior officials of their departments usually including the chief executive of the department.

Supporting the ministerial councils are meetings of the chief executives of the respective departments: the health officials meeting is the Australian Health Ministers' Advisory Council (AHMAC); the community services meeting is the Standing Committee of Community Services and Income Security Administrators (SCCSISA).

In the case of AHMAC, the membership consists of:

- the head and one other senior member of each state and territory health authority
- the Secretary plus two other members of the Commonwealth Department of Health and Aged Care
- the Secretary of the Department of Veteran Affairs
- the Director-General of the New Zealand Ministry of Health.

The Chair of the National Health and Medical Research Council, the Director of the Australian Institute of Health and Welfare, and the Managing Director of the Health Insurance Commission are able to attend AHMAC meetings as observers. The Commonwealth provides half of the funding for AHMAC, with the states and territories providing the remaining funds in proportion to their population. The New Zealand government also contributes to the cost of the Secretariat. AHMAC and its parent ministerial committee create a range of national working parties, usually of short duration. It also sponsors a small number of standing committees such as the National Drugs and Poisons Schedule Committee, the National Public Health Partnership, and the Australian Medical Workforce Advisory Committee. The secretariat arrangements for these subgroups vary from being undertaken within the state or Commonwealth bureaucracies (as an adjunct to existing roles) or more formalised and separate arrangements.

AHMAC usually meets twice a year and has a three-person executive consisting of the chief executive officer from a large state, one from a small state, and the secretary of the Commonwealth Department of Health and Ageing. The Chair of AHMAC is one of the two state members of the executive. The executive of AHMAC holds telephone conferences on a regular basis to finalise the agenda for AHMAC and the Health Ministers' Conference, as well as to consider matters that arise between meetings. Such matters can also be dealt with out-of-session by correspondence. The community services conferences function in ways analogous to the health ministers' conferences and AHMAC.

The ministerial council and the related meeting of officials provide for very senior consideration of Commonwealth–state issues. Although ministers and the chief executives are briefed by their own staff on matters coming before the meetings, they may be prepared to negotiate compromises on outstanding issues in the relevant meeting. Both the ministerial councils and the peak bureaucratic meetings form important decision-making points in the process of Commonwealth–state negotiations and reporting.

National Health and Medical Research Council

Another important coordinating mechanism at the national level is the National Health and Medical Research Council (NH&MRC). The NH&MRC was created under Commonwealth statute (the National Health and Medical Research Council Act 1992) and comprises ministerial appointees drawn from the health professions, together with appointees with knowledge in a range of non-health related areas such as business, trade unions, consumer issues, and social welfare. All are appointed by the Commonwealth minister for a three-year period. In addition, each of the states and territories has a nominee as a member of the Council. The NH&MRC has three broad functions: provision of policy advice, ethics advice, and recommendations about research funding. It is the NH&MRC's aim to ensure that its policy advice is informed by research, although the links between the research-granting functions and the policy advisory functions are often tenuous.

A 'principal committee', the Health Advisory Committee, supervises the policy advisory process. This committee establishes a range of working parties and other committees reporting to the Health Advisory Committee to provide advice on contemporary policy issues and to develop guidelines on best practice (for example, see Smallwood and Lapsley 1997). The ethics function of the NH&MRC is the responsibility of the second principal committee of council: the Australian Health Ethics Committee (AHEC). This committee is responsible for the guidelines and functioning of hospital and other institutional ethics committees (which ensure that research proposals are conducted in an ethically sound manner), as well as dealing with broad ethical issues relating to health care (for example, the committee has considered issues such as organ transplantation and assisted reproductive technology).

The research functions of the NH&MRC are under the aegis of its Research Committee, which sets overall policy directions for research, and also supervises the process of allocating NH&MRC research funds, including review and assessment of research grant proposals, awarding research training grants, and designating research subjects of strategic importance.

The NH&MRC also has statutory responsibility for regulation of research involving human embryos and has established a Licensing Committee to provide advice in this area.

Although the NH&MRC secretariat is situated within the Commonwealth department, the NH&MRC does not have a direct link to Commonwealth policy formulation and its advice is not directly linked into the policy processes of either Commonwealth or state governments. Nevertheless, the decisions of the NH&MRC are persuasive in terms of general policy direction and are taken into account by health professionals and policy makers.

The internal administrative structure of the NH&MRC broadly parallels its committee structure with 'Centres' for health advice, policy and ethics, research management, compliance and evaluation, and corporate operations.

Commonwealth Grants Commission

The Commonwealth Grants Commission plays a major role in intergovern-mental relations in Australia. The commission, established by an Act of the Commonwealth Parliament, provides expert advice on the formula for the distribution of Commonwealth funding to the states and territories (see Commonwealth Grants Commission 1995; see Mathews and Jay 1972 for the evolution of the Commission's role).

The Commonwealth Grants Commission's role has emerged because of the peculiarities of the Australian Constitution and the historical development of the Commonwealth's role in taxation. The Constitution grants the sole right to impose excise duties (including sales tax) to the Commonwealth. The High Court has interpreted excise quite broadly, and in 1998 ruled invalid state business franchise taxes on tobacco and petrol as illegitimately imposing an excise. The Commonwealth, using its wartime powers in 1942, assumed responsibility for income tax. Although this decision was challenged in the immediate postwar period, the Commonwealth's pre-eminence in taxation was upheld. As a result, both income tax and excise have become the preserve of the Commonwealth. As these are the most significant growth taxes in the Australian economy, this has limited the states' ability to impose taxes to meet burgeoning demands to provide for state services, including hospitals. The Commonwealth, however, provides both tied and untied grants to the states to assist in ensuring that service needs are met. The tied grants (known as Specific Purpose Grants or section 96 grants, because of the head of power on which they are based) are particularly prevalent in the health sector, and the most notable of these is the Australian Health Care Agreement. Although the agreements for Specific Purpose Grants include formulae for the distribution of funds, in general these formulae are overridden by the decisions of the Commonwealth Grants Commission. The untied grants (known as General Purpose Grants or Financial Assistance Grants) are distributed on the basis of Commonwealth Grants Commission assessments and can be allocated by the states according to their own priorities. The introduction of the GST on 1 July 2000 changed the form of these untied grants to automatic transfer to the states of GST revenue, although the Commonwealth Grants Commission still determines the allocation between states.

As a result of the different taxation powers and different responsibilities of service and provision, states are increasingly reliant on the Commonwealth for funding. A significant proportion of state revenues come from the Commonwealth government (including GST payments and Specific Purpose Grants), and thus a significant proportion of Commonwealth taxation is used to fund payments to the states. Effectively, this means that the Commonwealth is raising more money than it needs for its own purposes and states are raising far less money from their own taxation for their own purposes. This 'vertical imbalance' is more marked in the Australian federation than in other comparable federations such as Canada and Germany.

The other imbalance in Australian federalism is 'horizontal imbalance'. This derives from the fact that each state faces different circumstances in delivering services that in turn means that the states have different cost structures to deliver the same set of services. In addition, their revenue-raising powers to supplement the Commonwealth funding varies (for example, different abilities to impose resource taxes). Together, states thus face the need to impose different levels of tax to meet the same level of service provision, and may not have the ability to do so. The Commonwealth Grants Commission process is designed to redress this problem through what is known as a 'horizontal equalisation process'.

The Commonwealth Grants Commission (1999) defines the process of horizontal equalisation in the following terms:

> State governments should receive funding from the Commonwealth such that, if each made the same effort to raise revenue from its own sources and operates at the same level of efficiency, each would have the capacity to provide services at the same standard' (p. 4).

The process of equalisation involves assessment of states' revenue-raising capacity and the different costs of providing services. The Grants Commission assesses the needs for health expenditure in two broad categories, hospitals and other health services. The hospital category includes all inpatient services, patient transport, and research. Non-admitted patients are included in the other health services category. The hospital category accounts for 15.4 per cent of total states' standard budgeted expenditure and so it is a significant factor in determining interstate relativities. The states have different needs for expenditure to meet an equivalent standard for hospital provision because of a number of factors, termed 'disabilities'. The principal one is difference in state socio-demographic composition of the population, incorporating factors relating to age and gender distribution, Aboriginality, proportion of population in rural and remote areas, the income distribution of a state's population (because people on low incomes tend to have a high demand for public hospital services), and English fluency (because it costs more to provide services to people with low English fluency). The different proportion of people in each of these categories will affect the expenditure requirements of a state and thus, according to the Grants Commission methodology, the states deserve more for these purposes. The other factors that are taken into account by the Grants Commission include input costs (differences between the states in the price of labour, electricity, and so on); other hospital costs such as dis-economies of scale; within Diagnosis Related Group (DRG) case complexity variation; and the effects of dispersion, patient transport costs, isolation costs, and other administrative scale factors.

According to the Grants Commission assessment, South Australia, Tasmania, and the Northern Territory have a socio-demographic com-position which results in significant additional expenditure relative to all other states. Some factors have a relatively small impact, in particular, iso-lation. This is partly because, by definition, there are relatively few people affected in an isolated population. Overall, a significant amount of money is redistributed by following the Grants Commission assessments of relative hospital expenditure needs with Victoria, Queensland, and the Australian Capital Territory being significant losers through this component of the process and South Australia and the Northern Territory significant winners.

The other health services category includes assessments for nursing home care, mental health, community health (including emergency and outpatient services, dental services, alcohol and drug services), and public health. The factors used to assess expenditure needs are similar to those used for hospitals, including factors related to socio-demographic composition of a population, the economic environment (in particular, factors relating to the nonviability of private health services in some areas, which in turn put greater demand on state government provision), isolation, input costs, and so on.

The health factors in the Grants Commission calculations are merged with other factors such as law, order and public safety, and roads, to deter-mine overall expenditure needs, and together with revenue needs, these are used to determine how Commonwealth payments to the states will be distributed.

Specific Purpose Grants are classed into three broad categories according to the way in which the Grants Commission treats them for horizontal equalisation purposes as part of the assessment of revenue needs. First, some grants are deemed not to be within the standard budget of the states and are excluded from Grants Commission assessments ('exclusion method'). This applies to payments that are reimbursements for services provided on behalf of the Commonwealth (such as when a state instrumentality receives Medicare benefit type payments in the same way and for the same services as private medical practitioners).

Other grants are categorised into two further methods (the 'inclusion approach' and the 'absorption approach'). In both cases, expenditure financed from the specific purpose payment and any financing from state sources is included by the Grants Commission in assessing any expenditure standards in this area. The allocation made in the funding formula incorporated in the agreement that establishes the specific purpose payment is effectively overridden, and the revenue needs for providing the services covered by the specific purpose payment are taken into account by the commission in determining the overall revenue needs for the states. The difference between the two approaches is in the way the Specific Purpose Grant itself is treated in terms of equalisation. Under the inclusion approach, the specific purpose payment is assumed to meet part of the total financial assistance requirement assessed for each state. On the other hand, under the absorption approach, the specific purpose payment is treated as though it were part of a general revenue pool. The base health care grant in the Australian Health Care Agreement is treated by absorption. The Commonwealth can influence how particular grants are handled by directing the commission in its terms of reference. This affects a number of components of the Australian Health Care Agreement, including grants for mental health, which are treated by exclusion as a result of such directions.

Although the Commonwealth Grants Commission adopts this highly technical approach to determining its recommendations, its allocation process remains highly political as it involves distribution (and redistribution) of significant sums of money. Accordingly, the outcome of the Grants Commission processes and their consideration at Premiers' conferences is associated with significant political posturing. New South Wales, Victoria, and Western Australia most frequently question the process, as they are the states that benefit most from a per capita approach and hence are the states from which funds are redistributed to the other states.

6

Hospitals

Hospitals are without doubt the key institutions of the health sector, accounting for over one-third of total health expenditure, as well as playing a dominant role in professional education. The public often thinks of health care in terms of hospital care, and images of the hospital operating theatre or emergency department are regularly used to portray health care generally. However, the nature of acute health care services is changing. Patients are increasingly being cared for in the community with support from a hospital, and quite sophisticated surgical procedures can now be done without an overnight hospital stay. These changes lead to problems in defining precisely what a hospital is and in counting the number of hospitals, the number of hospital beds, and assessing hospital activity.

Table 6.1 Australia: Summary of hospital services and use

Provision	In 2001/02, there were 1306 hospitals (57 per cent public) with 78,868 beds (65 per cent public) which provided 23 million bed days (70 per cent public) to 6.4 million inpatients (62 per cent public). Of the patients, 47.6 per cent in public, and 59.9 per cent in private hospitals were treated on a same-day basis.
	The average length of stay for all patients was 3.6 days, for patients who stayed overnight it was 6.5 days.
	Public hospitals provide 39.5 million outpatient occasions of service including 5.7 million occasions of service in emergency departments.
Resourcing	In 2000/01, hospitals cost A$20 billion to run.
	In 2001/02, public hospitals cost A$16.3 billion to run, A$3059 per patient treated or A$749 per patient day.
	In 2001/02, public hospitals employed 192,187 equivalent full-time staff, 44 per cent of whom were nurses.

Although the general public has no difficulty in recognising a hospital physically, statisticians and health services researchers often confront tautological definitions of hospitals and hospital services. For example, the National Health Information Knowledgebase defines a hospital as: 'A health care facility established under Commonwealth, state or territory legislation as a hospital or a free-standing day procedure unit and authorised to provide treatment and/or care to patients' (AIHW web site: www.aihw.gov.au/knowledgebase/index.html).

This definition states that a hospital is something that Commonwealth, state, and territory legislation says is a hospital! In practice, statistics on hospital care are collected by state health departments that have developed working rules as to which institutions and services are incorporated within the scope of hospital services. Clear definitions, however, remain elusive.

The most contemporary and authoritative source of information on hospitals is the AIHW annual publication *Australian Hospital Statistics*; this is supplemented by the Australian Bureau of Statistics publication, *Private Hospitals* (Catalogue No. 4390.0). The data in this chapter are drawn from these publications. Table 6.1 provides a brief summary of hospital services and use in Australia in 2001/02.

Pathways to care

There are many pathways into hospital care; they involve decisions by both consumers and health professionals (see figure 6.1).

Choices are made at each point of the pathway, and there is a considerable degree of variability in what decisions are taken given the same 'facts'. Patients presenting to one general practitioner might be referred to a

Figure 6.1 Pathways to hospital admission

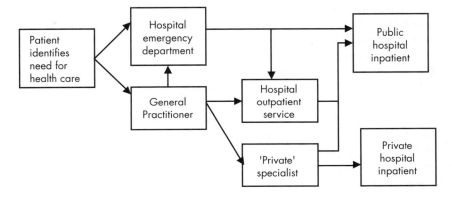

hospital for admission, but if they presented to another general practitioner, he or she might recommend more tests or might wait to see the course of an illness or disease before recommending admission. These differences in style result in considerable variation in admission rates to hospitals throughout Australia (Renwick and Sadkowsky 1991; Richardson 1998c).

Hospitals may be described in terms of a number of characteristics: proprietorship, location, services, and so on. The principal categorisation used in analysis of hospitals in Australia is that of proprietorship, with the key distinction being between 'public' and 'private' hospitals. It should not be assumed that these distinctions are easy to make or self-evident.

Simple definitions of 'public' hospitals, such as whether or not the board of management of a hospital is appointed by the Minister for Health, do not include all public hospitals (for example, religious hospitals would be excluded from that definition). The most common definition of a public hospital is one of those 'recognised' under the Australian Health Care Agreement. The major weakness of this definition is that there are a number of hospitals not 'recognised' but that would be classed as public on most tests of public ownership and administration, especially psychiatric hospitals. In recent years, states have supported development of private hospitals that provide 'public' services (such as care to public patients under the Australian Health Care Agreement) but that are owned and operated by independent operators (Productivity Commission 1999, p. 79). This policy approach is still controversial (Stockigt 1996; Collyer and White 1997; White and Collyer 1998).

Hospital inpatient capacity and utilisation

In 2001/02, Australia had 1060 hospitals and 246 day procedure centres providing 78,868 beds, of which 65 per cent were in public hospitals (see table 6.2). Public hospitals, which account for 57 per cent of all hospitals, are generally larger (mean: 69 beds) than private hospitals (mean: 49 beds).

Overall, Australia has 4.0 acute beds per 1000 population. There are substantial differences between the states in hospital provision, in terms of the relative role of the private sector (36 per cent of all beds in Victoria being in private hospitals compared with 30 per cent in New South Wales). Almost 50 per cent of beds in Tasmania are in private hospitals, in part reflecting the fact that one of the state's major public hospitals was privatised in the 1990s. There are also differences in overall level of provision between the states. South Australia has a bed:population ratio of 4.9 beds per 1000 population, 32 per cent higher than the Victorian provision of 3.7. The different level of provision is also associated with different levels of utilisation: South Australia has a separation rate of 352.7 per 1000 population (age-standardised) and bed day utilisation of 1310 per 1000 population, being 4 per cent and 12 per cent respectively above Victorian levels. (A separation is a discharge, death, or transfer.)

Just over half of all separations from hospitals in 2001/02 did not involve an overnight stay. The 'same-day' proportion was slightly higher in private hospitals (53 per cent; 60 per cent of all separations from private facilities, taking into account day procedure facilities) than public hospitals (48 per cent). The same-day proportion varies between states: 42 per cent of separations from New South Wales public hospitals are same-day compared to 53 per cent from Victorian public hospitals. In contrast, 62 per cent of separations from private facilities in New South Wales are same-day, compared to 60 per cent in Victoria.

Although the proportion of beds in larger private hospitals that are able to deal with more complex procedures is higher than it was a decade ago, the average complexity of cases treated in private hospitals is still less than in public hospitals. In 2001/02, the average 'DRG cost weight' (a measure of complexity derived from the mix of patients classified according to their Diagnosis Related Group, and the DRG average cost) was 9 per cent lower in private hospitals than in public (0.91 compared with 0.99).

Figure 6.2 shows the Major Diagnostic Categories (body systems) for which patients were admitted to hospitals in 2001/02, together with proportions of bed days and costs. About 13 per cent of all admissions were for diseases and disorders of the digestive system, the principal reason for admission being for an endoscopy, a procedure normally done on a same-day basis. This

Figure 6.2 Australia: Hospital separations, patient days, and costs by Major Diagnostic Category, 2001/02

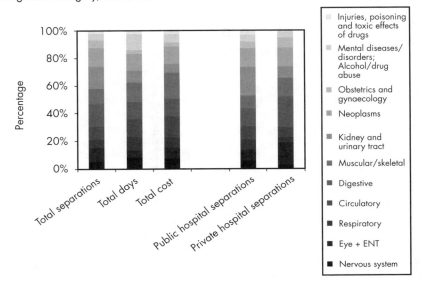

Table 6.2 Australia: Provision and utilisation of hospitals, 2001/02

	NSW	VIC	QLD	WA	SA	TAS	ACT	NT	TOTAL
Provision									
Public hospitals									
Number	218	144	181	89	80	26	3	5	746
Beds	17,402	11,641	9880	5142	5057	1109	670	560	51,461
Beds/hospital	80	81	55	58	63	43	223	112	69
Beds/1000 population	2.7	2.4	2.7	2.7	3.3	2.3	2.1	2.8	2.6
Private hospitals and free-standing facilities									
Number of private hospitals	99	80	57	28	37	9	3	1	314
Beds in private hospitals	6683	5804	6130	3158	2342	995	339	105	25,556
Beds/hospital	39	47	60	77	39	91	47	54	49
Number of private free-standing day-hospital facilities	92	57	49	14	26	2	5	1	246
Beds/chairs in private free-standing day-hospital facilities	711	642	266	73	115	9	33	2	1851
Total private facilities	191	137	106	42	63	11	8	2	560
Total private beds	7394	6446	6396	3231	2457	1004	372	107	27,407
Total private facility beds/1000 population	1.1	1.3	1.7	1.7	1.6	2.1	1.2	0.5	1.4
Total									
Number	409	281	287	131	143	37	11	7	1306
Beds	24,796	18,087	16,276	8373	7514	2113	1042	667	78,868
Beds/1000 population	3.8	3.7	4.4	4.4	4.9	4.4	3.3	3.3	4.0

Table 6.2 Australia: Provision and utilisation of hospitals, 2001/02 (cont.)

	NSW	VIC	QLD	WA	SA	TAS	ACT	NT	TOTAL
Provision									
Total									
Beds/hospital	76	78	67	71	63	60	168	111	73
% beds in public hospitals	70.2%	64.4%	60.7%	61.4%	67.3%	52.5%	64.3%	84.0%	65.2%
Utilisation									
Public									
Separations/1000 population	188.6	222.5	192.5	190.7	229.7	165.0	216.3	394.3	202.8
Same-day separations as % of total	41.9	53.1	47.3	48.0	48.7	47.7	53.7	54.3	47.6
Bed days/1000 population	870.2	827.3	726.4	752.6	950.1	732.0	804.2	1327.4	829.4
Private									
Separations/1000 population	103.4	118.2	165.5	143.0	123.0	145.3	93.9		124.8
Same-day separations as % of private hospital total	52.3	55.5	52.4	51.4	48.7		48.3		52.7
Same-day separations as % of private facilities total	62.1	60.1	62.2	56.1	53.4	54.1	48.3		59.9
Bed days/1000 population	278.2	339.5	492.4	417.5	360.0	446.5	309.1		356.7
Total									
Separations/1000 population	292.0	340.6	358.0	333.7	352.7	310.3	310.3	394.3	327.5
Same-day separations as % of total	49	55.6	54.2	51.5	50.3	50.7	52.1	54.3	52.3
% separations from public hospitals	64.6%	65.3%	53.8%	57.1%	65.1%	53.2%	69.7%		61.9%
Bed days/1000 population	1148.4	1166.7	1218.8	1170.1	1310.0	1178.5	1113.3	1327.4	1183.8
% bed days in public hospitals	75.8%	70.9%	59.6%	64.3%	72.5%	62.1%	72.2%		70.1%

Source: AIHW 2003a

Major Diagnostic Category (MDC) thus accounts for a much lower proportion of bed days.

The major reason for the kidney and urinary tract MDC admissions is renal dialysis, almost always involving a day-only admission. On the other hand, admissions for the MDCs relating to the nervous system, circulatory system, and mental health disorders have longer lengths of stay and so these MDCs account for a larger proportion of bed days than separations.

The distribution of costs, in part, follows bed days, but is naturally affected by other factors (such as use of operating theatres and intensive care units). The circulatory and musculoskeletal system MDCs, for example, both represent a higher proportion of total costs than either separations or bed days.

Figure 6.2 also shows the difference in the proportion of separations for public and private hospitals. Significant differences can be seen here, for example in the proportion of digestive system admissions, again probably reflecting the prevalence of day-only endoscopies in the private sector. The difference in relative importance of the kidney and urinary tract between public and private hospitals reflects the difference in relative importance of renal dialysis between the two sectors.

Differences between separations, bed days, and costs, and between the public and private sectors, are also shown in the relative ranks for the more detailed categorisation, adjacent Diagnosis Related Groups (DRGs), shown in table 6.3. (Adjacent DRGs are the groupings of diagnoses and procedures that are subsequently split into DRGs on the basis of co-morbidities, age, etc. A 'Z' in the description indicates that the adjacent DRG is not split, and that it is also a final DRG.) The most frequent reason for a separation from a public hospital is renal dialysis. The second most frequent reason for separation from a public hospital is vaginal delivery. Other top reasons are heavily weighted to same-day activity. Renal dialysis and vaginal delivery appear in the top three ranks using the three different public hospital activity measures. The second ranking adjacent DRG in terms of public hospital bed days, schizophrenia disorders, is ranked 32 in terms of separations. This reflects the long length of stay for this condition. The highest cost adjacent DRG is tracheostomy, also an infrequent cause for a separation, but ranked ninth in terms of bed days.

The importance of endoscopies in the private sector is shown in the high ranking for relevant adjacent DRGs (G44, G45, G67) on the ranking criteria. Surgical procedures such as major lens procedures, knee replacements, and dental extractions are all ranked highly on one or more of the private hospital activity criteria but somewhat lower in public hospitals. Injuries rank higher in public hospitals than private hospitals, reflecting the relative importance of hospital emergency services in the two sectors.

Figure 6.3 compares hospital utilisation rates (both in terms of separations and bed days) for males and females by age.

Table 6.3 Australia: Most common reasons (by adjacent DRG) for hospitalisation, 2001/02

Adjacent DRGs	Descriptor	Public Hospitals			Private Hospitals		
		Rank by separations	Rank by beddays	Rank by cost	Rank by separations	Rank by bed-days	Rank by cost
L61Z	Admit for renal dialysis	1	1	3	5	22	46
O60	Vaginal delivery	2	3	2	11	1	5
R63Z	Chemotherapy	3	20	32	2	7	12
G44	Other colonoscopy	4	24	21	1	2	4
O65	Other antenatal admission	5	23	35	58	70	67
G45	Other gastroscopy for non-major digestive disease	6	33	33	3	8	9
G67	Oesophagitis, gastroent, and misc digestive system disorders	7	13	18	42	27	53
F74Z	Chest pain	8	30	30	55	81	82
E62	Respiratory infection/inflammations	9	4	6	47	13	30
E65	Chronic obstructive airway disease	10	7	9	63	12	32
X60	Injuries	11	32	44	136	115	145
E69	Bronchitis and asthma	12	25	28	87	68	110
G66	Abdominal pain or mesenteric adenitis	13	39	52	69	91	132
O01	Caesarean delivery	15	9	5	16	4	7
C08Z	Major lens procedures	16	85	27	4	10	3
U61	Schizophrenia disorders	32	2	4	185	45	83
A06Z	Tracheostomy any age any cond	125	9	1	219	36	10
U63	Major affective disorders	116	46	10	33	6	1
I04	Knee replacement and reattachment	43	5	14	57	3	13
D40Z	Dental extraction and restorations	37	135	93	6	18	14

Figure 6.3 Australia: Hospital utilisation rate (separations per 1000 population; patient days per 100 population) by age group and gender 2001/02

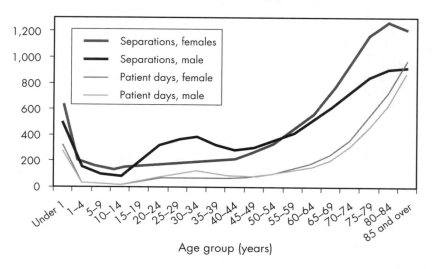

Figure 6.3 shows a dramatic escalation in utilisation rates in later years, with separation rates for people aged over 65 being more than double those of people aged 25 to 45. Bed day rates for the over 65 population are more than 10 times those of younger age groups. For most age groups the bed day rate is around twice to three times the separation rate; however, for the over 75-year-old age group, the relativity between bed days and separations is different, with bed day rates being about 10 times separation rates, reflecting the much longer average length of stay for this age group.

Figure 6.4 Australia: Proportion of separations and patient days by age group and gender, 2001/02

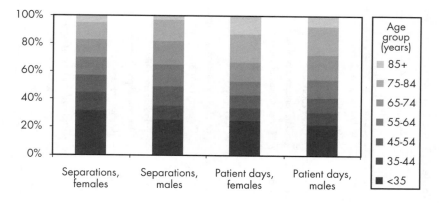

Figure 6.6 Australia: Trend in average length of stay, public and private acute hospitals, 1985/86 to 2001/02

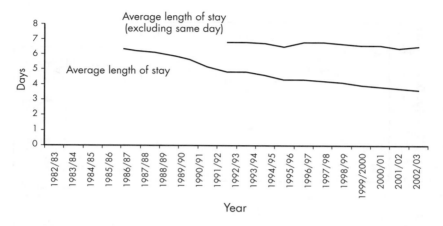

- from 1999, private health insurance growth
- a transfer of private patients from public hospitals
- improved efficiency through an increase in occupancy rates and reduction in length of stay (see figure 6.6)
- growth in the 'self-insured' population (that is, people without health insurance who seek hospitalisation in private hospitals or as private patients in public hospitals)
- increased adverse selection in the insured population, which increases the rate of use of services in that population (the privately insured population is, on average, sicker than previously).

Thus, despite the decline in health insurance prior to 1999, the private sector has not experienced a reduction in demand.

The dramatic increase in separation rates also reflects the growth of private day procedure centres. Since 1982/83, length of stay has almost halved (from 6.9 days to 3.9 days in 2001/02). However, this decline masks the contributing factors. The reduction in average length of stay has occurred principally because of the significant increase in the proportion of day-only patients. Very long stay patients are also staying in hospital for a shorter period. Both these trends have been facilitated by improvements in medical technology (for example, shorter-action anaesthetic agents and flexible endoscopy). For those patients who stay overnight, the decline in length of stay has been marginal.

Most states regulate the number of private hospital beds, and bed licences are tradable commodities. Thus, although there has been a redistribution of private beds, few private beds have been closed. The reduction in private hospital provision per capita has been caused principally by an increase in the population with only marginal changes in total private bed provision. Per capita provision of private hospitals in nonmetropolitan areas has increased, partly reflecting reductions in population but partly, also, the development of new private hospitals in major rural centres. Private hospitals have also experienced substantial growth (as reflected in increased admissions per 1000 population) with the increase principally occurring through reduction in length of stay and, to some extent, increased occupancy rates. About 55 per cent of all private hospitals are for-profit, and this sector of the industry is expanding in share. Over the period 1996/97 to 2000/01, the number of beds in for-profit hospitals increased by 15 per cent while beds in not-for-profits declined (by 3 per cent). Separations from for-profit hospitals increased faster than not-for-profits (41 per cent versus 13 per cent).

The 1990s saw a restructuring of the private hospital industry, with the emergence and increasing importance of for-profit hospital groups in the industry, and a corresponding reduction in the number of free-standing 'independent' for-profit hospitals (Productivity Commission 1999; O'Loughlin 2002). The for-profit groups ('chains') are often listed companies.

The most dramatic trend in service provision over the last decade has been in provision of distinct public psychiatric services, where there has been a reduction of over 60 per cent in provision of inpatient care. This has been caused by two key factors supported by policies at state and national level (Singh and McGorry 1998). First, advances in psychotropic medication have meant that patients who previously required very long stay care in psychiatric institutions can now be maintained in community settings. A second trend has been the 'mainstreaming' of psychiatric services: acute psychiatric care is provided in acute general hospitals with dedicated psychiatric admission wards.

Figure 6.7 Australia: Percentage change in total separations, largest Major Diagnostic Categories, 1997/98 to 2001/02

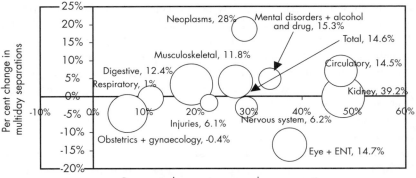

Per cent change in same day separations

NB: Size of circles indicates relative number of total separations, 2001/02, % is change from 1997/98

Figure 6.7 shows data on the change in separations for the largest MDCs over the period 1997/98 to 2001/02. The axes for the graph show the percentage change in same-day and multi-day separations. The size of the circles shows the relative number of total separations in the MDC in 2001/02 with the percentage in the label showing the change in total separations over the two-year period.

Overall, total separations increased 14.6 per cent over the four-year period, almost 4 per cent per annum. Almost all of this increase was in same-day separations (which increased 30 per cent) with the number of multi-day separations increasing only marginally (1.0 per cent). There are significant differences in patterns of provision between the various MDCs. Overall activity in maternity services was basically unchanged over the period, but with significant change in composition: multi-day activity was substituted by same-day activity. The 15 per cent increase in eye and ENT admissions also involved substitution (reduction in multi-day admissions). For most of the larger MDCs the number of same-day separations increased significantly, almost 50 per cent in the case of diseases and disorders of the kidney and urinary tract and in circulatory system diseases.

Non-inpatient services

Non-inpatient care is an important component of hospital provision accounting for about 25 per cent of all hospital expenditure. In recent years, many hospitals have broadened their range of activities such as domiciliary services, health education, and the like. This is especially the case in New South Wales where Area Health Boards, covering both hospital and community health services, have been established.

Specialist medical clinics run as part of hospital 'outpatient' services complement those provided by specialists in their private rooms. However, as will be shown in chapter 7, private specialist services usually require a substantial co-payment or patient financial contribution (moiety). The Australian Health Care Agreement precludes states charging fees for hospital outpatient services. Continued provision of outpatient services is thus important for equity reasons: consumers using outpatient services are generally elderly people of lower socioeconomic status with chronic conditions (Jackson et al. 1997).

Attendance at an outpatient department represents one of the most common reasons for contact with health institutions. In 2001/02 there were 39.2 million outpatient occasions of service Australia-wide, just over two occasions of service per capita, representing about 10 outpatient occasions of service for every public hospital inpatient admission, or six occasions for every public or private admission. Just over one-fifth of outpatient occasions

Figure 6.8 Australia: Non-admitted patients per capita, by state or territory and type of service, 2001/02

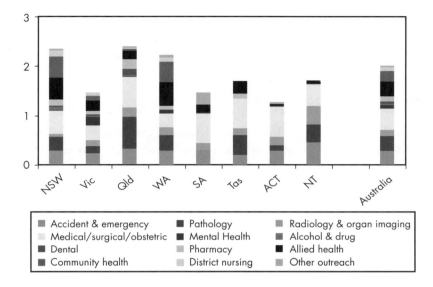

of service (0.45 per capita) are visits to the traditional medical/surgical or obstetric clinics. Many of these visits lead to a pathology test, diagnostic imaging investigation, or a pharmacy prescription. These 'downstream' services account for a further quarter of all occasions of service. About one in seven non-inpatient attendances are emergencies.

Figure 6.8 shows the composition and rates of outpatient occasions of service in each state, with rates ranging from 2.4 per capita in New South Wales and Queensland to 1.3 in the ACT.

Utilisation rates are significantly affected by the organisation of the health system in the different states and by practice pattern differences. There is a 50 per cent variation in the utilisation rate for emergency occasions of service across all states except the Northern Territory, with rates falling between 0.22 and 0.33 occasions of service per capita. The rate of provision for medical/surgical/obstetric clinics is more variable: from 0.29 per capita in Victoria to 0.60 in the ACT. This variation probably reflects the extent of privatisation of non-inpatient services rather than variation in demographic characteristics or variation in underlying clinical need. Other types of service show even greater variability. The ratio of the highest per capita rate to the lowest (called the Extremal Quotient) is 49 for mental health services (probably reflecting the extent to which these services are integrated into public hospital management and/or statistical systems). The Extremal Quotient for allied health is 19. Community health per capital utilisation varies from 0.41 in New South Wales to 0.05 in Queensland, with a number of states reporting zero activity (and hence an Extremal Quotient cannot be calculated). The allied health and community health differences reflect the integrated nature of the New South Wales health system (the largest per capita rates are reported in that state) relative to the separate organisation of community health in other states.

Home-based acute care

As was noted earlier in this chapter, defining the hospital is becoming increasingly difficult, as acute care, which previously could only be provided in hospitals, is now provided in homes (Iliffe and Shepperd 2002; Shepperd and Iliffe 2003). There are two main developments of home-based acute care: programs to avoid inpatient hospitalisation (typically referred to as 'hospital-in-the-home') and home-based post-acute care. Hospital-in-the-home programs have developed in Australia to provide care of a kind that would otherwise necessitate admission to a hospital, typically involving regular visits to the patient's home by nursing staff. The most common example of this is intravenous therapy. Admission to a hospital-in-the-home program is usually initiated in the hospital emergency department. Hospital-in-the-home programs are increasingly available in Australia (see Lowenthal et al. 1996; Caplan et al. 1999; Cooper 1999; Montalto 1999); patients in these programs often count for state government funding purposes as if they were hospital inpatients.

Home-based post-acute care normally does not involve patients with the same level of acuity as participants in hospital-in-the-home programs (although a distinction between the two types of programs is not always clear). Post-acute care is principally offered to ensure that early discharge from hospital to home can occur safely. It may involve hospital staff making home visits in the immediate post-discharge period, or can involve negotiated arrangements (including brokerage funding) to purchase care from existing community support agencies.

Interest in and funding of hospital-in-the-home programs is increasing program diversity across Australia, which can affect the relative efficiency of programs (Viney et al. 2001). There is also heightened interest in other 'diversion' strategies aimed at reducing demand for hospital admissions. One such strategy is based on telephone 'call centres', providing advice by telephone to potential patients to assist in determining the appropriate response to their health care needs. The most noteworthy of these internationally is NHS Direct in the United Kingdom. The first large-scale Australian call centre development was established in Western Australia (Health Direct) in 1999 with promising results (Turner et al. 2002).

Paying for hospital services

Currently, there are four broad approaches to paying for hospital activity: capitation; historical/negotiated payment; per diem; and per case funding. In the longer term, it may be possible to adjust hospital payment rates on the basis of their outcomes: the extent to which they contribute to improving health status. However, the technology to do this does not currently exist. Unlike the USA, where many hospitals have capitation-based contracts as a key source of funding, none of the Australian states or territories has adopted a capitation approach to funding public hospitals. Further, health insurance funds are prohibited from paying for private patients on a capitated basis. New South Wales hospitals are the responsibility of Area Health Authorities, with the authorities' budgets being in part determined by the weighted population for which they are responsible. However, this capitation approach is not used for hospital funding within the area; Area Health Authorities fund their hospitals on a historical or negotiated basis.

In the past, most states funded their hospitals, either directly or indirectly, on the basis of historical budgets (with marginal annual adjustments). Hospital budgets may have been approved on an input or 'line-item' basis: the central funding authority approving 'staff establishments' specifying the number of nurses, cleaners, doctors, and other categories of expense (such as food, supplies). The historical budget was occasionally renegotiated when the hospital had a major redevelopment or additional services approved. In the 1980s, hospital budgets were renegotiated on a more regular basis (usually annually) but with the historical allocation still the base. Typically, the negotiated budget was based on the prior year's budget, with or without a standard adjustment, increasing the budget for inflationary effects, or reducing budgets across the state for deemed productivity improvements. Historical budget setting is now rare, and standard across-the-board cuts have been replaced by tailored budget cuts. Similarly, an increased budget usually comes with some form of service rationale. The historical budgeting approaches have thus evolved to be equivalent to a negotiated basis.

Negotiated budgets for public hospitals are formalised in a contract or 'agreement' between the state health authority and the hospital. These agreements often also include negotiated goals covering a range of aspects of hospital administration, including broad targets about the number of patients treated and number of outpatient attendances, together with a specification of the funds that would be available to that hospital in that year. However, negotiated budgets do little to change historical funding arrangements either in terms of patient flows or efficiency. A Victorian parliamentary review of that state's late 1980s health service agreement process came to the damning conclusion that:

While health service agreements may have contributed to overall efficiency gains there is little tangible evidence to indicate that they have tackled the problems of discrepancies in hospital performance ... health service agreements have not achieved a significant move from historical patterns of funding.

(Economic and Budget Review Committee 1992, p. 11)

The third approach to paying hospitals is to base payments on the number of patient days. Per diem payment approaches are most commonly applied to nursing home or other non-acute institutional provision, and those acute services with longer lengths of stay (for example, rehabilitation services) where the bed day is an appropriate measure of the product of the institution. Private hospital reimbursement (and charges to private patients in some states) has been based on a tiered per diem approach since 1987. The Commonwealth government prescribed a tiered per diem model using differential bed day payments for patients in each of five treatment bands: advanced surgical; surgical/obstetrics; psychiatric; rehabilitation; and other. This funding model also recognises that longer stay patients in each of these bands have lower costs per bed day.

The Commonwealth-prescribed payment is the minimum payment that insurers must make for private patients, and these payments are probably lower than costs even in efficiently operating private hospitals. Most insurers make higher per diem payments in the early days of stay, and introduce multiple step downs of stay. These step down arrangements make long lengths of stay uneconomic for private hospitals, and provide similar incentives for efficient provision as are provided under the fourth form of hospital payment, per patient or case payments.

Under 'casemix funding' (per patient reimbursement policies), the funder or purchaser assumes the risk for cost variations caused by variations in the number and type of patient treated, by setting differential prices for different types of patients and allowing budgets to vary with volume of patients treated. The hospital therefore becomes more clearly accountable for variation in the efficiency of the services it provides (Palmer 1996). Hospital payment should include incentives on hospital management to provide appropriate care efficiently. Hospitals should assume responsibility for the number of days of stay and number of services provided (pathology tests, nursing interventions), as well as the costs of each day of stay and of each service (Saltman and Young 1981; Young and Saltman 1985).

Hospital budgets should reflect the number and mix of patients treated. A way of standardising for hospital 'casemix' is therefore required so that hospitals can be held accountable for efficiency variations in how they treat similar patients. One of the key advances in health economics and health services research over the last few decades has been the development of

DRGs. Because of their design characteristics, in particular resource homogeneity (patients in the same DRG are expected to consume similar amounts of resources), DRGs can be used to standardise for differences in the casemix of hospitals to allow comparisons of hospital efficiency and for payment purposes (Fetter 1991).

Australia has a long history of casemix development. The first research in this area in Australia was undertaken in 1985 aimed at testing whether the Diagnosis Related Groups (DRG) classification system as developed by Professor Fetter in the USA was relevant to Australian clinical practice (Palmer et al. 1986). The project also attempted to assign costs on a DRG basis in a sample of three Victorian hospitals. Since that small beginning, Australia has embarked on an ambitious casemix development program. The Commonwealth has funded a program to develop an Australian version of the USA's DRGs, and hospital services in Australia can now be described in terms of Australian Refined Diagnosis Related Groups, with 661 separate DRGs. A number of states have now implemented casemix funding of hospitals in a variety of forms.

A prerequisite for casemix funding is greater clarity in describing hospital activities. Typically, three broad streams of hospital care can be identified: inpatient services, outpatient services, and 'teaching and research'. These are not equally well suited to casemix funding and they do not specify the full range of other activities provided by hospitals, including home care services. These latter services are normally captured in 'specified grants' or 'site specific grants' made on a negotiated basis. (Examples of specified grants are home dialysis, and funds for special wards for treatment of prisoners.)

Casemix funding also requires that prices and volumes of activity be specified for each of the major types of care as well as specification of quality standards.

The key events in the transition to casemix funding occurred in 1993/94 when Victoria adopted casemix funding for public hospitals (for an analysis of the original Victorian funding policies, see Duckett 1995b and Health Solutions 1994; for a discussion of the policy process that led to the introduction of casemix funding, see Lin and Duckett 1997). South Australia introduced casemix funding in 1994/95 (for information on the 2000/01 casemix funding arrangements in Victoria, see McNair and Duckett 2002; for South Australia see Moss 2002).

The 'Lawrence' health insurance reform of 1995 provided the framework for the introduction of casemix payments in the private sector. The Lawrence arrangements were introduced by the then Commonwealth Health Minister, Dr Carmen Lawrence, and allowed private health insurers to pay hospitals on an 'episode' (casemix) basis rather than per diem. Health insurers would also be able to contract with medical practitioners to cover any gap between Medicare reimbursement and the fee charged for in-hospital services.

A second key element of the legislation was designed to change the role of health insurers from passive payers of hospital bills (and part payment of in-hospital medical bills) to more sophisticated purchasers and negotiators. Adoption of this new role (and acquisition of the new skills necessary) has been relatively slow and was politically contentious. Neither private hospitals nor medical practitioners welcomed the additional accountability and intrusion the new contractual arrangements potentially involved. Lawrence's Liberal successor as health minister, Dr Michael Wooldridge, agreed to legislative amendments to protect medical autonomy and promoted these arrangements to ensure that patients would face no out-of-pocket costs for their hospitalisation or, at worst, know the level of out-of-pocket expenses ('no gap or known gap' policies). The Senate also insisted on a regular review of the negotiation provisions by the Australian Competition and Consumer Commission (for the most recent report see the ACCC web site at www.accc.gov.au). These arrangements have slowly grown and a number of health insurers are now negotiating per case payments with hospitals. Insurers are also developing a network of 'preferred provider' arrangements with private hospitals, thus putting increased financial pressure on hospitals not within such a network. No gap policies are also increasing: in March 2003 81 per cent of in hospital medical services (there may be more than one service per hospitalisation) involved no gap; a further 3.5 per cent of services were covered by known gap arrangements (PHIAC web site: www.phiac.gov.au/statistics/medicalgapinfo/gapmar03/index.htm).

Casemix funding yields efficiency improvements more rapidly than negotiated funding. However, negotiated budgets could be based on a continual improvement approach with efficiency improvement targets being set for even the most efficient hospital in a jurisdiction with larger efficiency gains being expected of less efficient hospitals. Evidence from England, where the 'targets' approach has predominated, suggests that the use of targets was neither related to overall regional or national efficiency measures, nor acted to reduce measured efficiency differences over time (Jacobs and Dawson 2003). The overt justification for negotiated budgets may stress the potential for greater levels of efficiency improvements than a mechanistic casemix approach. However, such an overt justification may simply mask a covert need to allow government or the health authority more flexibility in budget setting to respond to non-economic factors, such as the perceived need to provide adjustments to hospital budgets for political reasons. In these circumstances an objective payment formula may limit the potential for political adjustments to budgets.

Inpatient services

Inpatient services have been the main focus of casemix development, partly because it is the core business of hospitals, accounting for over three-quarters of all hospital expenditure, but also because inpatient casemix classifications are the best developed.

Casemix funding normally provides for a statewide standard contract and a standard base price across the state or for broad classes of hospitals. The contract also provides the rules under which funding varies with volume. Under casemix funding, payments to hospitals are based on relative weights ('cost weights') estimated using cost modelling or data extraction from hospital clinical costing systems (Jackson 2001). Cost modelling is a relatively simple costing approach that uses general ledger data and patient activity data to estimate hospital specific prices by DRG (Chandler et al. 1991). It uses 'service weights' (for example, pathology weights, theatre weights) to estimate service costs in each DRG, which are then summed to yield an estimated cost and relative weight for each DRG. Initial cost modelling in Australia used US service weights but the Commonwealth government, through the Casemix Development Program, funded the development of Australian service weights to be used in calculating DRG relative weights for public and private hospitals at state and national level (KPMG Peat Marwick 1993). The alternative approach to deriving cost weights is to use data from hospital clinical costing or patient costing systems (Jackson et al. 1999). These systems, which are used for internal management purposes (Stoelwinder and Abernethy 1989), provide costing information at the patient level that can be aggregated by DRG to provide cost relativities on a DRG basis. Data from Victoria's 18 largest hospitals (accounting for over half of the state's separations) are used to set Victorian price relativities (Jackson 2001).

DRGs are developed to represent the 'normal case' for that grouping and, therefore, in addition to the standard or base payment, 'outlier' payments are paid for unusual cases. Outliers are those cases that are statistically different from the norm, falling outside high and low boundaries or 'trim points'.

Australian funding formulae generally set trim points using the 'L3H3' approach: the low trim point is one-third the average length of stay for that DRG, the high trim point is three times the average length of stay (McGuire et al. 1995). High outliers (cases above the high trim point) receive an additional per diem payment, while low outliers (cases below the low trim point) get paid less than the ordinary base payment. The outlier payments are converted to a payment unit called 'inlier equivalent separations' in the Victorian system. This simply counts each high outlier stay as a multiple (say 1.6) of the typical stay in that DRG.

Casemix funding of hospitals involves extremely low transaction costs. All discharges from all hospitals in Australia have diagnoses and procedures recorded in computerised databases, with diagnosis and procedure coding being undertaken at the hospital level. The development of a payment system relies on this routine production and transmission of data, and the low transaction costs of the payment system are possible because the

Table 6.4   Australia: Public hospital funding arrangements, 2001/02

State or Territory	Funding Arrangements
New South Wales	Adjusted population based funding to Area Health Authorities, area autonomy on funding to hospitals, hence different bases in use. Move towards comparing efficiency of hospitals on basis of their casemix.
Victoria	Casemix funding
Queensland	Historical, adjusted by casemix information
Western Australia	Casemix funding
South Australia	Casemix funding
Tasmania	Input basis
Australian Capital Territory	Casemix-based funding
Northern Territory	Casemix funding

information flow on which the system is based is already in place. Information on the number of patients treated is aggregated by the state health department, the relative weights and hence relative prices are applied on a monthly basis through a simple spreadsheet type program, and adjustments to cash flow to hospitals (and their budgets) are made on a quarterly basis. Because locally coded data are used for payment purposes, coding audits are conducted to monitor coding accuracy (Reid 1991).

Because of the strong efficiency incentives enshrined in casemix funding, most states now have adopted casemix funding or use casemix information to inform budget processes (see table 6.4).

Given the capped nature of public sector spending, casemix funding incorporates expenditure capping systems, either through declining marginal payment for additional volume or through explicit volume caps.

Outpatients

The second broad type of care provided by hospitals is 'outpatient' or 'non-inpatient' services. Relatively little national progress has been made in specifying the casemix within outpatient services with the result that the current approach in most casemix states is based on occasion of service counting within 10 to 15 broad areas (for example, medical, surgical, allied health, and so on).

There are two main strands of development work taking place in Australia on casemix categorisation for outpatient services: 'clinic' categorisation and individual patient-based classifications. The latter approach relies on substantial increased investment in data collection systems for outpatient services (including diagnosis coding) that may make it infeasible for introduction in the foreseeable future.

Victoria and Queensland use a systematic 'clinic' categorisation system as part of casemix funding arrangements for outpatient care; for example, the Victorian Ambulatory Classification System (VACS), developed using patient-level costing data, identifies 44 clinic types and associated relative weights (Jackson and Sevil 1996). Payments (and relative weights) for episodes of outpatient care in VACS incorporate the clinic visit and any associated investigation and pharmaceuticals ordered in a 30-day window around the clinic visit (O'Connell and Sharwood 1997). Because of poor activity recording in some clinical areas (especially allied health) and because of the distinct nature of the product of emergency departments, Victoria has only implemented a casemix funding system for medical and surgical clinics. Clinic-based systems involve an audit process to ensure homogeneity of clinic types between hospitals (Jackson and Sevil 1997).

Training and development

Teaching hospitals are more expensive than non-teaching hospitals. This difference is in part due to the fact that teaching hospitals are involved in another product variously called 'training and development' or 'teaching and research'. Generally, this has been measured in terms of the number of junior medical staff (interns and registrars) together with recognition that the first year on the job of many health professionals includes a training component.

Hospitals in Australia still participate in a range of post-registration educational programs for nurses and these, too, attract payments. Payment systems for undergraduate activity of hospitals vary. Victoria has developed an undergraduate payment based on 'placement weeks' of undergraduate students; other states provide a percentage add-on to other training and development activity payments.

Access to public hospital inpatient services

Although Medicare has eliminated financial barriers to access to hospital care, the existence of hospital waiting lists indicates that there are other barriers to access to care. Priority for treatment for public hospital care is determined on the basis of whether or not the patient can 'afford' to wait, with the costs of waiting being based on the 'risk' to the patient of delay. For many patients, any delay may prove critical, and immediate or emergency treatment is required. Rapid deterioration is less likely for patients in need of minor surgery or non-urgent elective procedures and it is these patients who may be judged to be able to afford to join a waiting list (Street and Duckett 1996).

There are a number of ways of measuring problems in access to elective surgery:

- *Waiting lists.* These simply measure total numbers waiting. This is a common measure used in the media but only gives a very crude figure uncategorised for urgency. It adds those waiting for convenience (e.g. booked to have an operation in the school holidays), those waiting for a week or so to optimise scheduling of operating capacity or beds etc, and those waiting longer times because of inadequate capacity.
- *Waiting times.* A more sophisticated measure than simply numbers waiting but needs to be categorised in some way by urgency and/or procedure.
- *Extended waits.* This is the contemporary preferred measure. It recognises that some minimal level of waiting list is useful for efficiency reasons but also that there are problems with people waiting too long (e.g. deterioration of condition). An extended wait measure relies on categorising patients to determine urgency and what is a reasonable wait, given the patient's clinical condition, social environment, etc.

For the two waiting time measures, data can be derived from those admitted (e.g. how long did they wait prior to admission?) and from those currently waiting but not yet admitted.

Waiting lists in Australia are typically classified in terms of Category 1, Category 2, and Category 3. The definitions of those categories are:

- Category 1 – admission within 30 days desirable for a condition that has the potential to deteriorate quickly to the point that it may become an emergency.
- Category 2 – admission within 90 days desirable for a condition causing some pain, dysfunction, or disability but that is not likely to deteriorate quickly or become an emergency.
- Category 3 – admission at some time in the future acceptable for a condition causing minimal or no pain, dysfunction, or disability, that is unlikely to deteriorate quickly and that does not have the potential to become an emergency (AIHW 2002e, p.5).

These categories are assigned by surgeons and are somewhat subjective. Improved objectivity can be obtained by using procedure-specific scoring systems (see Hadorn and Holmes 1997a, b; Hadorn and Steering Committee of the Western Canada Waiting List Project 2002, 2003; Taylor et al. 2002; Noseworthy et al. 2003).

Figure 6.9 shows days waited prior to admission for all elective surgery patients and for two specialties: cardiothoracic and ophthalmology. Two measures of waiting are shown, the median (50 per cent of patients waited more than this time, 50 per cent less) and the 90th percentile (10 per cent of patients waited more than this time, 90 per cent less).

Fifty per cent of patients requiring elective surgery in public hospitals in 2001/02 waited more than 27 days, in the ACT the median wait was 40

Figure 6.9 Australia: Days waited by patients admitted from waiting lists, 2001/02

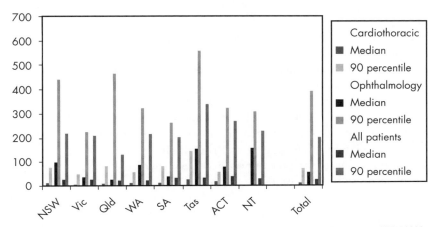

Data source: AIHW 2002e

days. Ten per cent of patients waited more than 203 days, with 10 per cent of patients in Tasmania waiting almost one year.

There are significant differences between the two specialties with significantly shorter waits (on both measures) for cardiothoracic surgery compared to ophthalmology. There are also significant differences between states. The 90th percentile for Queensland patients waiting for cardiothoracic surgery is more than one month longer than for similar Victorian patients; the median New South Wales ophthalmology patient waits slightly more than two months longer than their Queensland counterpart. Ten per cent of ophthalmology patients waited around a year or more in New South Wales, Queensland, Western Australia, and Tasmania. The wait was almost two years in the Australian Capital Territory.

Strategies to reduce excessive waiting times need to be carefully designed to avoid creating perverse incentives to reward hospitals with long lists or waiting times (Street and Duckett 1996). Contemporary supply strategies, which assume that current surgery rates are too low, include increasing funding; increasing productivity (through changing incentives, payment arrangements, or day-surgery rates); improving management of waiting lists; creating specialist elective surgery centres; use of private sector facilities; or transferring patients to facilities with lower demand or lower waiting times. Demand side strategies include use of explicit guidelines; and reducing pressure on public services by encouraging use of private services (Hurst and Siciliani 2003). Waiting list reduction strategies such as these have been shown to work (Street and Duckett 1996; Cullis and Jones 2000) and it should not be assumed that waiting lists are intractable or that demand is infinite (Frankel et al. 2000).

Elective surgery is not the only hospital service with access issues. In a number of states there are problems of access to hospital emergency services. The most common ways of describing inadequate access to these services are:

- waiting times in emergency departments for given 'triage' or urgency categories
- occasions of ambulance bypass, i.e. how often a hospital has notified the ambulance service that it is not available to receive ambulances with emergency cases. It is important to note that even if the hospital is on 'bypass', patients who arrive by other means of transport will be received
- number of patients retained in hospital emergency departments for extended periods (e.g. greater than 12 hours or 24 hours). Strictly speaking, this is not a measure of access to emergency services but rather of access to hospital wards.

State health authorities have responded to these urgent access problems by changing funding arrangements (Cameron et al. 1999; Duckett and Jackson 2001) and promoting change to hospital protocols and organisation through, for example, short stay units associated with the emergency department (Daly et al. 2003).

Public hospital operating costs

Operating costs of public hospitals in 2001/02 totalled A$17 billion, 62 per cent of which was for salaries and wages, with a further 5 per cent for superannuation, and 4 per cent for visiting medical officers, bringing the total for salary and related payments to 71 per cent (see figure 6.10). This relatively high proportion of costs spent on labour is typical of service industries.

About 45 per cent of salaries and wages expenditure was for nursing staff, reflecting the fact that nurses are the largest single category of employees in hospitals, providing 24-hour cover for all ward areas.

The relative composition of various items of expenditure will differ with the role of the hospital and, to some extent, the hospital's management and outsourcing arrangements. Referral hospitals, for example, would expect to have more 'diagnostic and health professionals' per patient, and thus a higher proportion of staffing (and expenditure) in this category relative to smaller hospitals dealing with a less complex case load.

There is little Australian evidence about optimal hospital size. (Butler's early study (Butler 1995) did not standardise well for casemix.) The overseas literature suggests that there are economies of scale up to about 100 to 200 beds and diseconomies of scale emerge in hospitals with more than 300 to 600 beds (Posnett 2002). The wide ranges referred to here reflect the weakness and uncertainty in the literature. It has also been suggested that analysis

Figure 6.10 Australia: Public hospital operating costs, by type of costs, 2001/02

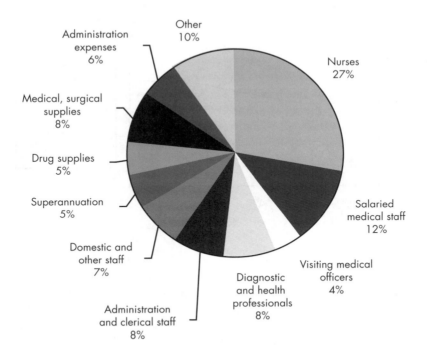

of efficiency should be undertaken at the DRG level (Eckermann 2002). The sole Australian study that has done this suggested economies of scale differ for different DRGs, and emerge at quite low levels of activity (Watts 2002). There is consensus in the literature that outcomes for patients are better in larger hospitals (Posnett 2002) and in teaching hospitals (Ayanian and Weissman 2002). Minimum volume thresholds have been developed in the USA for a number of conditions (Elixhauser et al. 2003). Failure to adhere to these thresholds may expose hospitals and referring physicians in the USA to increased litigation risk in the event of an adverse event (Mello et al. 2003).

Figure 6.11 shows trends in real per capita expenditure on hospital services since 1990. It can be seen that hospital expenditure has increased over that period in both public and private hospitals. The data presented in figure 6.11 is adjusted so that it is expressed in 1999/2000 dollars. Expenditure on hospital services is thus increasing faster than the growth in prices of the economy as a whole, and faster than population growth. The growth in expenditure, has, naturally enough, led to an emphasis on cost-saving strategies in hospitals, including strategies to change the basis of hospital payment (see later in this chapter).

One of the reasons for the growth in expenditure has been the effect of

Figure 6.11 Australia: Per capita expenditure on hospitals (1999/2000 dollars), 1990/91 to 2000/01

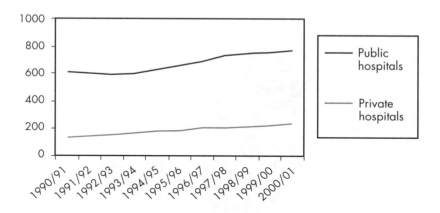

technological change: the introduction of new drugs, devices, and treatments. In contrast to the situation in many industries, where new technologies are labour-saving and cost-reducing, new technologies in the health sector are presented as quality-enhancing rather than cost-reducing. Diffusion of new technologies is a global phenomenon, at least in developed countries. Countries appear to differ in terms of when new technologies are first introduced and the speed of introduction (Technological Change in Health Care (TECH) Research Network 2001), with Australia being a relatively mid-range adopter but with rapid diffusion after adoption. The USA is an early adopter, also with rapid diffusion.

Increasing hospital costs is also a global phenomenon, although policy responses differ. In Australia, regulatory mechanisms have been used to require economic evaluation of new technologies prior to their introduction. States have also slowed technological change by constraining capital expenditure (Deeble 2002). In the USA there has been a strong emphasis on using competitive markets, and the resulting competitive price pressures, to slow hospital expenditure growth. Although this competitive strategy has been shown to be successful in price moderation, there has been an adverse impact on quality of care (Mukamel et al. 2002).

Comparison of efficiency of public and private hospitals

The question of whether the private sector is more efficient than the public sector or vice versa is regularly subject to debate. Data from the National

Figure 6.5 Australia: Trends in beds and separations, public and private hospitals, 1982/83 to 2001/02

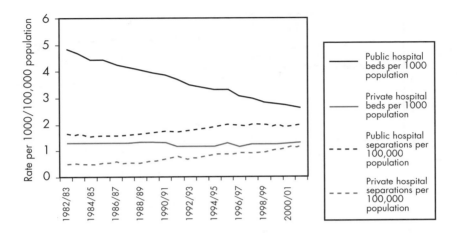

Even though the elderly are only a relatively small proportion of the population, these very high rates of utilisation also translate into high proportions of hospital activity. Figure 6.4 shows the proportion of separations and bed days by age group and gender in Australia.

It can be seen that the over 65-year-old population represents about one-third of all hospital separations but one-half of bed days (56 per cent of total bed days). These very high proportions emphasise the critical role hospitals play in care of the elderly and the importance of standardising for age and gender in hospital planning. However, these data do not support an argument that elderly persons' use is 'disproportionately large'; their use may indeed be proportionate to need (McKie et al. 1996).

Trends in inpatient provision

Figure 6.5 shows that since 1986 there has been a substantial decline (almost halving) in the number of public acute hospital beds per capita, with the number of private acute beds being relatively stable. The decline in public provision has been a result of specific government policies to reduce bed provision, particularly in rural areas.

Despite the reduction in beds per capita, there has been a 45 per cent increase in separations per capita (20 per cent in public hospitals, 135 per cent in private hospitals). There are a number of factors contributing to growth in private hospital activity over this period:

Cost Weights study (www.health.gov.au/casemix/costing/fc_r5.htm) can be used to clarify this issue. These data are derived from a sample of public and private hospitals and present robust estimates of the DRG costs in each sector. These data reveal apparent differences in costs between public and private hospitals when adjustment is made for the mix of cases. For example, in 2000/01 the estimated average cost for AR-DRG O60D Vaginal delivery without complicating diagnoses was A$2491 in public hospitals and almost A$500 more, A$2957, in private hospitals. In contrast, AR-DRG E69C Bronchitis and asthma age <50 without co-morbidity and/or complications is almost A$300 less expensive in private hospitals (public hospital cost A$1441, private hospital cost A$1161).

The average cost per weighted separation in public hospitals in 2000/01 was A$2707, about 22 per cent higher than if the same casemix had been treated using private hospital reported costs (mean cost = A$2214; the actual average weighted cost per separation from private hospitals was A$2030). This would imply that private hospitals are more 'technically efficient' than public hospitals, treating the same casemix.

However, these crude figures need to be adjusted for discrepancies in the way costs of care are met in public and private hospitals, reflecting in turn Commonwealth–state divisions in responsibilities for health expenditures. The most notable differences between the two sectors relate to medical, pharmaceutical, and depreciation expenses. Medical services (including pathology testing and imaging) in private hospitals are not incorporated in hospital expenditure, and bills are met by patients directly and reimbursed through Medicare and health insurance funds. Patients, reimbursed through the Pharmaceutical Benefits Scheme, also meet pharmaceutical costs. This is in contrast to the situation for public patients in public hospitals where all the costs are met by the state government through its funding of public hospitals. For the dwindling number of private patients in public hospitals, medical costs are reimbursed through Medicare, but pharmacy costs are still borne by the hospital. As a result of these differences in funding arrangements and hence cost-recording, the medical, pathology, imaging, and pharmaceutical costs per patient in public hospitals as reported in cost weight studies are substantially higher than those recorded in private hospitals.

The reverse is true for depreciation. Typically, capital costs in public hospitals have been provided separately from operating costs and thus depreciation costs have not been well attributed in the public sector. By contrast, stockholders in private hospitals require a full accounting of capital costs, and recorded depreciation costs are somewhat higher in the private sector relative to public sector.

The net effect of adjusting these elements to a common basis is that their combined contribution to total cost is somewhat higher in public hospitals (accounting for an average of 27 per cent of total costs) than in private hospitals (an average of 18 per cent). Removing the discrepant cost bases narrows the reported cost differential: the average adjusted cost per separation in public hospitals is A$1967 and, for treating the same casemix, is A$1882 in private hospitals (for private hospitals with their own casemix, the average adjusted cost is A$1803). Given the statistical variation around these estimates, it is probably reasonable to conclude that either private hospitals are only marginally more efficient than public hospitals or that there is no difference in efficiency between the two sectors.

Although this analysis is standardised for the casemix in the two sectors, not all differences can be taken into account this way. For example, to the extent that within-DRG variation exists, public hospitals are likely to have the more seriously ill cases because of referral patterns to tertiary teaching hospitals, provision of emergency services, and the like because of the 'safety net' or residual role of public hospitals. This further supports a conclusion of little difference in efficiency between the two sectors.

Hospital care for veterans

Prior to the mid 1990s, hospital care for veterans was centred on hospitals owned and operated by the Commonwealth government through the Repatriation Commission. There were large Repatriation General Hospitals in all states, which had university affiliations as teaching hospitals. Hospital care for veterans, paid for by the Commonwealth, was also available in state public hospitals and, with prior approval, in private hospitals.

A series of reports into the repatriation system in the 1970s and 1980s highlighted the need for change to this system, partly because the repatriation hospitals were often not well located to serve the dispersed veteran population. The reports also drew attention to the impact of the changing demographics of the veteran population: as the veteran cohort from World War II aged, demand for hospital care for veterans would increase but it would then decline precipitately as that cohort died. Demand for hospital care from subsequent veteran cohorts would not be sufficient to justify maintaining a separate repatriation hospital system.

Commencing in the late 1980s, the Department of Veterans' Affairs (DVA) began a process of changing the way it met its responsibility to ensure access to hospital care for veterans (Lyon 2000). First, it divested itself of the repatriation hospitals either to the states (in the case of the repatriation hospitals in Sydney, Melbourne, Adelaide, and Hobart) or to the private sector (Brisbane and Perth). The divestment arrangements ensured that the hospitals would still provide additional services for veterans, recognising the historic links between the veteran community and those hospitals. Second, it changed the nature of its contracts for hospital care. Rather than direct ownership and provision of hospital services, DVA became a purchaser of care. The current purchasing arrangements are of two kinds. DVA negotiates block contracts with states for veterans' use of public hospitals. These contracts provide for a payment covering the full cost of care and are usually structured on a casemix basis so that if demand for public hospital care by veterans declines, so too will DVA payments to the state. The second type of DVA purchasing arrangement covers veterans' access to private hospitals. This is done on a tender basis with tender payments on a full–cost basis. For a small group of private hospitals in each state, with contracts incorporating special provisions for monitoring the quality of care provided and veterans' satisfaction with care, veterans may be admitted to the hospital without prior DVA approval at the contracted tender price for an episode of care. Access to other private hospitals requires prior DVA approval.

The DVA arrangements represent a separate funding stream for both public and private hospitals. As DVA pays for the full cost of care for a significant group of hospital users, it can exercise significant power in the marketplace. Although the initial round of hospital contracts had some flaws (Auditor-General of Victoria 1998), current purchasing contracts are quite comprehensive in terms of quality and satisfaction measures. Further, the tender basis for the private sector contracts has also ensured that DVA is able to achieve very competitive prices for veterans' care.

Access to treatment for rare conditions

Given the relatively small size of Australia's population, situations will arise where there is no treatment available in Australia for a particular condition. The Commonwealth has a special program, the Medical Treatment Overseas Program, to assist patients in these circumstances to receive care in the United Kingdom, USA, or other countries. Treatments eligible for funding under this scheme must meet the following criteria:
• the treatment or effective alternative treatment must not be available in Australia (that is, the capacity, knowledge, skills, or facilities are not available)
• the treatment must be of a life-saving nature
• there must be a real prospect of success
• the treatment must be beyond the experimental stage and accepted as a standard form of treatment by the medical profession.

In addition to medical and hospital costs, the program provides return economy airfares for the patient (and, if necessary, an attendant or if the patient is under 18 years old, a parent). In 2002/03, three patients were approved for assistance from the program at a total cost of A$360,000.

Ambulance services

Ambulance services are managed independently of hospitals and area health services but are obviously an important part of the acute health infrastructure. In a number of states, ambulance services are not administered through the health portfolio but are administratively part of the emergency services portfolio (see table 6.5).

There are three major types of organisational arrangements for ambulance services in Australia: statutory authorities (New South Wales, Victoria); organisations incorporated within either the Department of Health or the Department of Emergency Services; and not-for-profit organisations, mainly linked to the St John Ambulance network. There are about 9000 paid

Table 6.5   Australia: Relationship of ambulance management agencies to government by state or territory

State or Territory	Name of service	Relationship to government
NSW	Ambulance Service of NSW	Statutory authority reporting to the Minister for Health
Vic	Metropolitan Ambulance Service Rural Ambulance Victoria Alexandra and District Ambulance Service	Separate statutory bodies reporting to the Minister for Health
Qld	Queensland Ambulance Service	A division of the Department of Emergency Services, reporting via the Director-General to the Minister for Emergency Services
WA	St John Ambulance	An incorporated not-for-profit organisation under contract to the WA Government
SA	SA Ambulance Service	An incorporated joint venture between the State Minister for Health and St John Priory Australia
Tas	Tasmanian Ambulance Service	A statutory service of the Hospital and Ambulance Division of the Department of Health and Human Services
ACT	ACT Ambulance Service	An agency of the ACT Emergency Services Bureau, reports to the ACT Minister for Police, Emergency Services and Corrections
NT	St John Ambulance	An incorporated not-for-profit organisation under contract to the NT government

Source: Steering Committee for the Review of Commonwealth/State Service Provision 2003

ambulance employees throughout Australia with these services supplemented by almost 6000 volunteers (Standing Committee on State Services Provision 2003). Almost half (48.1 per cent) of ambulance callouts require an emergency response with a further one-sixth being for an urgent response. About one-third of all ambulance service responses are nonemergency responses. Across Australia, 50 per cent of emergency responses occur with seven to eight minutes, with 90 per cent of responses within 15 minutes, although there are significantly longer response times in remote areas.

Unlike other areas of acute health where the Commonwealth government has a significant involvement, there is essentially no Commonwealth funding of ambulance services. Across Australia, about 60 per cent of total ambulance revenue comes from state governments (see figure 6.12).

There is a significant difference across Australia in the balance of revenue sources for ambulance services. The three main sources for ambulance services are state and territory governments, ambulance subscription schemes (on average 10 per cent across Australia), and transportation fees (on average 25 per cent across Australia). Ambulance subscription schemes do not exist in New South Wales and Tasmania and account for trivial proportions of revenue in Western Australia, the Australian Capital Territory, and the Northern Territory. Ambulance funding in Western Australia is principally sourced from transportation fees (61.3 per cent of revenue) with direct government assistance being around one-fifth of all revenue (21.7 per cent). In most states however, the fee revenue is around one-fifth of all revenue.

Figure 6.12 Australia: Sources of ambulance service revenue, 2001/02, by state or territory

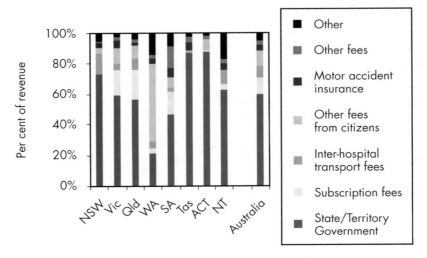

Source: Steering Committee for the Review of Commonwealth/State Service Provision 2003

Australia-wide, ambulance expenditure per head is around A$50, with significantly higher expenditure in Queensland (A$66.5) and significantly lower expenditure in Western Australia (A$31.2). These differences cannot be explained by demographic considerations and the low expenditure in Western Australia probably reflects the different funding arrangements in that state.

Blood and organ donation

An important part of acute health services is the availability of blood as part of treatment, and organs for transplantation. The basis for Australia's blood service is voluntary donation: about 3.5 per cent of Australians donate blood in any year. Blood services are supervised by the National Blood Authority, a Commonwealth statutory authority established under the National Blood Authority Act 2003. National blood services are also regulated by the National Blood Agreement between the Commonwealth and the states and supervised by a Ministerial Council. The National Blood Authority is responsible for managing a contract with the Australian Red Cross Blood Service, the division of the Australian Red Cross that is responsible for managing the voluntary donation of blood, and a contract with an independent company, CSL Ltd, for blood fractionation.

The National Blood Agreement provides that 63 per cent of the cost of blood services throughout Australia will be met by the Commonwealth with the remainder met by states and territories. For service operating costs and the costs of high cost patients, the state and territory share is determined on a per capita basis. For routine blood use, a state's share is determined on the basis of its use of blood services as measured by a National Blood Products Price List.

The Health Insurance Commission operates the Australian Organ Donor register that is available on a 24 hours per day, seven days per week basis to provide a national approach to distribution of organs. Donors can register with the donor register and, in the event of the death of a donor; the information can be supplied to hospitals and families to enable decisions about organ donation.

Quality of care

At the most basic level, the quality of hospital care is underpinned by state and territory regulations to ensure appropriate design, cleanliness, staffing, and so on. Inspectorial visits, however, only occur irregularly, generally following complaints. The standards themselves may also be inappropriate as inadequate staffing has been identified as a factor in the incidence of adverse events and of poorer quality care in Australia (Beckmann et al. 1998; Morrison et al. 2001) and in the USA (Aiken et al. 2002; Needleman et al. 2002; Hickham et al. 2003).

Regulation of minimum standards is supplemented by a number of mechanisms to encourage hospitals to attempt to improve their quality of care on a continuous basis. Although there have been many attempts to raise the profile of quality management in Australian hospitals, there is still a high prevalence of adverse events reported. Wilson et al. (1995), in the major Australian purposive survey, concluded that more than one in every six hospital admissions was associated with an 'adverse event': an unintended injury or complication or a prolongation of hospital stay where the injury or complication arose from health care management (rather than from the under-lying condition). About half of those adverse events were judged to be potentially preventable. According to Wilson et al. about six in every 1000 admissions to hospital end in a preventable death associated with an adverse event. The costs of adverse events were estimated, using the Wilson et al. data, at A$483 million per annum (Rigby et al. 1999). A subsequent reanalysis of the Wilson et al. data (Runciman et al. 2000; Thomas et al. 2000), using a tighter definition of preventability, found that the prevalence of adverse events was around 10 per cent, the now generally cited rate. Similar levels of adverse events have also been found in community surveys (Clark 2001).

A number of other approaches to measuring quality of care have also been adopted, including measures based on readmission rates, case fatality rates, continuity of care, and patient satisfaction (Boyce et al. 1997; MacIn-tyre et al. 1997; O'Hara and Carson 1997; Ansari et al. 1999; Bellomo et al. 2002). Detailed analysis of care following trauma suggests that a significant proportion of trauma deaths are also preventable or potentially preventable (McDermott et al. 1996).

Hospital accreditation

A key mechanism for improving quality has been the process of 'hospital accreditation'. Although other forms of accreditation now exist (for example, under the auspices of the International Standards Organisation in the form of the ISO 9000 series of standards), the principal hospital accreditation agency in Australia is the Australian Council on Healthcare Standards (ACHS). The ACHS has a two-tier governance structure consisting of an 11-member board elected from a larger council. The ACHS is composed of representatives of the two founding organisations, the Australian Hospital Association and the Australian Medical Association; and of the various Royal Clinical Colleges; the Australian Nursing Federation; the Royal Australian College of Medical Administrators; the Australian College of Health Services Executives; the Australian Council of Allied Health

Professionals; the Australian Private Hospitals' Association; and the Commonwealth and state Departments of Health. The underlying principles of the ACHS are continuous improvement, self-assessment, and peer evaluation.

Only in Victoria are public hospitals required by state authorities to be accredited. Elsewhere, it is a voluntary decision taken by hospitals wishing to indicate their compliance with a certain standard of hospital care. In 2001/02, 73 per cent of all hospitals in Australia were accredited, covering 93 per cent of all beds. Non-accredited hospitals are small with a mean size of 17 beds.

The ACHS accreditation process is cyclical, involving self-assessment and external peer review. The typical ACHS cycle is four years, involving two rounds of external reviews. Central to the ACHS process is a hospital-wide survey (between one and five days long, depending on the size of the organisation). The process involves between two and nine surveyors (again, depending on the size of the organisation). The core survey team normally consists of an administrator, a medical practitioner, and a nurse. The second hospital-wide survey in a cycle is called a 'periodic review' and is undertaken by the original survey team but the visit, except in large organisations, is only one day.

The survey team assesses the hospital (or group of hospitals) against 14 standards clustered into six organisational functions: continuum of care (four standards), leadership and management (four standards), human resources management (one standard), information management (three standards), safe practice and environment (one standard), and improving performance (one standard). Assessment of performance against the standards is made by reference to 43 separate criteria. Satisfactory performance on 19 specified criteria, including the nine criteria associated with the safe practice and environment standard, is essential for award of 'accreditation'. The survey leads to a 'survey report' that summarises the survey team's findings about each function, including recommendations and suggestions for performance improvement (Australian Council on Healthcare Standards 2002b). The second output of the survey is a quality action plan that is developed by the hospital to respond to the key issues raised in the survey report and includes strategies for addressing those issues. The quality action plan is the subject of follow-up from the ACHS, especially at the periodic review. The result of the organisation-wide survey could be four-year accreditation, two-year accreditation with the requirement to address specific recommendations, or no accreditation.

The self-assessment and continuous improvement components of accreditation are premised on organisations identifying and collecting relevant indicators against which they can track their own performance and compare it with other organisations. The ACHS stimulated the development of a range of specific clinical indicator sets through its Care Evaluation

Program (Collopy et al. 1995; Collopy 1996; Booth and Collopy 1997). This program was a cooperative development with a range of clinical colleges to identify and define clinical indicators covering most specialty areas such as internal medicine, surgery, obstetrics and gynaecology, anaesthetics, and emergency medicine. This work provided the basis for the contemporary ACHS Performance and Outcomes Service that produces indicators in most specialty areas. Indicators cover all aspects of quality, particularly focusing on safety, effectiveness, appropriateness, and timeliness. As well as providing feedback to hospitals on their relative performance, this service publishes aggregate national data for each of its almost 200 performance indicators (Australian Council on Healthcare Standards 2002a). The focus of the publication is on the potential to improve performance in Australian hospitals and ACHS has identified a number of indicators where improvement is clearly possible, because a number of hospitals report good results, but where average performance is poor (see table 6.6).

The ACHS indicators have been designed to assist hospitals to identify (and correct) quality management problems across most areas of clinical management. Examples of reported 2001 indicators include:

- 19 per cent of patients with acute myocardial infarction do not receive thrombolytic therapy within one hour of presentation at the hospital (an improvement on the 1998 result of 28.5 per cent)
- 0.29 per cent of patients acquired bacteraemia within hospital
- 35.1 per cent of non-procedural, non-urgent inpatient plain radiography reports were not available within 24 hours
- 69.5 per cent of primiparous women who delivered vaginally required surgical repair of the lower genital tract, with significant variation between states (South Australia 56 per cent compared to New South

Table 6.6   Key areas for potential quality improvement in Australian hospitals as identified by ACHS, 2002

Area	Comment
Delays in emergency department	Over 1 million patients not seen by a clinician within recommended time
Waiting time for radiotherapy treatment	Patients waiting more than 21 days increased over the period 1999/2001
Turnaround time for serum/plasma potassium reports	Turnaround within 45 minutes improving (58 per cent in 1998 to 61 per cent in 2001). Victoria (40 per cent in 2001) performing worse than other states.
Delays in the availability in non-procedural non-urgent radiographs	Proportion of x-rays not available within 24 hours is increasing
Documented immunisation status for infants	Documentation of status declining (to 80 per cent in 2001)

Wales, 75.4 per cent) and between public (66.4 per cent) and private hospitals (79.6 per cent).

Quality management processes are necessarily multifaceted, partly because of the many ways in which good quality can be defined. Measurement of quality of care should incorporate at least two distinct elements: technical quality ('cure quality') and satisfaction ('care quality'). Very often a discussion of quality focuses on one of these indicators to the exclusion of the other, implying, for instance, that either technical quality is the only relevant quality measure or consumer satisfaction should be the principal way of measuring care in health service organisations.

In terms of technical or cure quality, appropriate performance indicators include condition-specific measures, such as the case fatality rate, but indicators involving morbidity should also be used (for example, an indicator of the success of cataract operations could be the extent of handicap in vision-related activity after an operation). Although early work on quality measurement eschewed use of large-scale administrative databases in favour of specially collected clinically relevant data, more recent work has shown that administrative data can be used to standardise for casemix and hence measures of quality of care (especially quality of surgical care) can be constructed using routinely available data sets (Hannan 1998). A key measure of quality is whether the service provided was necessary at all ('doing the right thing' versus 'doing the thing right'). This aspect of quality, sometimes called 'appropriateness', can be measured using scales such as the Appropriateness Evaluation Protocol (Restuccia et al. 1987).

Technical quality is often tracked for individual cases as part of the treating clinician's ordinary processes for assessing outcomes of operations and treatment. Increasingly, however, systematic patterns of outcomes in terms of cure quality are being measured statistically, so that the average performance of an institution, a specific clinician, or the outcomes for particular subgroups in the population can be examined.

'Care quality' is appropriately measured by the experience or satisfaction of consumers. The two different measures relate in part to the phrasing of the questionnaires: patient satisfaction is usually measured on a Likert scale, in contrast to patient experience questionnaires which are based on asking patients about their experience with the institution, for example whether they were told when they could resume normal activities after discharge (Draper and Hill 1996). Patient experience can also be monitored through incidence of patient complaints.

Improving the quality of care is a cyclical process involving collection of data, analysis, action to improve performance, and evaluation (Wan and Connell 2003). Information technology is increasingly used as part of quality management processes to identify adverse events (Bates and Gawande 2003; Bates et al. 2003) and as an important facilitator of a safe environment for care delivery through use of electronic health records and computerised ordering of tests and pharmaceuticals (Committee on Data Standards for Patient Safety 2003). Ferlie and Shortell (2001) have suggested that quality improvement strategies can (and should) take place at four levels: individual (for example, feedback on performance); group/team (for example, clinical audit); organisation (for example, emphasis on a learning culture); and at the system environmental level (for example, legal system, payment system design). In many cases adverse events in hospital are not attributable to in-dividual failures, but rather are the result of failures of communication within the system (for example, failures to ensure availability of test results). Accountability for quality of care should be both institutional and individual and quality management processes should therefore be able to address these system level problems rather than solely focus on individual clinicians (Wilson et al. 1995).

In order to be accredited, hospitals must have systematic quality manage-ment processes, including processes to analyse adverse events using techniques such as Root Cause Analysis. Such techniques facilitate consider-ation of all the factors that might have contributed to an adverse event: materials (such as equipment unavailability or failure); human factors (fatigue, skills, number of staff); methods and processes (systems to identify patients, collect specimens, provide results), and environmental factors (nature of patient population, for example language).

The support hospital management gives to quality management processes is obviously important. The management culture of the hospital is critical to the operation of quality management systems and the processes for individual and group accountability.

Accountability pressures on hospitals are increasing through the public-ation of comparative performance measures, such as comparative case fatality rates; governments and the courts are also specifying the obligations of treat-ing practitioners to their patients/consumers.

The Australian Council on Safety and Quality in Health Care

The Wilson et al. (1995) study of adverse events described earlier led to the establishment of a national taskforce to develop recommendations on ways of dealing with the high rates of adverse events. The initial Task Force Report (Commonwealth Department of Health and Family Services 1996) was followed by the establishment of a National Expert Advisory Group whose report (1999) led to the establishment of the Australian Council on Safety and Quality in Health Care in 2000. The council is intended to:
• provide national leadership in system-wide approaches to quality improvement in health care

- develop an overall coherent plan for improving the quality of health care services
- facilitate action by appropriate organisations and agencies in priority areas.

The Council has established five main action areas: supporting health care professionals to deliver safer patient care; improving data and information; involving consumers; redesigning systems of health care to facilitate a culture of safety; and building awareness and understanding of health care safety. In its first years of existence, the council has placed a significant emphasis on medication safety, which is seen as one of the major causes of adverse events. It is also developing a medical device tracking system to facilitate notification and recall where devices may be suspected of leading to adverse events; and investigating the use of coronial data and hospital management data to identify adverse events.

The council has also promulgated a national set of sentinel events that should be used by states and health authorities for reporting. The sentinel events identified include procedures involving the wrong patient or body part, maternal death or serious disability associated with labour or delivery, and medication error that has led to the death of a patient. It is also developing national standards for credentialing and clinical privileges, and communication with patients about adverse events.

Governance and operation of hospitals

The governance structures of hospitals vary in part by type of ownership but also by the size and role of the hospital. Public hospitals typically are governed by boards of directors appointed by the state or territory minister for health, with most public hospitals being governed by boards of directors with responsibility for more than one hospital. In some states, these multi-hospital systems take responsibility for all publicly provided health services and substitute for regional offices of the health authority (for example, Area Health Authorities in urban New South Wales). In other states, for example, Victoria, boards in Melbourne are accountable only for a group of hospitals, with health department oversight of both hospital and community health services.

Although the formal roles and responsibilities of the governing authority of hospitals (be they health authorities or hospital boards) are similar, their *modus operandi* is often quite different. Boards with responsibilities for larger conglomerations of services, or hospitals with larger budgets, typically function in a corporatised manner similar to boards of private sector businesses, leaving day-to-day responsibility for management of the organisation to the chief executive officer and management staff. The corporatised governing authorities also use more business-oriented approaches to determining the services to be provided by institutions within their control and for decision making generally. In contrast, governing bodies with responsibility for smaller budgets typically become involved in a broader range of decisions including those at the operational level.

Religious hospitals (whether they are public or private) have developed quite complex management arrangements (see Gleeson 1989). Originally, religious hospitals were run directly by the religious organisation; in the case of Catholic hospitals, generally an order of nuns. With the decline in the number of sisters, religious hospitals are now managed by boards of directors appointed by the order. The board usually includes representatives from the order, and sisters may still hold key roles in the organisation. A number of orders have organised their hospitals into national chains governed by a single national board of management responsible for overall strategic directions for all of the order's hospitals.

Private hospitals also have mixed governance arrangements. As indicated earlier in this chapter, many private hospitals are owned by corporate hospital chains that generally have boards of directors, which function in the same way as boards of other major corporations. In some cases, the board of the hospital chain is a subsidiary of the board of the overall major holding company. As with larger public hospitals, such boards clearly function on a commercial basis in terms of style and scope of decision making.

There are many private hospitals that are still owned by individual investors or small groups of investors that own one or two smaller hospitals. The governance arrangements for these organisations vary in terms of their formality, and the nature of the decision-making process. Hospitals may also be run by partnerships including partnerships of doctors, or doctors and other investors. In general, the smaller organisations have less formalisation of decision-making processes compared with the larger corporatised boards. In smaller private hospitals the individual investor may also function as the chief executive, managing the hospital on a day-to-day basis.

Internal management of the hospital also varies according to its size and role. In larger hospitals, management involves general, nursing, and medical administrators. Increasingly, the roles of chief executive and director of nursing are combined in smaller hospitals, both public and private.

The relationship of the medical staff to the management and governance structures of the hospital is often complex. In the private sector the medical staff may be perceived as key clients of the organisation and the hospital's viability depends on attracting and maintaining high quality medical staff who admit patients to the hospital. Good consultative arrangements need to develop between the private hospital management and the medical staff. This will ensure that the hospital is meeting the expectations of the medical staff in terms of admission processes, scheduling, and equipment, and will also ensure appropriate structures for quality management and assessment of new medical staff.

The relationship between medical staff and managers of public hospitals is even more complex, involving salaried medical staff (both specialists and medical staff in training) and visiting medical staff who provide services to both public and private patients.

Unlike the procedure in private hospitals, where the medical staff are generally not paid directly by the private hospital (but rather bill patients directly or via the patient's insurer and Medicare), payments to medical staff make up a significant proportion of a public hospital's expenditure (see figure 6.10). Medical staff are paid by the public hospital for treating public patients but directly by private patients for their treatment. The public hospital thus has an employer/employee relationship with medical staff. However, because of their status and mobility, medical staff are often in a strong employment bargaining position and hence there are some similarities between the relationship of medical staff in public hospitals and those in private hospitals.

Internal structures for governance of medical staff in larger hospitals involve formalised groupings of medical staff by specialty (for example, medicine, surgery, obstetrics), or across specialties, grouping specialists treating patients with diagnoses in the same body system such as cardiovascular services or cancer services (see Duckett et al. 1981). These 'divisions' are headed by a director drawn from a relevant medical specialty.

The development of casemix funding arrangements together with the increased financial pressure on hospitals through budget reductions in the early to mid 1990s placed stresses on the traditional organisational structures of public hospitals. Traditional hospital management, which had often focused on managing the inputs into care (cleaning staff, cost per pathology test, and so on), needed to be supplemented by structures that could legitimately address processes of care and final rather than intermediate outputs (Fetter 1991; Duckett 1994a). The informal structures for involvement of medical staff in decision making in the hospitals gave way to more formalised arrangements such as 'divisional' structures (Duckett et al. 1981; Alexander 2000). Moreover, these divisional structures extended their roles from those that focused on professional management (for example, organising deployment of medical staff and 'peer review' activities) to those that assumed responsibility for budgets and other management priorities, such as waiting lists. Although these broader responsibilities did not necessarily require a change in structure, they certainly required a change in culture; a change that was not necessarily always welcomed or understood by medical staff (Degeling 1994; Parker and Dent 1996). The budgetary responsibilities were often accompanied by additional management staff support and a number of hospitals created middle management positions servicing the medical leadership of the divisions. These more elaborated divisions, with their clear budget responsibilities, began to take more definitive action to ensure achievement of negotiated hospital targets in areas such as inpatient activity, waiting lists, and emergency admissions.

In a number of hospitals, nursing structures were also revised and the centralised, hierarchical nursing organisations were replaced with 'nursing divisions' that paralleled the medical divisions. In a number of hospitals, divisional activities were managed with devolved budgets by a duumvirate of medical and nursing divisional directors (see Hickie 1994; McCaughan and Piccone 1994). The new divisional structures also led to a new generation of 'clinician managers', where the divisional directors continued with a major clinical role, thus maintaining legitimacy with their clinical colleagues. This was in contrast to the tradition of previous medical administrators who had pursued full-time training and development in medical administration from early in their career, and had not developed or maintained clinical qualifications or skills. In many cases, divisional directors were drawn from the ranks of the university professoriate (as this group was often the main group of full-time staff within a hospital).

A major distinction between the management of public and private hospitals relates to the nature of accountability for management processes in the organisation. Unlike private hospitals, public hospitals are generally covered by state or Commonwealth Freedom of Information legislation that provides for access to the records of hospitals by patients and other interested parties, including medical records under certain circumstances. In addition, public hospitals are generally covered by the judicial or administrative review processes established by the state and often by legislated requirements for more systematic and formalised complaints procedures.

The services of public hospitals are also subject to the normal accountability processes of the Westminster system of government, as the state or territory minister for health is accountable to parliament for the activities of those hospitals. As with all other aspects of parliamentary accountability, these processes are variable in their application and Ministers may seek to avoid parliamentary accountability by arguing that the activities or decisions under review are those of 'autonomous' areas or hospital boards of directors.

Evaluation of hospital services

An evaluation of Australian hospital services in terms of the four criteria identified earlier in this book (equity, efficiency, quality, acceptability) reveals mixed results. In terms of equity, financial barriers to access in Australia are addressed through the Medicare arrangements. In contrast to the USA, where a significant proportion of the population is not covered by insurance, all Australians are covered for the financial costs of hospital care in a public hospital. However, this coverage does not ensure equitable access. Those with health insurance are not subject to long waiting times for elective care compared to those who rely on the public hospital system. It is also the case that people with health insurance tend to have greater access to interventional technologies relative to those without insurance (Robertson and Richardson 2000), although it is unclear whether this increased intervention leads to improved outcomes.

In terms of efficiency, there is little persuasive evidence. The Australian hospital system is cheaper than that in the USA, but so too is every other hospital system in the world. The introduction of casemix payment arrangements focused attention on technical efficiency in the public sector in those states and so the design of funding arrangements gives some comfort about this aspect of efficiency. There has been no systematic work on evaluation of overall allocative efficiency in the hospital sector.

In terms of quality, the Australian public hospital system is often said to provide high quality care of a standard approaching the best in the world. However, about one in 10 hospital separations are associated with an adverse event. The risk level of complications of care cannot lead to complacency about the hospital system's success in ensuring the safety of its patients.

Finally, in terms of acceptability, patient surveys regularly report high levels of satisfaction with hospital care in Australia, and so this criterion may provide the most positive assessment of the overall performance of the system.

Hospital system issues

Hospitals in Australia have changed dramatically over the last two decades, in part as a result of changes in the proportion of same-day cases (as shown earlier in this chapter) and technology (Braithwaite et al. 1994, 1995; Braithwaite 1997). In more recent times, hospitals have also changed as a response to the move from historical to casemix funding in most Australian states.

The past decade has seen increasing use and specificity of payment incentives in hospital policy, in terms of both the relationship between Commonwealth and state governments and between states and hospitals, as evidenced by the introduction of casemix funding. This transformation has been made possible in large part by developments in the technology of measurement of hospital activity (especially casemix standardised measurement of inpatient activity using DRGs), and by the development of the necessary infrastructure for performance measurement. The next decade is likely to see a sharpening of the incentives on states and hospitals as part of a drive for improvements in the efficiency and effectiveness of the hospital system.

A much higher proportion of activity in hospitals of the future will be performed on an ambulatory basis. Further, a decreasing proportion of hospital activity will require immediate access to the expensive infrastructure associated with hospitals of today. More procedures will be able to be undertaken on a day-stay basis and ambulatory care centres will become increasingly important components of acute health care. Hospitals will need to develop close organisational arrangements with such facilities (Robinson 1994), either through organisational integration or tight contractual arrangements. Hospital planning should take account of this new environment (Edwards and Harrison 1999; Edwards 2002; Zajac 2003) and affected communities must be involved in the process as community perception of the role of and need for hospitals may be quite different from the perceptions of the planners (Haycock et al. 1999).

Economic pressures will not be relaxed. An increased reliance on economic incentives to drive efficiency improvements can only be achieved if the tools for measurement are developed at the same pace as organisational practice changes. Casemix measures, such as DRGs, were developed in the context of a particular structuring of health services and patterns of care. A critical factor that needs to be closely monitored is whether the very definition of the product of health care is changing; for example, whether hospitals achieve 'efficiencies' by changing the definition of when their portion of 'patient care' is completed, resulting in more recovery taking place post-discharge rather than in hospital prior to discharge. Operationally, it could mean transferring the costs of hospital care to community or rehabilitation providers or to the family. To the extent that these transfers of costs have occurred, the significant recorded improvements in efficiency associated with the introduction of casemix funding may, in part, record changes in who pays rather than true improvements in efficiency. It is therefore essential that measurement of hospital activity take into account these changing product definitions.

Improvements in measurement will also be necessary to respond to the ideologically inspired wave of privatisation of hospital care. The *sine qua non* of any contract is specification of what is being bought and sold. Hospital privatisation contracts must therefore specify in sufficient detail the services to be provided by the privatised organisation. Subject to the constraints outlined above, inpatient services can be well specified. This is not the case in many other aspects of hospital care such as ambulatory services, or the teaching and research activities of hospitals. To the extent that the services are not specified, these important aspects of the health care system may suffer through privatisation initiatives (Ashton 1997).

The changes in technology that underlie many issues of change in hospital practice will drive many aspects of hospital reform. State governments (the principal providers of public hospital capital) are now ideologically less disposed to using state capital funds for hospital refurbishment and upgrading and are increasingly turning to the private sector to capitalise public hospitals. The benefits of privatisation are often presented in terms of both capital (less money to be borrowed) and improvement in recurrent cost, as it is argued that private providers are able to operate more efficiently than public providers. The research evidence for these claims is in part based on artefacts of cost measurement, and privatisation initiatives can thus be regarded as high-risk deliberate experiments.

The focus of most hospital reform programs in Australia has been on improving hospital efficiency. Addressing this issue means that attention can be paid to addressing other critical issues of hospital performance such as measurement of quality of care. Quality measurement of hospital care is complex, and just as there have been improvements in measuring hospital product and efficiency over recent decades, so too has there been improvement in the ability to compare the quality of hospital care. This is an important issue in Australia, as Wilson et al. (1995) revealed substantial levels of iatrogenesis associated with health care treatment. A related issue will be the one of ensuring not only that what is performed in hospitals is of high quality, but that it is appropriate. This separate question of whether the admission or operation was necessary arises because of the high levels of unexplained variation in utilisation rates for a number of medical and surgical conditions (Andersen and Mooney 1990). Strategies for addressing this issue are extremely complex (Evans 1990a), but will need to be the focus of policy attention and of internal hospital management practices (Hensher and Edwards 2002).

7

Public Health

Public health is 'the organised response by society to protect and promote health and prevent illness, injury and disability'. This definition is taken from the Memorandum of Understanding for the National Public Health Partnership (1997), and highlights a number of important characteristics. Public health is an organised response, meaning directed and focused. The response is a societal one rather than fragmented activities of individuals. The focus of public health is on protection, promotion, and prevention.

The 'public' in public health blends three distinct meanings. First, it connotes programs that are 'for the public' in the sense that the objectives of the programs have a social or community-wide focus rather than a narrow focus on individual ('private') gain or benefit. Many (but not all) public health activities entail universal access or provision. Second, public health activities are principally developed in response to the 'public interest'. Although this meaning has some overlap with the preceding one, the public interest may be best served by limiting some public health activities to a specific subsection of the population on cost-effectiveness grounds (for example, only high risk babies might receive some forms of immunisation). Public health activities developed in the 'public interest' may also lead to infringement of private interest by prohibiting some activities by companies or individuals or by restricting personal freedom (for example, restricting movement because of quarantine concerns). Third, the definition of public health implies that it is 'publicly organised', planned, funded, and generally delivered by public institutions, particularly governments.

The National Public Health Partnership has endorsed the 'core functions' of public health as being to:
- assess, analyse, and communicate population health needs and community expectations
- prevent and control communicable and noncommunicable diseases and injuries through risk factor reduction, education, screening, immunisation, and other interventions

- promote and support healthy lifestyles and behaviours through action with individuals, families, communities, and wider society
- plan, fund, manage, and evaluate health gain and capacity building programs designed to achieve measurable improvements in health status, and to strengthen skills, competencies, systems, and infrastructure
- strengthen communities and build social capital through consultation, participation, and empowerment
- promote, develop, support, and initiate actions that ensure safe and healthy environments
- promote, develop, and support healthy growth and development throughout all life stages
- promote, develop, and support actions to improve the health status of Aboriginal and Torres Strait Islander people and other vulnerable groups.

Public health is distinguished from acute and chronic care in two key ways. First, the outcomes of many public health interventions can only be assessed over a long time frame. Although some public health activities have immediate benefits, many are aimed at increasing the likelihood of good health or reducing the risk of poor health in the future. Second, contemporary public health best practice emphasises interventions focused at a variety of levels ranging from identified individuals to asymptomatic

Table 7.1   A continuum of possible policy responses to premature death from heart disease

Points on intervention continuum	Population group
Rescue	
e.g. Coronary artery bypass surgery or thrombolysis	Sick individuals
Routine medical care	
e.g. hypertension control	Positively screened individuals
Access to health care	
e.g. 'free' care, increase supply of care	Potentially sick individuals
Traditional public health	
e.g. immunisation, lifestyle modification programs	Worried individuals
Family and support services	
e.g. child welfare, home visitors, social support	Needy individuals and families
Social cohesion	
e.g. subsidised clubs, reduced income inequality	Community structure

populations. Lomas (1998) has outlined a continuum of possible policy responses to premature death covering the acute care–public health spectrum. His continuum uses examples of premature death from heart disease, although any other condition could be used as the focus (see table 7.1).

The focus of the interventions on the Lomas continuum involves continually expanding populations from sick individuals in need of acute care through to those who have been positively screened for heart disease and people who are at risk of heart disease (called 'worried individuals' by Lomas). Importantly, Lomas moves beyond a traditional health system focus and identifies that wider elements of the social structure can have an impact on health status, and thus intervening at a broader community level can reduce premature deaths from heart disease. Indeed, he argues that interventions at the social cohesion level 'are at least as worthy of exploration as improved access or routine medical care'. In contrast to the individual focus of acute care, public health interventions can involve any of the (sub) populations identified by Lomas.

Public health incorporates five broad strategies: creating a safer environment; creating a healthier environment; reducing risks of transmission; encouraging healthier behaviour; and enabling functions (see table 7.2)

Table 7.2   Examples of public health strategies

Strategy	Examples
Creating a safer environment	Primarily regulatory: air and water quality; occupational health and safety; food handling/manufacture Road design Insect (vector) eradication
Creating a healthier environment	Community development Social support initiatives Developing social capital
Reducing risks of transmission	Immunisation (supported by compulsion, e.g. school entry certificates or reminder systems) Quarantine, school exclusion Contact tracing Reducing risky behaviours Outbreak investigations
Encouraging healthy behaviour	Advertising regulation/prohibition Price/tax strategies Campaigns with or without support groups (smoking, alcohol, exercise) Food manufacturing (sugar content)
Enabling functions	Information/data development and dissemination Workforce development Research

Most public health strategies are not directed at changing individual behaviour (the exception is the fourth function, encouraging healthier behaviour) but rather are targeted at changes in the wider environment. Encouraging healthier behaviour is often focused on individual behaviour but public health interventions can also be directed at the broader environment (for example, changing advertising regulations or price of products). Individually focused messages need to be carefully designed to ensure consistency of messages across programs, and have a number of weaknesses, for example a message that suggests illicit drugs constitute a principal health problem versus tobacco may be seen as hypocritical, as would the conflict between food manufacturers promoting unhealthy food versus health promotion campaigns to reduce food intake, etc. It is also important that the messages do not reduce self-esteem in recipients. Further, as was argued in chapter 2, individuals are not entirely free to make their own choices because of the pervasive effects of the family and social environment, etc.

Public health interventions can be grouped into five broad categories:
- regulation (of businesses or individuals through quarantine and immunisation)
- economic incentives (fines, taxes, prices)
- screening and early detection
- education and behaviour change
- social capital creation.

These interventions can be appropriately directed to any of the underlying causative factors affecting ill health. Interventions can be directed at changing institutions (social and cultural) as well as being more specifically targeted at settings such as workplaces, schools, and so on. Public health activities designed to influence social institutions are characterised by political action and advocacy, often organised as movements or campaigns that may proceed over long periods of time.

Public health action usually requires collaboration across economic sectors (health, transport) as well as across state (or even national) boundaries. It requires global scanning, because of the speed of international travel and the potential impact of global environmental changes on public health (McMichael 1993). Broad global environmental changes might have direct effects on health in the short term. Ozone depletion, for example, will increase the likelihood of sunburn and, over the longer term, will have an impact of increased incidence of skin cancer. These interactions between global and environmental effects highlight the importance of multisectoral action in public health and environmental issues.

Public health interventions have an impact on many areas of society and it is consequently difficult to place clear boundaries around 'public health' and its constituent parts. Public health also suffers from definitional disputes, with particular terms and definitions waxing and waning in popularity.

Figure 7.1 Key elements of public health activity

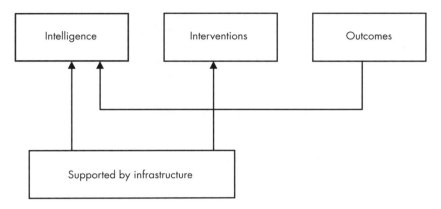

Many public health terms can be phrased negatively or positively with the same public health strategies being described as aimed at 'preventing disease' or 'promoting health'. The more detailed discussion of public health interventions later in this chapter uses the three broad (positively phrased) categories above: health protection; early detection; and health promotion. Disease prevention activities can be classed with either health protection or health promotion.

Public health involves more than interventions, including support through 'intelligence' and 'infrastructure' (see figure 7.1).

A fundamental element of the public health approach is an 'intelligence' function: the use of data to inform and monitor progress on addressing public health issues. Public health intelligence involves analysis of local, regional, and national data in order to identify events and trends that need to be addressed.

Public health interventions lead to outcomes. There is also a feedback loop from the outcomes to the intelligence function. Importantly, both public health intelligence and public health interventions need to be supported by an appropriate infrastructure, including an appropriately trained public health workforce (Beaglehole and Dal Poz 2003), a policy development capacity, information collection and analysis, and so on.

Infrastructure

Public health issues often evolved from local concerns (such as waste, soil contamination, and nuisance). Public health infrastructure grew from this local base and, given the constitutional framework of Australia, legislation was state-based and the delivery infrastructure was defined at the state level.

States often jealously guarded this autonomy to the detriment of national systems or coordination. As with railway gauges, a highly diverse delivery infrastructure developed across Australia, creating difficulties in harmonisation. Even in the 1980s, different states developed very different approaches to organising public health. New South Wales, for example, incorporated public health into its area-based structures for health services (see chapter 5) with the creation of area public health units. Victoria, on the other hand, followed a more centralised approach, albeit with a more active role for local government, reflecting the stronger tradition of local government involvement in public health in that state.

The importance of developing an appropriate public health infrastructure has been especially recognised in the mid to late 1990s. Provision of acute health services is based on a system of hospitals with recognised roles, including roles in research, and in training the next generation of the workforce. The public health infrastructure does not have such a widely disseminated and systematic system of support. The state-based nature of public health has also contributed to lack of leadership in public health as leadership has principally been concentrated in state bureaucracies and suffered under bureaucratic restructuring in the 1980s and downsizing in the 1990s.

A key strategy to develop public health infrastructure has been the Public Health Education and Research Program (PHERP) which, since 1994, has funded expansion of public health training (principally through Masters degrees in public health) in most Australian states. In the 1990s, the NH&MRC has also recommended strategies to build public health infrastructure (NH&MRC 1995, 1996), and promoted public health research infrastructure through its Public Health Research and Development Committee, but the main vehicle for improving infrastructure is the National Public Health Partnership, discussed later in this chapter.

Phases in conception of 'public health'

'Public health' is a broad term that has had different meanings in different societies over time (see Tesh 1988 for a review of some of the different meanings of the term). In ancient Greek mythology the god of healing, Asclepius, had two daughters, Hygiea (from whom we have the word 'hygiene') and Panacea: distinguishing a 'health' focus from a curative one. Hippocrates' writings also highlighted the importance of healthy environments and influenced 'public health' practice for two millennia. In practical terms, the ancient Romans built extensive infrastructure to protect public health by ensuring clean water (some of their aqueducts still stand) and through the construction of sewers. In Anglo-Celtic societies, the foundation of modern (scientific) public health is usually traced to the action of

John Snow (a London public health physician) who, in 1854, removed the handle from a pump supplying water in Broad Street, London, because he had deduced that water drawn from that pump was a major source of transmission of cholera (Holman 1992 and Baum 1998 argue that the more significant influence was the work of Edwin Chadwick, a nineteenth-century Poor Law reformer, whose advocacy led to legislation to regulate unsanitary sewers and drains).

The early emphasis of public health was on the control and containment of infectious diseases (Susser and Susser 1996; Beaglehole and Bonita 1997). The early public health paradigm (and that of epidemiology) was primarily mono-causal, based on the 'germ theory of disease': the critical research task was to search for the single microbe that caused each specific disease. The strategies that were available to public health practitioners included legislative ones of regulating industry and the water supply, and containment or quarantine. Immunisation subsequently became available as another public health strategy.

In the early part of the twentieth century, public health interventions focused on infectious diseases and the development of maternal and child health services. Strategies to control infectious disease were primarily associated with regulation or mass immunisation programs. Public health focused on transmission of vectors through means such as food handling and waste water. These hazards often arose locally, which led to an emphasis on local control through local government.

The development of maternal and child health services (variously termed 'baby health' or 'infant welfare' services) in the first decade of the twentieth century was the first major 'public health' intervention that focused on and was affected by changing the behaviour of individuals, in this case through providing advice and support. A 'universalist' service in the sense of being available to all mothers of new children, the new programs were introduced in the context of debates about declining fertility and high maternal and infant mortality (Hicks 1978; Kewley 1973 argues that the contemporary introduction of a maternity allowance was in fact not designed to increase the birth rate but to assist mothers). Maternal and child health services quickly spread throughout Australia and, until the development of community-based aged care services in the 1950s and a generalist community health service in the 1970s, were the only public sector networks of personal health services.

The importance of traditional public health containment strategies waned from about the middle of the twentieth century with the advent of penicillin. However, new public health challenges began to be identified. In particular, aided by the development of 'chronic disease epidemiology', public health practitioners recognised that infectious diseases were contributing less to the overall burden of disease in the community, and that new diseases, including chronic diseases, were important causes of ill health. Probably the most notable event in this development was the publication, in 1962, by the Royal College of Physicians of its concern about the link between tobacco and lung cancer (Royal College of Physicians of London 1962).

Unfortunately, the public health response to the new findings from epidemiology involved a focus on individuals, rather than the societal, structural, and regulatory approaches traditionally used for public health improvement. The main (although not exclusive) focus became one of attempting to change individual behaviours (sometimes called 'lifestyles'), rather than changing environments. This emphasis on 'lifestyle' change was exemplified in a 1974 report by the Canadian government on factors affecting ill health (named after the issuing Health Minister, Marc Lalonde) which was influential in many developed countries, including Australia. Although the Lalonde Report recognised the importance of environmental causes of ill health, policy prescriptions following Lalonde tended to emphasise 'lifestyle' rather than environmental strategies (Redman 1996). However, as was argued in chapter 2, individual behaviours are shaped and patterned by environments: taking up smoking is only in part an individual choice because the choice is shaped by peer groups and the broader social environment through advertising, availability, and social norms.

A third phase in the development of public health has been the rediscovery of the importance of the social environment in determining health and ill health, symbolised by the publication of the Declaration of Alma Ata (1978) which highlighted the role of community interventions in primary health care in achieving improved health (Declaration of Alma Ata 1978) and by renewed interest in differences in health status in different geographic areas and between low and high income groups.

Despite extensive positive rhetoric about the importance of these new community interventions, they challenged the dominant orthodoxy within society and hence have come to be seen by those in power as illegitimate. In contrast, traditional public health is seen as a legitimate part of the social infrastructure, despite scientific and political debates about the thresholds for appropriate and safe water supply and air quality. The 'lifestyle' focus does not challenge any significant interests in the community because of its focus on individual behaviour rather than environmental causation. The community approach, however, challenges the distribution of power in society by proposing restrictions on advertising and polluting industries, and is perceived to lead to a short-term conflict between health goals and economic development or profit accumulation goals.

The evolution of public health policy in Australia paralleled these historical phases. The early stages of public health and health promotion can be characterised as a period of (public health) professional dominance. Initially, this involved a focus on traditional public health protection areas including quarantine and environmental health or health protection, but over time this phase incorporated the wider public health roles arising from the focus on chronic diseases.

The NH&MRC played a key role in this process because it provided a forum for the state officials involved in public health to meet and agree approaches to standard setting and priorities, relatively independent of direct political and territorial considerations. It also was seen by the community generally and by the key professionals within the public health movement as a legitimate, authoritative body to promulgate such standards. The NH&MRC has an important continuing role in prevention by developing and authorising immunisation schedules and, jointly with environmental agencies, by standard setting in environmental health.

This period of professional dominance and a command or control 'protection' approach began to break down with the more general democratisation of social institutions in the 1960s and 1970s. Government activities in the 1950s and early 1960s, especially at state level, were reactive, focused on a relatively narrow and traditional view of public health. The Commonwealth also did not exercise leadership in responding to the emerging epidemiological challenges. This Commonwealth and state inaction created a policy vacuum in public health.

By the mid 1960s, a number of interest groups emerged articulating dissatisfaction with the existing health service delivery orthodoxy, including the contemporary approach to public health and health promotion. These interest groups challenged the professionally dominated approach to standard setting, service delivery, and health promotion even in the relatively core areas of environmental health policy (see Hutton and Connors 1999 for a history of the Australian environmental movement and associated local campaigns). Community-based interest groups also organised around a number of weaknesses in the service delivery system, including, for example, women's health (see Broom 1991) and questioned the single-minded orientation of the service delivery system towards cure, to the neglect of patient dignity and other aspects of the microprocesses of care. In the early 1970s, the newly established community health centres often took a broader view of strategies to promote public health. They began to operationalise community-based approaches to public health (Owen and Lennie 1992; Sindall 1992) and stimulated local health education or health promotion activities (Jackson et al. 1989). The existing structures for development of public health policy were not able to address these new challenges coherently. Public health responses to newly identified problems were fragmented, with new programs established for each (for example, policies on drug and alcohol services).

The most notable community approach to prevention came with the advent of AIDS in the early 1980s, where the gay community was particularly successful in advocating a community approach to preventing the spread of AIDS, relying very heavily on the involvement of the community in prevention activities. Very often community groups were able to enlist sympathetic professionals both inside bureaucracies and in the community to assist in their campaigns. Interest groups were often able to achieve the creation of specific program funding at the Commonwealth (or state) level with bureaucratic and political guardians.

Because public health policy had neither an analytic framework nor practical skills to pursue structural and social sources of ill health, the common underlying causative factors that might contribute to more than one policy area were de-emphasised. Thus, for example, drug and alcohol policy and AIDS policy developed separately, despite obvious overlap relating to the risk of reuse of needles in both areas.

By the late 1980s and the 1990s, there were increasing attempts to stimulate public health nationally and to impose some form of coherence and coordination on public health policy in Australia. This was accompanied by an attempt to provide an economic justification for investing in prevention (see Segal and Richardson 1994; Richardson 1998a; Segal 1998; Abelson 2002; Applied Economics 2003) and proposals to use economic tools to evaluate acute versus primary care choices (Edwards et al. 1998; Peacock 1998).

Public health is still a relatively neglected area of health policy, which is largely dominated by acute health issues. The pre-eminence of hospital and medical services is partly because of the 'excitement' and hyperbole associated with stories about advances in medical technology; the high proportion of health expenditure in these areas; and the political issues associated with resource allocation in hospitals, including waiting lists. A further reason for the lack of policy attention to public health is that the structures of provision are poorly integrated; also, public health policy is still a state responsibility and, as a result, different approaches are followed with different emphases in each of the states and territories. Despite these characteristics, there have been a number of successes. Tobacco smoking was identified in the early 1950s as being associated with cancer and heart disease and there has been a major effort, principally at state level organised by Anti-Cancer Councils, to reduce smoking in Australia. Importantly, the campaigns against smoking have involved a multi-faceted approach including regulatory approaches (to ban the advertising and promotion of smoking products (Saffer and Chaloupka 2000), and to ban smoking in public places, for example; see Borland et al. 1997), taxation strategies, mass media advertising aimed at behavioural and cultural change, as well as groups to support individuals' attempts to stop smoking. The state campaigns have been supplemented periodically with additional national funding for anti-smoking advertising programs. The

Figure 7.2 Australia: Smoking prevalence (percentage population smoking) 1945–2002

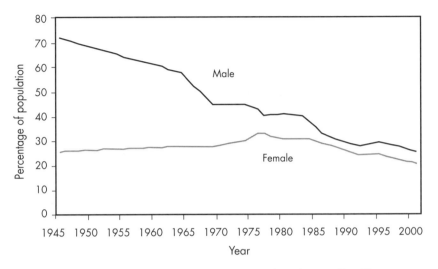

Data source: Winstanley et al 1995 and http://www.quit.org.au

campaigns have resulted in a significant reduction in smoking rates in Australia and smoking prevalence is now around one-quarter of the population aged 14 and over for males and one-fifth for females (see figure 7.2).

The anti-smoking campaigns have, to some extent, recognised that smoking behaviour is only in part an individual 'lifestyle' choice and the risk of smoking is in part shaped by the social and family environment. However, despite this recognition, the decline in smoking prevalence has been greater among the higher rather than lower income groups (and among males relative to young females), highlighting the importance of underlying social and environmental factors in influencing health behaviours.

Australia has had a remarkably successful program in reducing road trauma through a combination of public health intervention requiring people to wear seat belts (an initiative stimulated by the Royal Australasian College of Surgeons) and campaigns against speeding and drink driving. Advertising programs aimed at changing individual behaviour have been supplemented by legislative change (seat belt and random breath testing legislation) as well as programs to enhance law enforcement to contain speeding, drink driving, and other behaviours that increase the risk of motor vehicle crashes. Injuries are, however, still the leading cause of death in males aged between 15 and 44 (see table 2.3).

Health protection

Health protection is at the traditional core of public health and involves use of two of the main interventions: regulation and economic incentives. There are four major foci of health protection activity:
- environmental regulation (such as air and water quality)
- food safety
- the work environment (occupational health and safety)
- other transmission of communicable diseases.

For each of these foci, there are four generic regulatory interventions:
- setting standards
- regulating harmful activities
- surveillance to ensure that the standards in regulations are adhered to, and
- enforcement.

Immunisation is also available as a protection measure against some communicable diseases.

The protection function is normally focused on hazards occurring in the environment. These hazards can be chemical or microbiological in nature and can be naturally occurring or the result of manufacturing, extracting, or other industries. Government health protection can constrain both business and individuals. Public health legislation often gives public health officials wide powers, including powers of detention and quarantine. The legislative framework for these health protection functions varies quite significantly across Australia, with different states and territories adopting quite different models of control and regulation (see Bidmeade and Reynolds 1997; Australian Institute of Health, Law and Ethics 1998, p. 27). All public health legislation, however, deals with the four generic components discussed below.

The first component of protection, the standard setting process, involves a complex set of trade-offs, which can lead to significant controversy (Mazur 1981; Hammond and Coppock 1990; Bates 1994). In Australia, public health standards are normally promulgated by the NH&MRC, or by a Commonwealth–state ministerial council (such as the Foods Standards Council or the Environment and Conservation Council). The controversial nature of the standards relates to a number of factors. Very often the dose–response relationship (the relationship between environmental exposure to a chemical or other hazard and its impact on human health) is linear, that is, each additional increment of the chemical or other hazard causes an impact on health and the incremental impact is the same at what-ever level of the hazard in the environment. (An alternative assumption is that there is an s-shaped dose–response relationship, with small levels of the pollutant being of little hazard to humans but with a threshold above which there is significant hazard.) A linear dose–response relationship makes it difficult to set an absolute standard for exposure because the marginal impacts for exposure above and below the threshold are the same.

The trade-off is this: the lower the thresholds the more expensive the necessary mitigating works by manufacturers, but the higher the threshold the greater will be the risk to human health. Very low thresholds may also make it impractical for certain products to come onto the market. A further aspect of the controversy is that the benefits of a higher versus lower threshold fall in different places. Although entry of a new product into the market may be seen to benefit all consumers, the manufacturer or owner of a patent would particularly benefit (Benn 1997). Further, the costs of the hazard may fall in a particular geographic locality or on employees. As Mazur (1981) has pointed out, experts can be marshalled to advocate on either side of debates about appropriateness of the standards.

The second generic component of health protection is regulating harmful activities. This involves ensuring that certain activities that might have harmful impacts on health can only be undertaken in licensed premises, particular work environments, and so on. Regulations may also specify work practices, protective clothing, and warning signs and labels. Regulation can be proactive by requiring potential future activities to be subject to a health or environmental impact assessment prior to their commencing (see NH&MRC 1994 for a review of contemporary assessment requirements and guidance on conducting assessments). These assessments can be linked to approvals at any level of government (Commonwealth approvals for exports, or state or local planning approvals). As with standard setting, the regulation process can also be controversial (see Chapman and Wutzke 1997).

The third step in the protection chain is surveillance to ensure that the regulatory environment is being maintained. Surveillance is the basic public health tool, both in terms of ensuring appropriate preventive actions are taken (for example, with respect to food manufacturing and handling), and in terms of investigations following disease outbreaks. Public health legislation usually provides for two main methods of surveillance: government inspectorates (particularly local government inspectors), and compulsory notification. Notification, particularly relevant to surveillance of communicable diseases, may place requirements on primary care practitioners and/or laboratories that receive specimens and identify certain specified communicable diseases. Surveillance (and follow-up action) often also relies on consumer reports of pollution or disease outbreaks to alert public health officials of a breakdown in regulatory standards.

The final element of the chain is one of enforcement. The enforcement process can have a series of graded steps including:

- warnings, to provide a notice that a contravention has occurred and it must be attended to before the next inspection
- a notice to improve, specifying the time limit for contraventions to be corrected
- a notice to stop, an order that an activity must cease until the contravention is corrected (MacArthur and Bonnefoy 1998, p. 85).

The balance between the more educationally based (warnings) versus punitive (notices to improve or stop) approaches may change over time, and is one of the differences between the approaches of states and territories to regulation. Legislation redrafted in the late 1990s has seen a greater emphasis on industry self-regulation, and educationally based approaches rather than detailed inspection. The rationale for this change is in part a deregulatory political environment, in part a belief that the education approach will lead to systematic change not achievable by fear of inspection, and in part a desire to reduce the overall cost of government through reducing the number of inspectors.

There are a range of sanctions that can be applied if regulations are breached, most commonly fines, but in many jurisdictions regulation may provide for permanent closure of a facility. In some cases, a manufacturer may be liable to pay compensation to consumers affected by poor manufacturing processes, or clean-up costs for environmental contamination.

Expenditure

Australian health expenditure data show that about 0.4 per cent of GDP is spent on community and public health activities (5 per cent of total health expenditure), with about half on three main activities: communicable disease control, health promotion, and organised immunisation (see table 7.3). These figures underestimate public health expenditure in that they focus on identified health expenditure according to the system of National Accounts and exclude 'environmental protection expenditure'. As will be discussed below, about a further 0.5 per cent of GDP is spent on measures related to public health but classified as environmental protection.

Important components of health protection activity are recorded in the National Accounts not as health expenditure but as environmental protection expenditure, including expenditure on waste water and waste management and on protecting air quality. Other aspects of health protection, such as improving road safety, may be recorded as expenditure on justice (random breath testing) or transport (improving road design).

Total environmental protection expenditure in 1996/97 was A$8.6 billion. (The data in this section are derived from ABS 1999c.) Three domains of this expenditure are particularly relevant to public health, specifically environmental health. About one-fifth of total environmental protection was for sewerage, with most of this expenditure incurred by households and local government.

Table 7.3   Australia: Expenditure on core public health categories by funding source, 1999–2000 (A$million)

	Commonwealth Government	State and Territory governments	Total	Proportion of total (%)
Communicable disease control	21.4	132.1	153.5	16.5
Selected health promotion	36.0	129.9	166.0	17.8
Organised immunisation	49.1	104.3	153.3	16.5
Environmental health	18.7	42.7	61.4	6.8
Food standards and hygiene	10.8	14.2	25.1	2.7
Breast cancer screening	2.1	95.1	97.2	10.4
Cervical screening	57.9	23.0	80.9	8.7
Prevention of hazardous and harmful drug use	27.3	96.0	123.2	13.2
Public health research	58.0	14.3	70.3	7.5
PHOFAs and other general public health grants	0.3	-	0.3	-
Total expenditure	279.5	651.7	931.2	-
Percentage of total (%)	30.0	70.0	100.0	100.0

Data source: AIHW 2002c

Just over 10 per cent of expenditure was on garbage removal, and an additional 5 per cent of expenditure related to the air and climate. Thus, in total, over one-third of environmental protection expenditure can be regarded as being associated with protection of public health, suggesting that about a further 0.5 per cent of GDP is spent on public health activities. A broader definition of public health may include all waste disposal costs, further increasing the public health component of environmental protection expenditures.

Air quality

Although there is an obvious and direct impact of air quality on health, leadership on air quality monitoring primarily rests with environmental protection agencies rather than health authorities. Nevertheless, air quality is a focus of public health action in Australia and the National Environmental Health Forum has released a number of monographs on this topic covering various contaminants in the air (for example, see Salisbury and Ferrari 1997 on ozone: other monographs have also been issued on benzene, nitrogen dioxide, and sulphur dioxide).

The contentious nature of the standard-setting process in health protection is reflected in air quality standards. There is considerable variation in air quality standards: for example, the Australian permissible ozone standard is 50 per cent higher than the Canadian standard (Salisbury and Ferrari 1997). Australia has adopted a consistent set of standards to measure air pollution. These are known as the National Environment Protection Measures for Ambient Air Quality. Consistent national data on adherence to these standards has not yet (September 2003) been published.

Water quality

Indicators for drinking water quality are set in three broad areas: health criteria, aesthetic criteria, and amenity criteria but, again, the standard setting process involves trade-offs and policy choices (Lewis 1996). Responsibility for regulating water quality was generally moved from health portfolios in the 1970s to the portfolio responsible for water supply. This alignment of regulation and provision is clearly inappropriate in the context of privatisation of water supply and a realignment of responsibilities may be necessary in those states that privatise.

Public health issues relating to water quality are broader than simply drinking water quality: for example, recreational use of water. Regulation of recreational water quality involves similar criteria as drinking water quality, but different thresholds. Overall, there is a high level of compliance with drinking water quality guidelines, although the rate of compliance differs by location: metropolitan supplies comply with bacterial guidelines in 98 per cent of instances, whereas supplies in nonmetropolitan areas comply in 83 per cent of instances and remote areas in only 40 per cent (ABS 1996a).

Food safety

Australia's arrangements for food safety involve health, primary production, trade, and consumer affairs interests. The peak policy development body is the Australian New Zealand Food Regulation Ministerial Council, which is a ministerial body comprising ministers from Australian states and territories, the Commonwealth, and New Zealand (Yeatman 2002). The council is the determining body on standards. Recommendations to the council are made through the Food Standards Australia New Zealand (FSANZ), a statutory body established under the Commonwealth's Food Standards Australia New Zealand Act 1991. A Commonwealth-State Inter Government Agreement regarding a new food regulatory system, and a treaty with New Zealand, support the Act. A Food Regulation Standing Committee, consisting of Commonwealth, state, and New Zealand public servants, and a representative of the Australian Local Government Association, provides policy advice to the ministerial council. FSANZ sets standards for labelling of foods and develops standards for food handling, including safety practices, cleanliness of food premises, and so on. Monitoring adherence to these standards is principally undertaken through local food inspection/surveillance programs, commonly auspiced by local government, although the regulatory framework differs from state to state (Smith 1997), leading to differences and inconsistencies in regulation and enforcement practices (Office of Regulation Review (Industry Commission) 1995; Food Regulation Review Committee 1998). FSANZ also monitors the composition of foods, including the extent to which pesticide residues and contaminants occur in foods, through the Australian Total Diet Survey, which also estimates the Australian public's dietary exposure to these hazards.

The Australian Total Diet Survey, conducted about every two years, reports on a range of contaminants and pesticides using four broad standard setting approaches (see table 7.4).

The 20th Survey (2000/01) demonstrated that pesticides and contaminants within sampled food were all within the acceptable safety limits.

Contamination can occur at any point of the food processing and handling chain. State and local public health officials (including environmental health officers) monitor each of these steps. As outlined earlier, there are a number of approaches to surveillance, and increasingly local health officers are encouraging good practice through 'food safety audits' to prevent contaminants entering the food chain. Despite these protective measures, outbreaks of illness caused by microbiological or chemical contamination are increasing (Crerar et al. 1996). These outbreaks require careful epidemiological investigation. Public health officials identify and isolate the source of the contamination by interviewing those affected, and follow

Table 7.4   Standard setting approaches used in food regulation

Term	Definition
Acceptable daily intake (ADI)	'The level of pesticide intake at or below which there should be no appreciable risk of adverse health effects over a lifetime of consumption.' Usually measured in milligrams per kilogram of body weight per day (see p. 9).
Provisional tolerable weekly intake (PTWI)	The maximum weekly intake, based on current knowledge (hence 'provisional') for substances such as heavy metals (e.g. arsenic, lead, mercury) that have a cumulative impact on the body (see p. 10).
Maximum residue limit (MRL)	The 'limit on the amount of pesticide residue permitted in an agricultural commodity' (see p. 10).
Maximum permitted concentration (MPC)	The 'limit placed on the level of a contaminant in food … expressed on the edible portion of the food' (see p. 11).

Source: Hardy 1998

up, possibly across state boundaries. Although in many cases the source of the contamination is readily localised (uncovered or unrefrigerated food at parties), in some circumstances there may be faults in the food manufacturing process. Public health legislation provides very broad powers over food manufacturing, including the enforcement steps outlined earlier in this chapter.

Food regulation faces emerging challenges from new technologies. In particular, consumers (and retailers) have different interests from producers in respect of genetically modified foods. Food labelling laws may become a much more significant subject of public debate than they were in the last part of the twentieth century.

Occupational health and safety

Regulation of occupational health is covered by state and territory legislation. As with any work-related activity, the extent of involvement of government, employer, and consumer varies across jurisdictions (see Industry Commission 1995 for a review of different state approaches to occupational health and safety). Priorities for occupational health and safety interventions are affected by perception of risk, perceptions that vary according to role (Holmes and Gifford 1997).

At the national level the peak body is the National Occupational Health and Safety Commission (NOHSC, also known as Worksafe Australia), established under the National Occupational Health and Safety Commission Act 1989. NOHSC consists of 18 members, including the chair and chief executive officer of the commission, three nominated by the Australian Council of Trade Unions, three nominated by the Confederation of Australian Industry, and others nominated by Commonwealth and state ministers. It is a facilitatory and advisory body that aims to improve Australia's occupational health and safety performance. Although it has a standard-setting and educational role, it does not have an enforcement role. The enforcement role is vested in state government departments and workers compensation authorities.

Occupational health and safety performance can be measured (negatively) using data from workers compensation claims. In 2000/01 there were 319 fatalities compensated under state workers compensation systems (National Occupational Health and Safety Commission 2002). This is an incidence rate of four fatalities per 100,000 employees. The number of fatalities Australia–wide has declined from 441 in 1996/97 (a reduction of 28 per cent over that period). The distribution of fatalities is uneven across industries with four industries accounting for more than half of all fatalities (manufacturing, and transport and storage each with 16.3 per cent; construction 12.2 per cent; and agriculture, forestry, and fishing 11.4 per cent).

As figure 7.3 shows, the distribution of fatalities and non-fatal injuries is not the same. Although labourers account for a similar proportion of both types of

Figure 7.3 Australia: Work-related fatalities and non-fatal injuries, by occupation, 2000/01

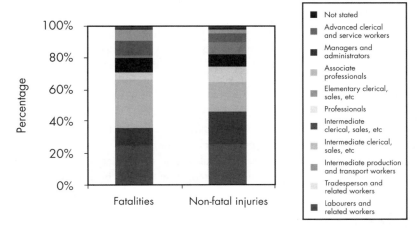

Data source: NOHSC, 2002

adverse events, intermediate production and transport workers account for a higher proportion of fatalities, as do managers. Tradespeople, clerical, and salespersons account for a higher proportion of non-fatal injuries relative to fatalities. Overall, 41 per cent of new workers compensation claims in 2000/01 were for body stressing, with a further 19 per cent for falls and trips. Mental stress accounted for 4.3 per cent of all new cases, but these cases resulted in the longest lost time (median nine weeks, average 17.8 weeks) and the highest costs per case. The high percentage of new claims for injury is partly because these events are acute and obvious. Other work-related disease may have a long latency period that makes identifying the causal factor(s) difficult. Labour mobility in many industries also makes assigning responsibility to a particular workplace difficult, inhibiting lodging a workers compensation claim.

In the early 1990s there was an increase in number of compensation cases, the incidence rate, and average cost per case. The more recent data show a decline in workers compensation incidents, which may be the result of successful prevention and protection strategies, or decreasing rates of reporting of minor incidents.

Other aspects of environmental health

Content areas for environmental health or health protection also include ionising and non–ionising radiation, noise control, regulation of pesticides and pest control generally, and other areas of injury prevention and control. As with many areas in public health, a number of government departments may need to be involved in developing health protection programs in these areas.

Communicable diseases

Strategies to address communicable diseases are framed by reference to the classic public health triad of agent/host/environment. In particular, public health practitioners (and public health policy) classifies diseases according to the route of transmission or risk factor (for example, food-borne, vector-borne, water-borne, blood-borne, vaccine preventable, and so on).

Reducing the incidence (and prevalence) of infectious diseases is an important focus of health protection. There are three main strategies used in this regard: immunisation; reducing exposure to transmission through changing individual behaviour; and quarantine. Protection against communicable diseases is also one of the objects of other aspects of health protection (such as regulation of air and water quality, and food safety).

Immunisation is the cornerstone of the public health approach to prevention of most childhood communicable diseases. Although immunisation is effected by providing a service to individuals, higher levels of immunisation lead to 'herd immunity': the communicable disease is not able to achieve widespread transmission because the prevalence of non-immunised individuals is such that there is a relatively small likelihood of their coming into contact with each other at the time that the disease is in its contagious period. Immunisation is particularly important against the contagious childhood diseases, although it is also relevant for the elderly who are increasingly being encouraged to be immunised against influenza each winter.

The Australian Standard Vaccination Schedule lists those vaccines endorsed by the NH&MRC as being effective and cost-effective. Although most of those vaccines are incorporated within the National Immunisation Program, and provided free according to an age-related schedule, since 2000 a number of vaccines on NH&MRC-endorsed vaccines have not been funded under the program. This leads to an equity issue where some children will be able to be protected against the relevant diseases and some will not have access because of financial barriers.

Australia's immunisation policy has been controversial. Immunisation itself carries a very slight risk of an adverse reaction that can lead to death or severe disability in the child and this tragic possibility affects perception of the risks and benefits of immunisation (Bond et al. 1998; Marshall and Swerissen 1999). This has led to occasional campaigns in the media, the effect of which is to attempt to discourage immunisation (Leask and Chapman 1998).

Immunisation is encouraged by government in a number of ways:
- Commonwealth subsidies of vaccine costs through the National Immunisation Program
- the Australian Childhood Immunisation Register, managed by the Health Insurance Commission, which registers all children who are immunised and then provides reminders at appropriate ages for subsequent immunisation

- payment of Childcare Assistance and the Child Care Rebate (two Commonwealth programs that provide financial assistance for families for the cost of child care) are conditional on the child being up-to-date with recommended immunisations
- the Commonwealth pays a Maternity Immunisation Allowance of A$200 at 18 months if the child is fully immunised (there is a limited range of exemptions from the immunisation requirement)
- a number of states require children to be fully immunised prior to school entry (see Thompson et al. 1994 for the Victorian experience in enacting this provision).

According to the Australian Childhood Immunisation Register, 91.2 per cent of children 12 to 15 months old were fully immunised as at 30 June 2003, with 89.3 per cent of two-year-olds fully immunised at the same date. These figures are higher than reported in the Australian Bureau of Statistics child immunisation surveys, but ABS surveys are based on parental recall and report differential prevalence of immunisation for vaccines that are delivered simultaneously. The register figures are based on actual reporting by immunisation providers, so they provide a more accurate estimate of immunisation in Australia. They may, however, still underestimate coverage because of failure to register immunisations (Lawrence et al. 2003).

There are significant differences in the way in which immunisation is provided in different states and territories of Australia (see figure 7.4).

Figure 7.4 Australia: Source of immunisation, by state or territory, 2001/02

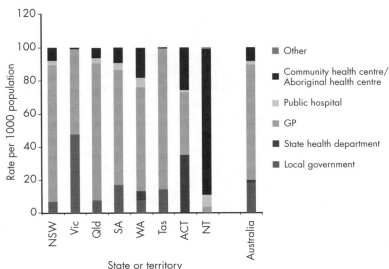

Source: Health Insurance Commission 2001

Figure 7.5 Australia: Measles notifications per 100,000 population, 1991–2002

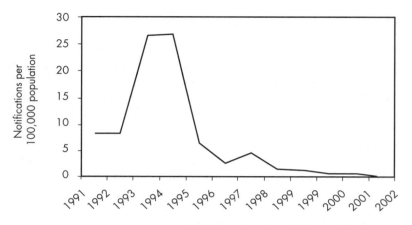

Data source: National Notifiable Diseases Surveillance System

In New South Wales, Queensland, and Tasmania over 80 per cent of immunisations are provided by general practitioners. In Victoria, in contrast, local government has a significant role in immunisation provision, a situation that is also common in South Australia. Community health centre provision is also common in other states. Although the Australian Capital Territory reports a very high level of state health department provision, this is essentially through its maternal and child health program, which is a local government function elsewhere in Australia.

An example of a vaccine preventable disease is measles. Figure 7.5 shows the incidence of measles in Australia from 1991 to 1999.

The very high peaks in 1993 and 1994 were associated with measles outbreaks in New South Wales and Queensland respectively. Prevalence of measles immunisation increased in the late 1990s, and this probably means that the relatively low incidence of measles will continue into the future.

The response to communicable diseases in Australia is coordinated through the Communicable Diseases Network of Australia and New Zealand, a collaboration of public health officials from Australian states and territories, the Commonwealth government, and New Zealand. The National Notifiable Diseases Surveillance System, established in 1990, publishes data about the incidence of communicable diseases on its web site, providing national surveillance of more than 40 communicable diseases (see www.cda.gov.au/surveil/index.htm).

For many communicable diseases there are no vaccines (most notably AIDS and sexually transmissible diseases, and some childhood diseases). The most high-profile contemporary communicable disease is HIV/AIDS, which has been the subject of specific national strategies (see Ballard 1999

Figure 7.6 Australia: HIV and AIDS notifications, and AIDS deaths, 1988–2001

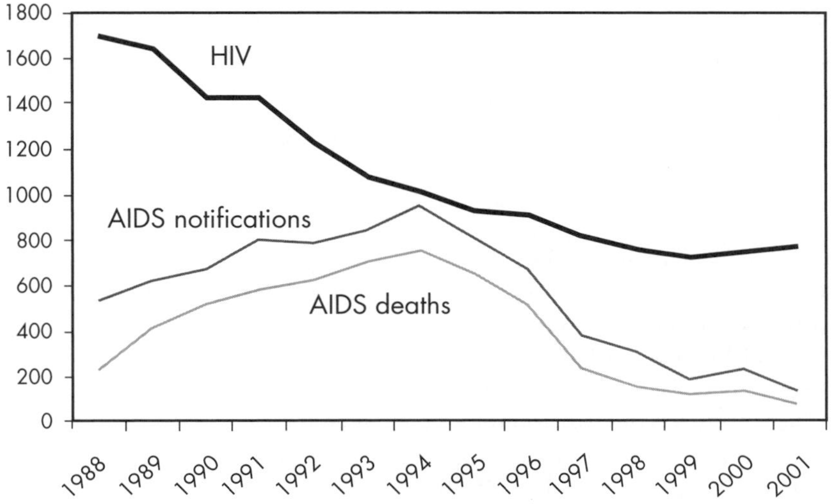

Data source: National Notifiable Diseases Surveillance System

for an account of the development of AIDS policy in Australia). Australia's HIV/AIDS strategy has attracted international attention for moving away from more traditional regulation and enforcement approaches to public health. It has been widely applauded because of its emphasis on involving the community particularly affected by HIV/AIDS in the development and implementation of policy. Figure 7.6 shows the incidence of HIV/AIDS in Australia since 1988.

It can be seen that annual HIV notifications have declined dramatically since 1988 with HIV notifications in 1998 being 42 per cent of those a decade earlier. Progression of HIV to AIDS, on the other hand, has increased from 1988 peaking at 950 in 1994. AIDS progression has slowed since then, reflecting the decline in HIV incidence. AIDS deaths parallel the trend in AIDS notifications: the peak year for AIDS deaths was also 1994 (735 deaths). Since 1999 the uniformly downwards trend in AIDS and HIV appear to have reversed (although the patterns are still not clear). The increases in AIDS and HIV seen in 2000 and for HIV in 2001 suggest that prevention effectiveness may be waning and a re-emphasis on community education may be required.

Early detection

An increasingly important public health intervention involves either early detection of disease or identifying whether an individual is genetically

Table 7.5   Types of screening

Mass screening	Comprehensive, organised testing of an entire population
Selective screening	Organised testing of a selected population
Case finding	Routine medical check-up
Opportunistic screening	Screening conducted as part of other interactions with the health system
Self-screening	Self-examination

predisposed to a disease. Tests have been developed to aid in early detection of many diseases, although not all of these are cost-effective (Russell 1994; for the economics of prevention more generally see Kenkel 2000; see Peckham and Dezateux 1998 for a review of issues in evaluation of screening programs). Screening efforts vary in intensity (see table 7.5).

Screening carries risks with it, including increased anxiety for those identified (both true and false positives). In order to ensure that only appropriate screening is undertaken, WHO has developed guidelines for effective screening programs (see Wilson and Junger 1968). The public health approach to screening focuses on mass screening and selective screening, but primary health care practitioners are also encouraged to undertake opportunistic screening where it has been shown to be effective or cost-effective. Advice on relative effectiveness is issued both by professional organisations and the NH&MRC (see NH&MRC 1997).

One of the first early detection programs was childhood screening organised through 'baby health' or maternal and child health centres in the early 1920s, discussed earlier in this chapter.

A more recently developed screening or early detection program is mammographic screening for breast cancer in women, known as Breast-Screen Australia, which provides for women aged 50 to 69 to be screened every two years to detect breast cancer at its earliest stages. BreastScreen provides a good contrast between an organised, public health approach to screening and idiosyncratic or opportunistic screening. BreastScreen's population of 50- to 69-year-olds, is the age group where screening has been shown to be most cost-effective in reducing mortality in a healthy population, based on international randomised controlled trials. (Women with a familial history of breast cancer form a different population.) It is an 'organised' approach in the sense that women in the relevant age group are notified when screening/rescreening should occur; an effort is made to ensure services are geographically and culturally accessible and that services are subject to a systematic quality assurance process. BreastScreen is also able to achieve economies of scale in its operations. Figure 7.7 shows information about breast screening rates in Australia.

Figure 7.7 Australia: Percentage of women aged 50 to 69 participating in breast screening, by state or territory, 1997/98

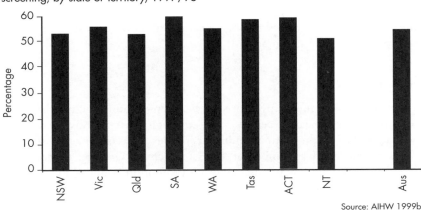

Source: AIHW 1999b

There is a significant difference in breast screening rates by state with the Australia-wide rate of 54 per cent. More importantly, all state rates are well below the BreastScreen target of 70 per cent.

As diagnostic tests that facilitate early detection of disease are developed, there is increasing pressure to screen for new diseases on either asymptomatic populations or populations at high risk because of familial or other factors. Progress on describing the human genome has also provided the basis for a new form of public health screening to identify those people who have a higher genetic predisposition to particular diseases.

Public health screening for genetic predisposition is controversial because it involves a broad range of ethical, economic, and public health considerations. Unlike traditional public health screening, screening for genetic predisposition does not involve early detection of an existing disease, but rather identifies whether a person has the genetic composition which increases their vulnerability to a future disease. The genetic predisposition may only increase the risk of the disease by a small percentage or it may indicate that the likelihood of acquiring the disease in the future is near certainty. The actions that can be taken to respond to these increased risks vary depending on the state of knowledge of the disease, the extent to which it is preventable, and the change in risk associated with the identification of a genetic predisposition (see Hall et al. 1998 for issues in evaluation of genetic screening).

Health promotion

The WHO has defined health promotion broadly: 'The process of enabling people and communities to increase control over the determinants of health and thereby improve their health' (Nutbeam 1998, p. 351).

This definition encompasses a broad range of activities. State health promotion efforts are organised through a variety of funding streams (some disease specific, some more generalist).

State initiatives

The main delivery mechanism for state health promotion funding has been via community health centres and through special, disease-focused campaigns. Health promotion funding at state level was enhanced in the mid 1980s by moves in a number of states to increase taxes on tobacco and hypothecate the funding to a state 'Health Promotion Foundation'. Victoria established the first such foundation (VicHealth) and similar foundations were established in other states (for example, Healthway in Western Australia; others in South Australia, Queensland, Tasmania, and the Australian Capital Territory). These foundations were originally established as autonomous statutory authorities able to pursue more challenging funding strategies than might be acceptable in a standard government department. Their autonomy, however, has often led to conflict with state departments who have responsibility to coordinate policy and this led to the abolition of the foundation in South Australia. All state taxes on tobacco were struck down by the High Court in 1997 as unconstitutionally imposing an excise and so the hypothecation basis of the foundations came to an end. (Hypothecation ended in Victoria in 1995 when the state government capped funding for VicHealth.)

National health promotion initiatives

The first major stimulus to health promotion nationally was the Whitlam Government's 1974 proposal to establish a community health program (see table 7.6). Although the main focus of this program was the creation of a broad basis for primary health care, the original Green Paper on the community health program proposed one of the key roles for the community health program as being in health promotion (Hospitals and Health Services Commission 1974). Specific Commonwealth funding for community health was subsequently discontinued by the Fraser Government in 1981 and the primary health care system is still relatively underdeveloped (see chapter 8). Subsequent reports (Davidson et al. 1979; Leeder 1993) proposed national funding schemes in health promotion but neither led to any policy action.

A number of other reports have attempted to specify key goals against which governments could be held accountable (Leeder 1995). This

Table 7.6   National policy reports focusing on health promotion

Year	Report	Issues
1974	A Community Health Program for Australia (Hospitals and Health Services Commission)	Proposes establishment of community health centres which would have a role in prevention and health promotion
1979	Report on Health Promotion in Australia (Davidson)	Proposed national health population program
1986	Looking Forward to Better Health (Better Health Commission)	Proposed funding in three priority areas: injury control, cardiovascular disease, and nutrition
1988	Health for all Australians	Identified need and framework for a 'National Program for Better Health'
1991	Pathways to Better Health (National Health Strategy)	Proposed a National Health Promotion Authority funding program with legislative base
1993	Goals and Targets for Australia's Health in the year 2000 and Beyond	Proposed goals and targets in terms of: • prevalence of mortality and morbidity • health lifestyle and risk factors • health literacy and health skills • healthy environments
1994	Better Health Outcomes for Australians	Proposed four 'focus' areas for action: • cardiovascular disease • cancer • injury • mental health

paralleled similar millennial attempts in the USA and other countries to achieve the WHO-inspired 'Health for All by the year 2000' (Nutbeam and Wise 1996), as well as local target-setting activities (for example, Brown and Redman 1995). The most ambitious of Australian examples was the 1993 report on goals and targets in health promotion/disease prevention, which presented a comprehensive menu of goals and targets covering a broad range of health areas. Unlike subsequent reports, the goals and targets report was not primarily organised on the basis of diseases, but rather tried to identify common principles for goal setting such as prevalence of mortality and morbidity, and cross-cutting strategic areas such as health literacy and health skills improvement that might lead to reductions in prevalence across a range of specific diseases.

Many of these reports have attempted to identify priorities: three in the 1986 Better Health Commission (injury control, cardiovascular disease, and nutrition); four 'focus areas' in the 1994 Better Health Outcomes report (cardiovascular disease, cancer, injury, and mental health). By 1999, a further two 'national priorities' had been added: diabetes mellitus and asthma. The current six national priority areas are the subject of biennial reports by the AIHW on progress towards achieving the goals and targets specified for these conditions. There are a number of problems involved in the focus on 'priority areas', discussed later in this chapter.

The 1986 Better Health Commission report stimulated the National Better Health Program, a national funding program, which included in its remit national funding for health promotion. However, the National Better Health Program had very broad goals, and evaluation of the program (Malcolm 1994) found that there was a need for: clearer strategic direction and coordination at the national level; and clarification of the role of a national health promotion program vis-à-vis a national Health for All strategy.

Confusion between these two latter concepts had led to unrealistic expectations of what the program could achieve.

Funding under the National Better Health Program was time-limited and the program was terminated at the end of its original cycle. There is currently no national comprehensive health promotion funding arrangement. The Commonwealth has not so far succeeded in developing a systematic and organised approach to health promotion at a national level leading to action at state and local levels.

The 1994 'focus' areas of the Better Health Outcomes report has led to the development of National Health Priority Areas. From 1995 onwards, the Commonwealth and states also agreed to take steps to establish greater cohesion in funding programs (through Public Health Outcome Funding Agreements) and improved policy development and coordination (through the National Public Health Partnership).

Public Health Outcome Funding Agreements

By the mid 1990s, states had become critical of the mushrooming of separate funding lines associated with public health initiatives, each with its own reporting and accountability requirements and with defined program boundaries. In the late 1990s, the Commonwealth and states took a major step to rationalise funding through the Public Health Outcome Funding Agreements. These Commonwealth–state agreements define broad bands for funding into which many pre-existing smaller grants were collapsed, with a single agreement as well as performance indicators covering the pre-existing areas. The programs covered by the 1999–2004 agreements are:

- National Drug Strategy
- National HIV/AIDS Strategy
- National Immunisation Program
- BreastScreen Australia

- National Cervical Screening Program
- National Women's Health Program
- National Education Program on Female Genital Mutilation
- Alternative Birthing Program.

Although the broadbanding helps to reduce the disjunctions caused by the separate funding streams, and introduces a more contemporary focus on outcome/output controls rather than inputs, the Public Health Outcome Funding Agreements are still characterised by separate reporting for each of the main funding streams, and may still entail separate programmatic responses to each of the strategies at local level.

National Public Health Partnership

The second pillar of the 1990s approach to establishing coherence within the public health/health promotion program was the creation of the National Public Health Partnership (NPHP) designed to 'integrate the public health system [by bringing] together key stakeholders who had a contribution to make in strengthening the public health sector' (Lin and King 2000). The partnership was created in 1997 through a formal Commonwealth–State Memorandum of Understanding. The aims of the partnership include:

- improving the health status of all Australians, in particular population groups most at risk
- improving collaboration in the national public health effort
- developing better coordination and increasing sustainability of public health strategies, and
- enhancing the capacity of states and territories to respond to local priorities.

The partnership group of the NPHP is a subcommittee of AHMAC and makes recommendations to health ministers via AHMAC. Its membership consists of the chief health officers/directors of public health in each state and territory, together with the Head of the Population Health Division of the Commonwealth Department of Health and Aged Care, representatives of the NH&MRC and AIHW, and an observer from New Zealand.

The NPHP is serviced by a small secretariat based in Melbourne and has adopted a workplan that involves:

- public health practice improvement (for example, benchmarking)
- public health information development
- national public health regulation and legislation
- national coordination of specific public health strategies (for example, HIV/AIDS strategy)
- public health research and development
- public health workforce development
- development of resource allocation strategies in public health.

Health promotion: individual versus environmental approaches

Despite the broad WHO definition of health promotion quoted at the start of this section, health promotion is more often operationalised in terms of changing individual behaviour. The underlying assumption of this approach to health promotion is that the best way to improve the health of populations is to focus on 'risk factors', in particular behaviours identified as precursors of the main causes of hospital admission or premature mortality. Programs are then developed specifically addressing those behaviours. This emphasis on particular risk factors handicaps planners' and policy makers' ability to address the complex, multicausal nature of ill health and leads to an automatic limitation of policy and research to a monocausal approach. This emphasises individual life choices that might be seen to be associated with these risk factors, rather than underlying social conditions that lead to certain patterns of behaviour.

Behaviour is a relevant and important factor in health promotion: data from the Australian Health Survey (Mathers 1994) show that female smokers have a 40 per cent greater chance of reported fair or poor health relative to nonsmokers, and male smokers have almost two-thirds higher rates of reporting poor health. Similar relativities are shown for people who are overweight and for those who are inactive, females having a 50 per cent higher chance of reported fair or poor health if they are inactive, and males 34 per cent higher. However, policy and research needs to move beyond simple single risk factors to take into account the complex environmental factors underlying patterns of mortality and morbidity highlighted in chapter 2.

The importance of environmental factors can be seen in Mathers' work analysing the Australian Health Survey (Mathers 1994). He analysed the relative contribution of the various factors that affect self-reported fair or poor health.

Figure 7.8 shows the cumulative effect of standardising for the various factors that might explain the health differentials for males in terms of employment status.

Clearly such differences need to take into account the age of respondents and other variables that may confound the relationship between employment and ill health. Thus, a substantial difference exists in age-standardised rates of self-reported fair or poor health between males who are unemployed relative to those in employment. Those in full-time employment have the base rate of 1. Unemployed males have five times the rate of reported poor health, and those employed part time for less than 15 hours per week have twice the difference in reported poor health, after standardising for age. Some of this difference is explained by differences in education levels and some by family composition: after standardising for these factors unemployed males have a risk of reported poor health of about 3.5 times the rate for employed males.

Figure 7.8 Australia: Rate ratios of fair/poor health by employment status, standardising for various factors, males

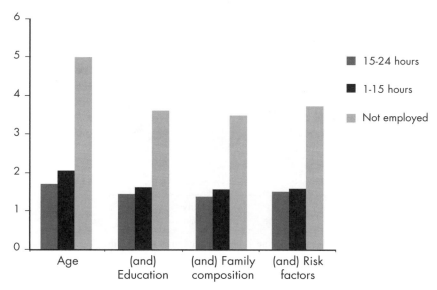

Environmental factors contributing to fair or poor health

Data source: Mathers 1994

What is striking about Mathers' analysis, however, is that even when standardised for the effect of the various behavioural risk factors such as smoking, inactivity, risk drinking, and so on, there is still a significant difference between unemployed and underemployed males and those in full-time employment. A more interesting finding is that after standardising for age and education, there is little further improvement in explaining the underlying factors which contribute to these differentials: family composition and the adoption of risky behaviours do not explain much of the difference in self-reported fair and poor health between the employed and unemployed population. (Figure 7.9 shows similar results for females.)

These data suggest that focusing our health promotion efforts solely on changing risk factors (such as smoking rates) will not substantially change the differential health status of the unemployed relative to the employed. Unemployed nonsmokers are still going to have much poorer health than their fully employed counterparts. Although the various risk factors used in this analysis are individually and collectively important, and do lead to differences in health status, their importance is overshadowed by a complex set of factors in the socioeconomic and physical environments that lead to major differences in health for the employed and unemployed populations.

Figure 7.9 Australia: Rate ratios of fair/poor health by employment status, standardising for various factors, females

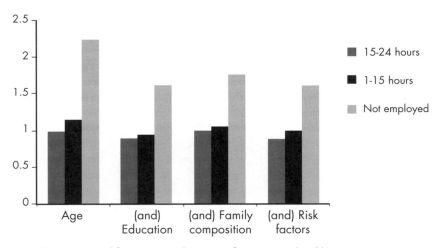

Environmental factors contributing to fair or poor health

Data source: Mathers 1994

Environmental, social, and community factors are thus critical in creating healthy and unhealthy environments (Anderson et al. 2003). Table 7.7 shows how social and physical factors can impact on health.

Reduction of income inequality is likely to lead to overall health status improvements, and would be welcomed by most in the health sector, but the policy levers for this are not within the purview of the health sector. Health sector workers and policy makers can design strategies to redress health inequalities (NHS Centre for Reviews and Dissemination 1995; Arblaster et al. 1996; Connelly 1999; Mackenbach and Bakker 2002). What has been argued here is that the simple risk factor approach to developing strategies for improving the population's health is not adequate to achieve real reductions in health inequalities. The emphasis on environmental factors proposed has been an increasingly dominant aspect of health promotion thinking over the last decade (see Yen and Syme 1999 for a review of the literature on the importance of the social environment on health), stimulated in part by the work of the WHO and reflected in the Ottawa Charter (WHO 1986b) and the need to be part of future planning for health promotion (Wise and Signal 2000).

There is now a developing literature that identifies the public health benefits of improving social cohesion, through increasing participation in clubs and associations and so on (for example, see Siahpush and Singh 1999). However, such 'participation' interventions are not normally seen as core public health activities, despite lip service to the importance of the social and economic environment as a determinant of health. Social cohesion and social capital, the concepts fundamental to the broader approach to public health, are appropriately measured through indicators such as community involvement in associations, clubs, and other networks (Hall 1999; Leeder and Dominello 1999).

Participation in voluntary work affirms the interrelatedness of individuals in a society. On average, people spent 22 minutes per day providing voluntary work and care (see table 7.8).

Approximately 20 per cent of the population participates in this process; for participants, the average contribution to voluntary work was 109 minutes per day. Participants have contributed an additional 20 minutes more per day on average in 1997 compared with 1992. However, over the same period, there was a marginal decline in the participation rate, with the decline slightly larger for males than for females.

Social participation creates a stronger sense of community and, among other benefits, helps the community deal with health issues.

The classification community participation includes attendance at meetings, civic ceremonies such as naturalisation, civic obligations including voting, and community participation generally. Although this aspect of social capital involved only eight minutes per day for all people, for participants in these activities it involved on average about half an hour a day. Importantly, 7 per cent more of the population were involved in community participation in 1997 relative to 1992 (23.5 per cent versus 15.2 per cent). Females had a significantly higher participation rate than males, and the participation rate for females increased by more than 10 per cent between 1992 and 1997.

Attempting to change either social institutions or individual behaviour is a complex task with long lead times for success (Nutbeam 1997). These lead times often mean that programs lose political support and are abandoned before they can come to fruition. The complexity of health promotion programs is underscored by the multifaceted and multifactorial nature of the programs, and the fact that changing environments often involves confrontation with established interests currently benefiting from the environments that shape the individual behaviours (for example, tobacco manufacturing companies and tobacco growers are obviously affected by strategies to reduce tobacco smoking). The changes in behaviours that are sought as part of health promotion programs may also be inconvenient or not seen as sufficiently valuable in the context of alternative uses of time.

Cohen and Henderson (1988) have highlighted the complexity of the health promotion endeavour by identifying two objects of health promotion: prevention goods, which reduce the risk of ill health; and hazard goods, which increase the risk of ill health.

Part of the health promotion endeavour is to change the balance of these two types of goods by increasing consumption of prevention goods (healthy behaviours) and reducing the demand for hazard goods (such as smoking).

Table 7.7 Conceptual framework for social and physical environmental factors' impact on health

	Factors	Protective Factors	Risk Factors
Social and economic environment	Neighbourhood socioeconomic level.	Economically stable communities are healthier than poor communities.	Racial and economic segregation, concentrated poverty lead to higher stress, higher levels of premature mortality.
	Cultural characteristics: norms, values, and attitudes deriving from race/ethnicity, religion, or nationality, as well as from other types of social and cultural groupings.	Cohesion and a sense of community, with access to key cultural institutions with healthy cultural norms/attributes.	Racism, language barriers, and acceptance of unhealthy behaviours. Absence of community norms and expectations that promote healthy behaviour and community safety.
	Social support and networks.	Friends, colleagues, and neighbourhood acquaintances provide access to social supports and economic opportunities, as well as to certain health services and resources. Adult role models, peer networks are influential in young people. Networks exist within the community and beyond it.	Lack of social supports. Potential role models have left the neighbourhood and have not remained connected to current residents or institutions. Residents do not have access to networks outside the neighbourhood that would assist in providing access to employment and other key opportunities. Sometimes referred to as absence of 'bridging' social capital.
	Community organisation: level of capacity for mobilisation, civic engagement, and political power.	Community organisations provide needed supports and services. Political power allows needed resources to be leveraged into neighbourhood.	Lack of organisation and political power impedes the flow of resources needed for neighbourhood problem-solving and hampers community leadership development.

Table 7.7 Conceptual framework for social and physical environmental factors' impact on health (cont.)

	Factors	Protective Factors	Risk Factors
Social and economic environment (cont.)	Reputation of the neighbourhood perceptions by residents, outsiders may affect behaviour towards the neighbourhood.	Perceived as 'good' or 'improving' neighbourhood with shared community and important regional attributes. Environment conducive to investment of new effort and resources.	Poor and 'bad' neighbourhoods are shunned subject to negative stereotypes and discriminated against, limiting success of isolated improvement efforts.
Physical environment	Physical features of the neighbourhood: air, water, climate, etc. shared across a wide area.	A healthy physical environment.	Presence of and exposure to toxins and pollution.
	Physical spaces such as housing, parks and recreation, and workplace.	Access to affordable, high-quality housing, local parks, and safe workplaces.	Exposure to lead paint, problems with inadequate sanitation and pest infestation, dangerous types of work (e.g. industrial in urban areas or logging/fishing in rural), and unsafe work environments.
	Public safety.	Desired and necessary amount of police and fire protection. Little crime, lots of street/sidewalk activity and interaction.	Prevalence of violence breeds fear, isolation, and a reluctance to seek even needed services, as residents avoid leaving their homes and spending time outside.
	Physical access to opportunities.	Good location and mobility for access to resources and new opportunities throughout the region.	Isolation of homes from job centres, particularly new suburban areas without public transit access. Distance from recreational facilities or safe parks for health-promoting activities such as exercise.

Source: Adapted from Bell et al. 2002 Reducing health disparities through a focus on communities. Policy Link. Accessed from Web at http://www.policylink.org/pdfs/HealthDisparities.pdf (24.9.2003).

Table 7.8   Participation in voluntary and community activities, 1992 and 1997

	Mean minutes/day all persons		Participation rate %		Mean minutes/day participants	
	1992	1997	1992	1997	1992	1997
Voluntary work and care						
Males	20	19	19.4	16.2	101	117
Females	20	24	25.2	23.4	80	104
Persons	20	22	22.4	19.8	89	109
Community participation						
Males	5	7	14.3	19.9	35	33
Females	6	9	16.1	27.0	35	34
Persons	5	8	15.2	23.5	35	34

Source: ABS 1998b

Both types of goods have two important attributes that influence their demand. First, they have a utility or benefit associated with the consumption of the good; in the case of prevention goods, for example consumers might derive pleasure from healthy behaviours (such as some forms of exercise) or community participation. Second, consumers may feel rewarded about the long-term benefit that is being accrued. Cohen and Henderson distinguish between these two forms of benefit (or utility), labelling one as 'utility in use' and the other 'utility in anticipation' (Salkeld 1998 makes a similar argument). Obviously, consumption of many popular hazard goods brings a direct utility to the consumer (except in the case where they have become addicted to the hazard good and they are receiving no benefit but cannot cease consumption). Unless health promotion programs come to terms with the way ordinary people evaluate the balance of risks and benefits for these two sorts of goods, little progress will be made towards a healthier society.

Implications for national policy

The complexity of forging national health policy across Commonwealth–state constitutional responsibilities and interests was highlighted in chapter 5. This is exacerbated in health promotion because while there may be broad aspirational goals for health promotion, it is very often not clear how these goals are to be achieved. The barriers to achievement of health promotion goals are as much intellectual and knowing what the right policy should be as they are to do with funding. Further, unlike hospital services, where the Commonwealth makes a direct payment to states who have the levers to implement the policy, health promotion normally requires a more personal intervention, and thus involves not only state governments but often local delivery agencies as well. However, as will be discussed further in the next chapter, the local level structures for delivery of health promotion are uneven (in the case of public structures) or uncoordinated (in the case of private providers, especially general practitioners). Together, these factors continue to handicap the effective delivery of health promotion programs. Advertising campaigns are often the instrument of choice for national and state level campaigns because their implementation can be directly achieved by central government.

A key component of national health promotion policies has been the identification of 'national priority areas', an approach that introduces further weaknesses into policy formulation. The structure de-emphasises the multifactorial or multicausal nature of disease creation, for example many of the risk factors of cardiovascular disease are shared in common with those of cancer. Further, by focusing on individual diseases, the approach automatically de-emphasises some of the social and environmental factors involved in disease creation as discussed in chapter 2.

The goals and targets specified for national priority areas cover a range of issues focused on changing individual behaviours, but in some cases include changes in the organisation of treatment, early detection, and rehabilitation. In common with many other broad social initiatives, there is often a mismatch between the identification of the problems and the development of strategies to respond to those problems. The strategies are rarely able to develop specific interventions at national, state, and local levels that will lead to specific consequences leading, in turn, to the achievement of the goals. Moreover, specification of interventions needs to recognise that they take place within a particular context, and (as was shown in figure 2.10) need to affect the environments that often determine individual behaviours.

Given the very large component of behaviour that is shaped by environmental factors, including peers and families, the development of strategies to achieve changes in a way that will have an impact on the goals is often difficult. It needs to be understood that the context of an intervention influences the ability to achieve specified goals; consequently similar interventions have different outcomes depending on their context. These are continuing challenges for contemporary public health policy.

8

Primary and Community Care

Although hospitals are the most expensive component of the health system, most interaction with the system occurs outside institutional settings. Forty per cent of the Australian population took some form of health-related action (other than taking medication) in the two weeks prior to the Australian Health Survey interview in 2001 (see figure 8.1). One-quarter of the population visited a doctor in the survey period. Only 1 per cent of the population was hospitalised in the period: care in the community represents the dominant form of interaction with the health system.

Primary health care services also provide an important foundation for other services: they can function as 'gatekeepers' to ensure that patients only progress when necessary to other parts of the system (secondary care in hospitals, tertiary care in teaching hospitals). Easy access to primary care services can also ensure that health problems are dealt with early in the progression of a disease. International evidence has demonstrated that stronger primary care systems are associated with reduced premature mortality (Starfield and Shi 2002; Macinko et al. 2003).

There are a number of ways of describing health services in the community. First, they are funded from multiple sources including the Medicare Benefits and Pharmaceutical Benefits Schemes, Public Health Outcome Funding Agreements, private health insurance (which funds a component of dental services, physiotherapy services, and so on), state and territory programs, and consumer payments (either for the full cost or as co-payments). Second, services can be described in terms of the health care provider. The providers include general practitioners, pharmacists, nurses (including maternal and child health nurses), naturopaths, and other health professionals. A range of non-health professionals are involved in care, for example home-help staff. Family, volunteers, and other nonpaid carers also provide a significant amount of care. The services can be organised in terms of private practice or other for-profit organisations, not-for-profit

Figure 8.1 Australia: Health-related actions in previous two weeks, 2001

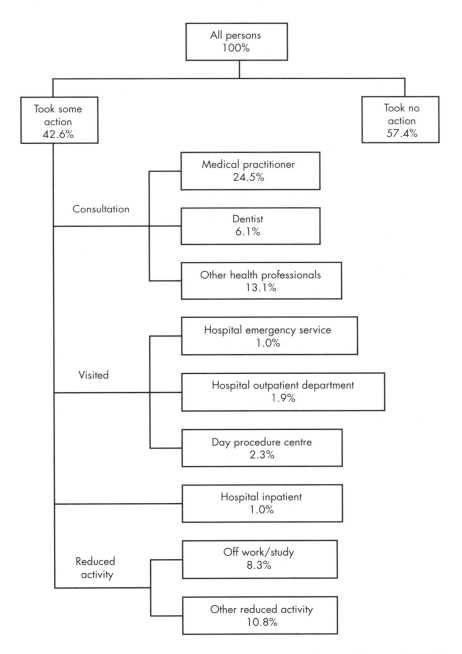

Data source: ABS 2002

charitable organisations, or organisations established by government. Services and providers are not a precise match, that is, the link between providers and services is not one-to-one. Nurses, for example, provide a broad range of services, but there is almost no single 'nursing' service that is not also provided by another profession. Third, services can also be described in terms of function: screening (designed to reduce the incidence of a specific disease), episodic or acute services (designed to resolve an immediate problem), health promotion services, and services for the chronically ill. This last group includes both residential services for the elderly or disabled and detoxification services for people with alcohol and drug problems. A range of nonresidential services is also provided for the chronically ill or for other specific population groups (for example, specialist community mental health teams).

The provision of these services is intended to lead to improved outcomes but these also vary. Objectives of primary health or community care at the individual level include improving health status, improving individual quality of life (including an individual's ability to perform activities of daily living), and improvement of quality of life for carers. At the community level, primary health or community care services are aimed at strengthening community ties which both protect against ill health and provide needed supports for those who require care.

Because of its multiple objectives, the primary and community care sector involves a complex array of funding, services, and professionals. For reasons that will be discussed later in this chapter, the sector is relatively underfunded.

Medical services

A critical component of Australia's primary health care system is medical services provided in the community. As was discussed in chapter 4, there are over 50,000 registered medical practitioners in the medical labour force, 90 per cent of whom are in clinical practice. Of those in clinical practice, 45 per cent are primary care practitioners and 34 per cent specialists, with the rest hospital-based nonspecialists and trainees. General practitioners manage a range of problems (see figure 8.2).

Figure 8.2 shows that consumers have on average one and a half problems to be managed by a general practitioner at each encounter, that is, every 100 encounters are associated with 151 reasons for those encounters (Britt et al. 2001). Almost one-fifth of the encounters are for general and unspecified reasons with a sixth of encounters being for respiratory conditions. Importantly, over two-thirds of encounters lead to at least one medication. Most of these medications are prescriptions: for every 100

Figure 8.2 Australia: General practice activity, 2000–01

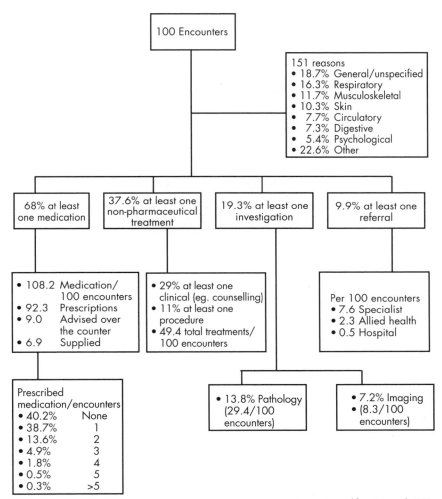

Source: Derived from Britt et al. 2001

encounters with a general practitioner there are 92.3 prescriptions written. In 40 per cent of encounters there are no prescriptions written, 38.7 per cent have one prescription, and in almost a quarter of cases there is more than one prescription provided. Medical practitioners also prescribe non-prescription medication, including natural medications (Eastwood 2000).

A significant number of encounters involve nonpharmaceutical treatment (suggested or provided) including counselling, often with a preventive focus, an area where general practitioners have a key role (Harris and Mercer 2001). One-fifth of encounters have a diagnostic investigation such as a pathology test

Figure 8.3 Australia: Percentage distribution of MBS benefits expenditure by type of service, 2002/03

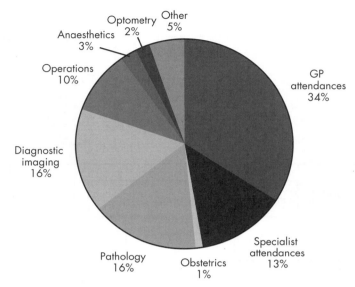

that is ordered in about 14 per cent of encounters. Generally, more than one pathology test is ordered so the overall rate of pathology test ordering is almost 30 pathology tests per 100 encounters. In almost 10 per cent of cases the general practitioner makes a referral to a specialist, allied health professional, or hospital.

Since 1984, Australians have been covered by a universal health insurance scheme, Medicare, which provides government rebates against the cost of medical services (see chapter 3). In 2002/03 a total of A$8.1 billion was paid for Medicare benefits, with about one-third of that amount paid for general practitioner attendances (see figure 8.3; data about Medicare in this section are drawn from the relevant web site <www.health.gov.au/haf/medstats/index.htm>).

In addition to direct expenditure on primary care, many pathology and diagnostic imaging services (which together account for about one-third of Medicare benefits) may be generated following a general practice visit. As noted above, about 20 per cent of all general practice encounters lead to an investigation, 13.8 per cent to a pathology service, and 7.2 per cent per cent to diagnostic imaging (Britt et al. 2001).

Utilisation of medical services has increased since the reintroduction of Medicare. In 1984/85 there was an average of 7.2 services per head, and by 2002/03 this had risen to 11.1 per head (see figure 8.4).

Figure 8.4 also shows the change in expenditure on Medicare services, showing a 356 per cent increase in expenditure from A$2.3 billion in 1984/85 to A$8.1 billion in 2002/03. The annual growth rate has varied

Figure 8.4 Australia: Trends in MBS expenditure and services per capita, 1984/85 to 2002/03

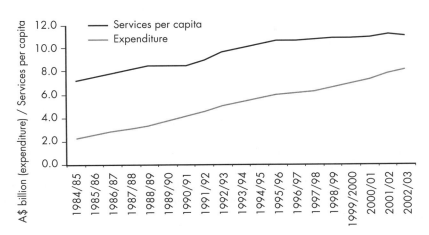

since 1985, peaking at 12 per cent in 1989/90. Later rates of growth have been much lower: around 4 to 5 per cent since 2000. Growth rates in expenditure for different types of services vary significantly (see figure 8.5).

Per capita expenditure growth has been slowest in obstetrics, the 25 per cent growth paralleling inflation over the period. In contrast, there has been a sevenfold increase in expenditure on radiation oncology, from A$0.51 per capita in 1984/85 to A$3.67 in 2002/03. This probably reflects significant change in the organisation of services: in the early Medicare years there were few privately provided services, whereas by 2002/03 there were private radiation oncology services in most states. Diagnostic imaging

Figure 8.5 Australia: Per cent growth in per capita MBS expenditure by type of service, 1984/85 to 2002/03

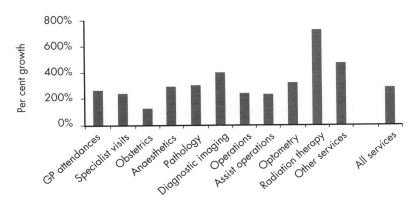

services have also increased rapidly: a fourfold increase over the period. This may reflect the introduction of new imaging modalities (for example, computed tomography, CT, and magnetic resonance imaging) that are more expensive than plain film radiography, or simply greater use of diagnostic imaging generally.

There are significant differences in per capita use between the states. For example, in 2002/03 people resident in New South Wales used an average of 11.85 Medicare services per head compared with 11.2 in Victoria and South Australia and 10.1 in Western Australia. (People resident in the Northern Territory used only 6.3 Medicare services per head. This is partly the result of the younger population in the territory, but is also the result of use of alternative ways of funding Medicare services, especially for Aboriginal and Torres Strait Islander peoples.)

The average figure of services per head masks a very wide distribution. In 2000/01, for example (the latest data available), about 18 per cent of the population did not use any Medicare services at all, with a further 9 per cent only using one service. Just over 2 per cent of the population used more than 50 Medicare services per annum. (This does not mean a weekly visit to a general practitioner as Medicare services include private inpatient services and pathology and diagnostic imaging.) Many of these very high users may have had one or more hospital inpatient episodes.

Importantly, 18.7 per cent of all services (translating to over 20 per cent of all Medicare benefits paid) were used by the 2.4 per cent of people who used more than 50 services in 2000/01; 50 per cent of MBS expenditure was consumed by the 11 per cent of the population who had more than 25 services in the year. Although about 71 per cent of all MBS services were direct billed in that year, only 65 per cent of services were direct billed for those in the highest utilisation group (those who used more than 50 MBS services), belying any argument that direct billing is associated with excess utilisation.

Some of the differences in utilisation are due to age and gender effects, as use of Medicare services follows the same pattern as hospital utilisation.

Figure 8.6 shows services per capita for males and females for 1984/85 and 2002/03. It can be seen that MBS use has a similar U-shaped curve to hospital use, with particularly high use by the elderly (Haas et al. 1996) and also increased use by women in the child-bearing years. The increase in per capita use between 1984/85 and 2002/03 is highest in older age groups.

The Commonwealth government publishes a fee schedule for the Medicare scheme annually. The schedule lists medical services and procedures and defines the rebate that will be payable by the government for these services. Most items listed on the schedule are surgical procedures, pathology investigations, or diagnostic imaging procedures. Most of the MBS expenditure, however, is for 'attendances'. The schedule distinguishes four levels of complexity for general practitioner attendance items:

Figure 8.6 Australia: Number of MBS services used per capita, by age and gender, 1984/85 and 2002/03

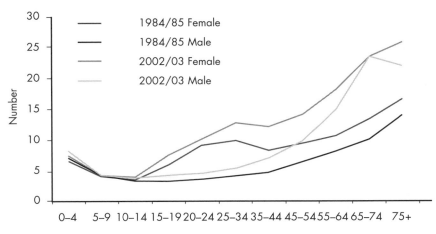

Source: Commonwealth Department of Health and Aged Care 2000

- Professional attendance for an obvious problem characterised by the straightforward nature of the task that requires a short patient history and, if required, limited examination and management.
- Professional attendance involving taking a selective history, examination of the patient with implementation of a management plan in relation to one or more problems.
- Professional attendance involving taking a detailed history, an examination of multiple systems, arranging any necessary investigations, and implementing a management plan in relation to one or more problems, and lasting at least 20 minutes.
- Professional attendance involving taking an exhaustive history, a comprehensive examination of multiple systems, arranging any necessary investigations, and implementing a management plan in relation to one or more complex problems, and lasting at least 40 minutes; or a professional attendance of at least 40 minutes duration for implementation of a management plan.

It can be seen that these items attempt to distinguish complexity of the interaction between the general practitioner and the patient. However, the items also incorporate a time-based element. Supplements are paid for home visits, attendances in hospitals and residential care facilities, and out-of-hours consultations.

Fee-for-service payments provide a strong encouragement to increase activity, with relatively weaker incentives for other desirable aspects of primary care provision (Gosden et al. 2001). A fee-for-service model is implicitly based on a 'professional' paradigm, where an individual professional has an individual relationship with an individual patient for which there is an individual payment. This is not the dominant situation in general practice today. Group practices are more common than solo practice and large for-profit chains are increasing their share of the general practice market (Catchlove 2001). Doctors working for these chains are changing their behaviour and self-perception (White 2000) and are exposed to ethical risks (Fitzgerald 2001). The increasing role of for-profit chains, motivated to ensure a return on equity, calls into question whether uncapped fee-for-service payments, extensively subsidised by government, provide the appropriate reward mechanism for the emerging industry structure.

The structure of the Medicare Benefits Schedule effectively encourages atomised practice, that is, the payment is structured to encourage short, individual patient interactions and thus de-emphasises managing the care of a single patient over months or years. Management of long-term conditions is increasingly important and this calls for a different approach to funding. Government and the medical profession have recognised the importance of introducing other modes of payments for general practitioners so as to encourage different practice patterns, the current scheme being known as the Practice Incentives Program (PIP).

Under this program, the total income for a general practice is based on a combination of fee-for-service income and other income not directly related to the number of individual consultations. This combination approach is known as 'blended payment'. Funding under the program is based on the size of the general practice, in terms of how many individuals the practice looks after, rather than the total number of separate consultations. The size measure is based on a 'Standardised Whole Patient Equivalent' (SWPE), which has two components. First, a Whole Patient Equivalent is calculated by assigning to each general practice a value of one if that general practice is responsible for all of the unreferred consultations received by the patient within a 12-month period. If the patient visits two different general practices, for the same number of consultations at each general practice, then each of those general practices would receive a half of a Whole Patient Equivalent. Each consultation is weighted by the schedule fee value for the consultation. This component of the formula thus rewards practices that provide all the care for an individual, rather than practices that typically only provide a component of care.

The Whole Patient Equivalent measure is standardised with a weighting factor according to the patient's age and gender. The weighting factor varies from a minimum of 0.57 for a five- to 14-year-old male, to a maximum of 2.29 for a female aged 75 or over. The program is premised on the expectation that the average full-time equivalent general practitioner treats about 1000 SWPEs per annum.

Eligible practices, which must meet overall quality or accreditation standards (Hays et al. 1998; Mott et al. 2000), receive a payment for each SWPE for a number of factors. The payments are designed to assist in the repositioning of general practice, to reward quality, and to recognise other important policy objectives such as enhancing use of information technology which can improve patient management (Celler 2003) and quality of care (Treweek 2003). Incentives are provided for six types of initiatives under PIP:

- upgrading of information management/information technology (for example, a payment of A\$2.00 per SWPE for use of prescribing software for the majority of prescriptions in a practice)
- after-hours care (for example, a payment of A\$6.00 per SWPE if the practice provides 24-hour coverage from within the practice)
- participating in teaching medical students
- participating in practices to encourage improved prescribing (for example, rewards for participating in clinical audits)
- employment of practice nurses (A\$7 to A\$8 per SWPE depending on location)
- disease-based incentives to provide annual check-ups, care planning for people over 65, registers to facilitate recall for follow-up, and improvements in screening rates. These incentives apply for diabetes, asthma, cervical screening, and mental health care.

Practices in rural or remote areas attract a loading of between 15 and 50 per cent on payments under PIP.

In addition to PIP, there is a separate program of general practice immunisation incentives that provides additional payments to the general practitioner for each child notified to the Australian Childhood Immunisation Register, and a tiered series of payments to practices that achieve targeted proportions of full immunisation.

Separate items (known as 'Enhanced Primary Care') are available for annual health assessments for the elderly and participation in multidisciplinary care planning and case conferences (Blakeman et al. 2001). These items, like PIP, are designed to reorient general practice away from the episodic payment approach. They have not been universally welcomed by general practitioners and are seen as detracting from professional autonomy (Marjoribanks and Lewis 2003); and in part because they are perceived to involve bureaucratic intrusion into the care process, thus deprofessionalising general practice (White 2000).

There is no restriction on what a medical practitioner can charge for a medical service provided the consumer is adequately informed. However, the Medicare rebate is based on the government's 'schedule fee'. The rebate level is 85 per cent up to a maximum gap between the rebate and the schedule fee for non-inpatient services, and 75 per cent (with no maximum gap)

Figure 8.7 Australia: Percentage of general practitioner attendances bulk billed, 1984/85 to 2002/03

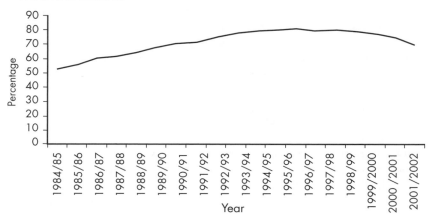

for inpatient medical services. The total patient co-payment may be greater than the maximum gap if the medical practitioner charges above the schedule fee. Medical practitioners can 'direct bill' the Health Insurance Commission (the agency responsible for administering the Medicare payments) for this full 85 per cent (or 75 per cent) of the schedule fee. Direct billing (more commonly known as bulk billing) increased each year since the introduction of Medicare up to 1996 where it peaked at around 80 per cent for all general practitioner services across Australia (see figure 8.7).

The subsequent decline in direct billing to the contemporary level of under 70 per cent of general practitioner services has been politically contentious and evinced a government policy response. As of September 2003 the government's proposals had not passed through Parliament and were the subject of review by a Senate Committee. Overall, 74.5 per cent of all medical services are charged at or below the schedule fee.

Direct billing is an important means of ensuring that consumers do not face financial barriers to access to medical care. Figure 8.8 shows the level of direct billing and observance of the schedule fee by type of service.

It can be seen that while around 70 per cent of general practitioner services are bulk billed, less than one-third of specialist attendances are direct billed. There are similarly low bulk billing and schedule fee observance rates for obstetrics, anaesthetics, and surgical operations. Consumers have a choice about whether to use private surgeons for these in-hospital services (such as operations), or have the alternative of surgery through the hospital Medicare arrangements (see chapter 6). However, for non-inpatient specialist services, the low level of bulk billing and schedule fee observance appears to affect access for people with low incomes (Scott 1997) and is a matter of concern, especially as hospitals reduce their provision of specialist outpatient services.

Figure 8.8 Australia: Percentage of services direct billed or billed at or below the schedule fee, by type of service, 2002/03

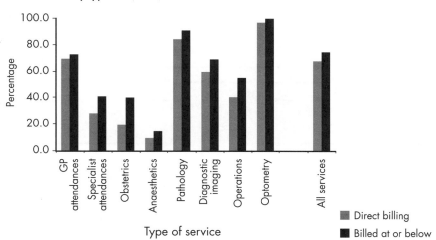

Constraining Medicare expenditure growth

The high rates of Medicare spending growth in the 1980s and early 1990s led a number of commentators to claim that Medicare spending was out of control and unsustainable. It is important to note that the MBS expenditure growth rate has substantially reduced in recent years, and these claims, if they ever were appropriate, cannot now be sustained. High expenditure growth is frequently attributed to population ageing and technology. However, analysis of trends in growth of expenditure in the past does not suggest that ageing is a critical factor. Figure 8.9 gives a breakdown of growth in expenditure on general practitioner services over the period 1985 to 2003 (see Barer et al. 1990 for an analysis of the period 1976 to 1986).

From 1984/85 to 2002/03 Commonwealth expenditure on benefits for general practitioner services (unreferred attendances) increased more than threefold (230 per cent). The main reason was the cost for each Medicare service that increased by an average of about 123 per cent, most of which is the general inflation (Consumer Price Index) effect. There was a 50 per cent increase in the number of services, attributable to an increase of 25 per cent in the population and an increase of 20 per cent in services per head. Little of the increase in per capita utilisation is due to the ageing of the population or changes in the male:female ratio.

The most critical factor in service growth is essentially unexplained practice pattern changes. Economists have suggested that medical practitioners do not simply respond to exogenous market demand, but are able to generate their own demand (see Richardson 1998b, 2001; but see Bickerdyke et al. 2002 for a more sceptical view). This suggests that as the

Figure 8.9 Australia: Factors affecting growth in expenditure on general practitioners, 1985–2003

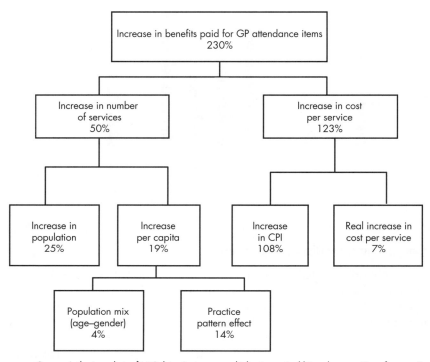

Source: Author's analysis of MBS data. Factors are multiplicative, not additive; decomposition of per capita increase in service based on all MBS items

supply of medical practitioners increases, so too will the demand for their services. Demand increases may not be accompanied by an improvement in benefit (such as improved health status) and, indeed, there is some evidence that additional supply has a perverse effect of increasing mortality rates (Richardson and Peacock 2003). Constraining supply then becomes critical to constraining service and cost growth.

Government has developed a number of strategies to constrain supply, including restrictions on internationally qualified practitioners (see chapter 4). Government has also restricted the number of medical graduates from Australian medical schools who can bill Medicare, by limiting Medicare provider numbers (which are required for billing) to those who have completed specialist postgraduate training, including training for the Fellowship of the Royal Australian College of General Practitioners (FRACGP). Previous policies had introduced higher rebates for general practitioners with the FRACGP compared to 'non-vocationally registered' practitioners.

In related moves, it has promoted accreditation programs of general practices to improve quality of care and consumer responsiveness (Hays et al. 1998; Mott et al. 2000).

Government has also undertaken a series of negotiations with different segments of the medical profession, in particular general practice, pathologists, and specialists in medical imaging (principally radiologists), to engage the profession in the effort to moderate growth in Medicare expenditure in these areas. The precise arrangement for each of these specialties varies but the common element is that the government estimates an expenditure growth factor, and if expenditure is projected to increase faster than the negotiated funding envelope (because of unexplained growth in the number of services or other reasons) then the government may adjust the schedule fee to bring the expenditure back within projections (or, in the softer version, discuss with the profession what action ought to be taken). The fact that professional groups have been willing to enter into these compacts with government is a positive sign of their willingness to address the issues in growth in per capita utilisation and in spending. The negotiated agreements with the profession also involve obligations on government such that the funding envelope would be increased for factors outside the control of the relevant specialty areas (for example, an increase in the number of internationally trained doctors being registered in Australia). These negotiated agreements represent the first examples of the medical profession sharing the risks of expenditure in terms of the risk pooling options discussed in chapters 1 and 4. These 'engagement' strategies appear to be more successful than previous strategies of using the structure of the Medicare Benefits Schedule and associated regulations to limit outlays. The structural changes were often contested politically and through the courts (Wheelwright 1994); nevertheless, the possibility or threat of structural change remains a useful component of the government's negotiating position with the professional groups.

A further strategy to restrain funding growth in the Medicare Benefits Schedule has been the development of processes to evaluate the cost-effectiveness of new technology for inclusion on the schedule (similar strategies are used in a number of other countries, see Banta 2003). Initially, this involved the Commonwealth establishing the National Health Technology Advisory Panel to give advice to government on the phasing-in of new technologies. The panel came into being in 1982 following the advice of a government committee that highlighted the possible cost implications of new technologies (Sax 1978) and the uncontrolled introduction of CT scanning into Australia. This body was subsequently replaced by the Australian Health Technology Advisory Committee with marginally different reporting relationships. The processes for technology assessment were built on the lessons learned from CT scanning where the Medicare Benefits Schedule paid a rebate based on the full average cost of a scan. Incorporating a capital component into the fee with no limit on the number of scans that could be billed for each machine allowed older machines to recoup capital payments well after the capital cost of the machine had been amortised. Funding for new technologies was revised to prevent this. Magnetic resonance imaging (MRI) was introduced in a phased way with initial Commonwealth funding only to a limited number of machines in public hospitals. Linear accelerators were regulated in a somewhat different way by separating out the capital and recurrent component of the cost and capping the amount of benefits for the capital component, based on the expected life and cost of the machine.

These processes had only limited success in regulating the introduction of new technologies (Hailey 1993, 1994, 1997; Kearney 1996), and they were not integrated into the routine processes for approval of new items on the Medicare Benefits Schedule, unlike the process for introduction of pharmaceuticals into the Pharmaceutical Benefits Scheme.

Technology assessment mechanisms were further revised in 1998 with the Commonwealth's introduction of the Medicare Services Advisory Committee, which is charged with providing advice on all proposals for new items to be added to the schedule. Advice is given on the safety, effectiveness, and cost-effectiveness of the new services and procedures. The situation faced by the Medicare Services Advisory Committee is somewhat different from the Pharmaceutical Benefits Scheme in that, unlike pharmaceuticals, there is no single advocate for a new item (a pharmaceutical manufacturer is normally required to demonstrate the cost-effectiveness of a proposed new item). Individual surgeons or professional societies may wish to propose new surgical technologies for incorporation on the schedule without the backing of a large manufacturer. The costs of undertaking rigorous evaluation and cost-effectiveness analysis thus cannot be borne by the proposer. The Medicare Services Advisory Committee has the power to recommend provisional inclusion on the Medicare Benefits Schedule to enable additional data to be collected over a defined period to facilitate cost-effectiveness analysis. Although the Medicare Services Advisory Committee has not attracted the same political attention as the Pharmaceutical Benefits Advisory Committee, its decisions are inherently political, in the sense they are about allocation of resources, and attention will need to be given to ways of managing value conflicts involved in rationing and determining levels of public subsidy (Syrett 2003).

Community health and care

Medical services and access to pharmaceuticals are complemented by a range of other community services. Some have a 'health' orientation, focusing on preventing or curing disease, while others focus on provision of other sorts of personal care. Some services, of course, do both. These services have a long history in Australia, dating back to the establishment of maternal and child health services in the early part of the twentieth century.

Development of community-based services has been patchy, and generally they have emerged in response to specific needs, rather than in response to the broader goal of providing a comprehensive first line of contact for health care. Services involving a range of professionals, such as nurses, physiotherapists, and occupational therapists, have been provided to respond to specific conditions (for example, beginning in the 1960s, community mental health teams). A generalist primary care platform only existed for primary medical care, the traditional method of providing first line access into the health system.

From the late 1960s, however, a number of reports articulated the need for a strengthened 'community health' base for the health care system (see Crouch and Colton 1983 for a New South Wales chronology; also see Sax 1972). Political expression was given to these developments in a Labor government initiative for a community health program (Hospitals and Health Services Commission 1974; De Voe 2003). The community health program was planned with extremely broad and ambitious objectives. These included the provision of:

- services that incorporate the most up-to-date knowledge and techniques available, provided by an appropriate range of medical, nursing, and allied staff
- services with an emphasis on prevention
- readily accessible primary services available equally to all, and a comprehensive range of facilities, back-up resources and supportive services coordinated according to function at local, regional, and state levels
- continuity and coordination of service
- efficient management to support the professional teams and to ensure courteous and prompt care for the public.

These community health services were expected to provide a number of components such as:

- programs of information and counselling to improve the habits, conditions, and environment that may precede disorders of health
- direct preventive action
- disease detection procedures to discover incipient or preclinical phases of disease
- information and counselling programs to motivate individuals to seek care once departures from normal health are perceived
- specific diagnostic and treatment services
- rehabilitation and supportive services for those with continuing disease and disability

- provision of help for those with chronic disability who have to adapt to sheltered living or working conditions.

The Hospitals and Health Services Commission (1974, p. 6) argued that while prevention and an emphasis on primary health care had long been recognised:

> Action to highlight preventive aspects of primary care has been inadequate and fragmented. The public clinical services that have been introduced to foster prevention are scattered, and operate in isolation from other clinical services and often from each other. They include public maternal and child health services, child guidance clinics, school health programs, family planning, occupational health, mental health, health education, venereal disease and tuberculosis services. Sporadic efforts are being made to develop counselling services aimed at particular problems such as obesity, alcoholism, or sports injuries.

The Hospitals and Health Services Commission also indicated its scepticism about the adequacy of existing primary medical care to meet these tasks:

> However, we do not have, and are never again likely to have, enough family doctors for them to undertake all the preventive tasks that are necessary—leaving aside any question as to whether they are the appropriate persons in all circumstances (1974, p. 6).

The community health program was introduced with generous cost sharing arrangements (initially 90 per cent Commonwealth funding for every 10 per cent state funding for operating costs). Despite this, states were reluctant to take up the program. In order to make it more attractive to the states, the Commonwealth developed very flexible funding guidelines. As a result, the program developed quite differently around Australia, funding community health centres with local committees of management in Victoria and South Australia, specialist mental health teams in Victoria and New South Wales, public service provision by community nurses in all states, and so on. The characteristics of the community health program were thus unique to each state, as state agreement was necessary for Commonwealth funds to flow. Although this flexibility in the program enabled the Whitlam Government to establish it, the diversity in the program between and within states left a negative legacy: the program was perceived to lack cohesion.

Following the election of the Fraser Government, expansion of the program was halted and eventually responsibility for it was transferred to the states. Prior to its election in 1983, the Labor Party promised the redevelopment of a national community health program, but implementation of this policy simply restored funding to pre-existing levels with no further expansion (Milio 1992). The new Labor Government's policy on community services focused on developing a targeted program for the aged, known as the Home and Community Care program (see below). Despite a number of subsequent efforts (for example, see National Centre for Epidemiology and Population Health 1992), there is still no coherent generalist community health or primary health care program at the national level.

Primary health care has thus developed differently in each state with different links to specialist services (such as alcohol and drug services and mental health), different regional structures, and different relationships to state government. The situation at the new millennium has returned to that identified by the Hospitals and Health Services Commission in the early 1970s of poor coordination and underdevelopment of services.

The major exception to this lack of national coherence has been the development of community services specifically for the aged. The Commonwealth government has a long-standing policy interest in provision of residential aged care facilities (discussed later in this chapter), partly stemming from its clear policy responsibility for aged pensions (and aged pensioners). Although a number of community services were funded by the Commonwealth in parallel with the residential schemes (for example, community nurses from the 1950s), there was very little policy emphasis on these services. Responsibility for community services was often placed in a different government department from that responsible for residential care. Following a series of reports in the early 1980s (see Gibson 1996 for a history of developing Commonwealth interest in this area), the Commonwealth revitalised its interest in community-based services through the establishment of the Home and Community Care program (HACC). This program was specifically designed to provide adequate community-based services in order to reduce the need for institutionalisation. It was argued in the process leading up to the funding of the HACC program that people were being accommodated unnecessarily in nursing homes because there were inadequate community-based services to maintain them in their own homes. The new emphasis on home and community care was consistent with contemporary policy directions in many countries (Baldock and Evers 1992) and represents an example of policy convergence in aged care, even though countries may have different starting points (Healy 2002). Evidence from the USA suggests that home health care contributes to reducing admissions to nursing homes and use of hospital emergency departments (McCall et al. 2002).

Community care for the aged and disabled

The HACC program provides a range of services, including community nursing, meals on wheels (delivered meals), and home help with approximately 50 per cent of expenditure sourced from the Commonwealth government and the remainder being funded by state and local government or through user charges.

Table 8.1   Australia: Instances of HACC services by assistance type, 2001/02

	Number of services	Per cent of services
Domestic assistance	196,521	15.3%
Assessment	165,085	12.8%
Case management/review	144,919	11.3%
Community nursing	132,371	10.3%
Centre-based care	123,097	9.6%
Transport	99,302	7.7%
Home maintenance/modification	95,913	7.5%
Delivered meals	87,281	6.8%
Allied health	75,519	5.9%
Personal care	55,887	4.3%
Other	111,489	8.7%
Total	1,287,384	100.0%

Source: Commonwealth Department of Health and Ageing 2002

Domestic assistance (home help) accounted for about 15 per cent of HACC services. Assessment, case management, case planning, and review together accounted for almost one-quarter of services. This high 'overhead' activity may indicate a shift into tight gate-keeping of HACC services and/or a brokerage model of service delivery.

In 2001/02 about two-thirds of HACC users were female, and 3.7 per cent were Indigenous. Fifty per cent of clients were in the age range 70 to 84, with a further 20 per cent 85 or over. Three-quarters of clients were in receipt of an age or Veterans Affairs pension, with a further 11 per cent in receipt of a disability support pension. Only 7 per cent were not in receipt of some form of government income assistance.

The community care sector is characterised by a large range of very small organisations. For example, in 1997/98 there were 2367 organisations in receipt of funding under HACC with almost 60 per cent of all HACC-funded organisations employing fewer than three staff for HACC-related activities. Such a large number of organisations can lead to problems of continuity of care. Again in 1997/98 (the latest year for which these figures are available), although 64 per cent of clients had their service needs met by one organisation, almost one-sixth of all clients were seen by three or more separate organisations.

One of the aims of any primary care service, including programs such as HACC, is to allow people to stay in their home environment as long as possible. There are two broad strategies that could be used to facilitate this objective: provision of a small amount of assistance that might be critical in assuring carers and the older person that it is possible to stay at home, or to provide intensive assistance. HACC statistics for 2001/02 suggest both strategies are at play. Just over half the HACC clients (51.8 per cent) received less than 10 hours of service; these clients accounted for 3.4 per cent of all HACC services. In contrast, 1 per cent of clients (around 5800 people) had an average of more than 10 hours of HACC services per week, and these clients consumed 21.1 per cent of all HACC services.

Unlike the market-based development of primary medical services, HACC funding is subject to planning guidelines. The allocation process involves both Commonwealth and state departments and their respective ministers, and so the potential for political priorities to enter the decision-making process is high. The program aims to achieve an equitable provision of HACC services across Australia by 2011. Since 1995 the program has established service provision targets or 'benchmarks' for evaluating allocation of resources (see Alt Statis and Associates 1994). However, there is considerable variation between and within states for many of these target areas.

Not all HACC services are reported on an hourly provision basis (for example, food services are reported in terms of meals provided, home maintenance in terms of expenditure). Figure 8.10 shows the per capita provision of HACC service types measured in hours. The base is the HACC target population: non-Indigenous people over 70 years, together with Indigenous people over 50 years.

It can be seen that overall rates of provision vary: Tasmania provides 11,739 hours of HACC service per 1000 HACC population, about 20 per cent below the national average. South Australia provides 18,843 hours per

Figure 8.10 Australia: HACC services received by state/territory, 2001/02 per 1000 HACC target population

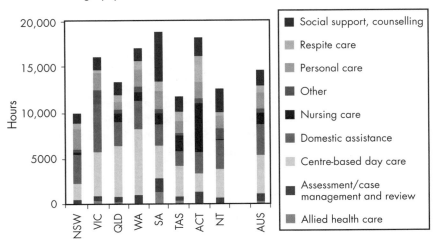

Data source: Commonwealth Department of Health and Ageing 2002

1000 HACC population, about 30 per cent above the national average and about 60 per cent greater provision than Tasmania. There are both absolute and emphasis differences in the mix of HACC services provided. Over 5000 hours of domestic assistance per 1000 HACC population is provided in Victoria, 2000 hours more than the next highest provision state (Western Australia). Almost one-third of all HACC hourly provision in New South Wales and Victoria is domestic assistance. Other states place a relatively higher emphasis on nursing care (Tasmania and the Australian Capital Territory) and centre-based care (Queensland and Western Australia).

Community Aged Care Packages (CACPs) provide a second strand of community care that parallels the HACC program. CACPs provide funding for clients who have been assessed as needing residential care but who, with a package of community services, are able to remain in the community. CACPs are thus seen administratively as direct substitutes for residential facilities and the level of provision of packages is counted in residential provision ratios for planning and funding purposes. Provision of CACPs has grown rapidly since they were introduced in 1992, and in 2002 there were 14.7 CACP packages per 1000 population over 70 (AIHW 2003b), with higher provision in remote (30 per 1000) and very remote areas (65.6 per 1000) than in major cities (13.9 per 1000). About 45 per cent of CACP clients transfer to a residential aged care service.

Evaluations by the Commonwealth Auditor-General (2000, 2002) have found deficiencies in HACC planning processes and in coordination between HACC services, and planning and other community-based programs, including CACPs.

Other specialist services

There have been several attempts to develop national programs of community services to address specific policy areas (other than the aged) including programs to assist in services for people from non-English speaking backgrounds (Kelaher and Manderson 2000), women's health services (Broom 1991), mental health services, youth services, and alcohol and drug services. Generally, these have come about in response to governmental reports, such as the Human Rights Commission Report on Youth Homelessness that led to the funding of youth health workers.

Alcohol and drug services

Alcohol and drug issues are of increasing importance as a major component contributing to the burden of disease in Australia (see Collins and Lapsley 1991, 1996 for an assessment of the cost impact of alcohol and drug use; see

Figure 8.11 Australia: Alcohol and other drugs: use, impact, and services

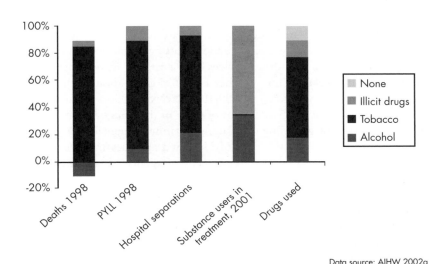

Data source: AIHW 2002a

also Senate Community Affairs References Committee 1995). The most significant alcohol and drug related risk factor is tobacco smoking which has a far greater impact on potential years of life lost than all other alcohol and drug factors combined (see figure 8.11).

Despite this, policy attention has often been directed to the scourge of 'hard' drug use and alcohol consumption, particularly among youth (for example, through the National Illicit Drug Strategy).

In 1998, almost 20,000 (19,019) deaths were attributable to tobacco consumption (Ridolfo and Stevenson 2001). There were only 1023 deaths attributable to illicit drugs. Alcohol was deemed to have a net mildly protective effect saving 2071 lives (alcohol was seen to cause over 1000 deaths from cancer, almost 1000 deaths from alcoholism and 400 deaths from road injuries but the protective effects of alcohol were seen to save almost 5000 lives yielding the net figure). Because of the different age distributions of smokers and illicit drug users and the time for smoking-related disease to impact on health, potential years of life lost from drug use was distributed quite differently from mortality. Again, tobacco was the leading cause with almost 185,000 potential years of life lost. Alcohol and illicit drugs were associated with similar levels of potential years of life lost (21,000 and 25,000 years lost respectively). Tobacco also dominated in terms of hospital separations with over 142,000 hospital separations in 1997/98 (accounting for 940,000 bed days) compared to 43,000 separations attributable to alcohol (287,000 bed days) and 14,000 separations for illicit drugs (95,000 bed days). In terms of the impact on health and burden on the health system, tobacco is the drug that causes the greatest burden.

Consumption of heroin appears to be increasing, possibly associated with increased alienation and perceived lack of opportunity among the young. A number of national campaigns have been developed to address this issue and similar strategies have been developed at state level (for a review of the 1993–97 National Drug Strategy see the report by Single 1997).

Specialist alcohol and drug services have emerged in response to these funding streams, resulting in a further lack of coordination in the primary and community care sector. In 2000/01 there were 393 specialist alcohol treatment services, about 52 per cent of these in the nongovernment sector. The distribution of government to nongovernment agencies varies significantly by state with 100 per cent of identified agencies in Victoria being nongovernment compared to 100 per cent of agencies in Tasmania being government (AIHW 2002a). A total of 83,529 clients were registered for treatment in alcohol and drug agencies with just over half being people under 30. In 2000/01, about one-third of clients were addressing problems related to alcohol, about two-thirds were related to illicit drugs, with less than 1 per cent being treated for tobacco issues. Of course, treatment for tobacco can be initiated by general practitioners or through QUIT programs. In terms of community use, a recent drug survey suggested that about 23 per cent of the community used alcohol, about 83 per cent used tobacco and about 17 per cent used illicit drugs. About 15 per cent of the population used none of those drugs.

Mental health services

As noted in chapter 6 there has been significant change in mental health services over the last decade. Specialist free-standing psychiatric hospitals have in most states been closed with services incorporated into general acute hospitals (mainstreaming). The other important mental health trend has been to increase the relative emphasis on care in the community (deinstitutionalisation). Figure 8.12 shows data on ambulatory mental health services per 1000 population (AIHW 2003e).

The most common form of interaction with the health system for mental health care is with general practitioners, at about 520 general practitioner attendances for mental health problems per 1000 population in 2000/01. The rate of general practitioner consultations is much lower in the Northern Territory and the Australian Capital Territory. In the Northern Territory this possibly relates to different provision arrangements for the Indigenous population, and in the Australian Capital Territory possibly because of the younger age distribution of the population. Specialist mental health services, for the more seriously mentally ill, are available from public and psychiatric hospitals and from private psychiatrists. There are about 100 psychiatric attendances billed on Medicare per 1000 population. Again, the Australian

Figure 8.12 Australia: Per capita provision, non-admitted mental health services, by state or territory, 2000/01

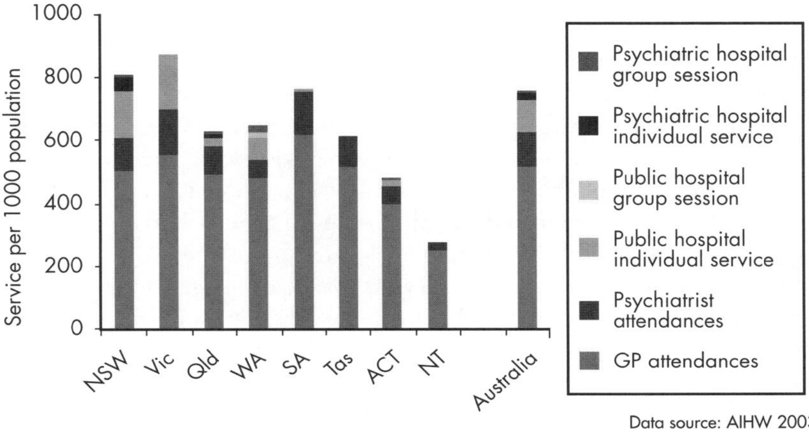

Data source: AIHW 2003e

Capital Territory and Northern Territory have somewhat lower rates than the other states but, in contrast to the rate of general practitioner attendances, Western Australia also has a low rate and Victoria a relatively high rate of private psychiatrist attendances. There is no apparent explanation for this variation.

In terms of hospital-provided services, there are significant differences in both the rate of provision between states and the mix of public acute hospitals and specialist psychiatric hospital provision. In Victoria, there are no services recorded as being provided in specialist psychiatric hospitals because all specialist psychiatric services are now part of a public acute hospital. There is again a significant difference in rates between states with New South Wales and Victoria providing around 190 and 170 services per 1000 population respectively, twice the rate in Western Australia and more than four times the rate in Queensland.

Dental services

In the two weeks prior to the National Health Survey in 2001, one in 20 Australians consulted a dentist. Dental services are provided in both the public and private sectors. Private dental practice has changed significantly over recent decades (Brennan and Spencer 2002a, 2002b) with the number of patient visits per year declining across the period. The type of visits is also changing with an increased emphasis on diagnostic and preventive services and endodontic services.

Public sector dentistry has also been subject to change. Traditionally, public dental services have been directed towards two separate subpopulations:

children and disadvantaged adults (Spencer 2001). Services for children were provided through state-based school dental services. From about the mid 1970s these services were provided by dental therapists, under the supervision of dentists. School dental services, however, vary significantly between the states. Figure 8.13 shows the extent to which dental providers have seen primary school children in the 12 months prior to December 2000.

It can be seen that the two larger states, New South Wales and Victoria, have about half the rate of school dental service visits compared to the other states. Further, school children are about 10 to 20 per cent less likely to visit any dental provider compared to other states. This can lead to substantial differences in dental health outcomes.

States provided residual dental services for disadvantaged adults for many decades, primarily associated with state dental hospitals and similar facilities. Following a review by the National Health Strategy (National Health Strategy 1992), the Commonwealth government initiated a Commonwealth dental health program in 1994 that attempted to address the contemporary problems of very long waiting lists for dental services. This program was discontinued in 1996 with the change of government (Senate Community Affairs References Committee 1998; Lewis 2000). The result has been a substantial deterioration in access to dental services for low-income adults (Spencer 2001). The Commonwealth continues to provide assistance for dental services through the Health Insurance Rebate resulting in a regressive assistance program with the insured population (generally wealthier than the uninsured population) having better access to dental services than the un-insured. The 1999 National Telephone Interview Survey revealed that 33

Figure 8.13 Australia: Primary school children dental visits in previous 12 months, 1999, by state or territory

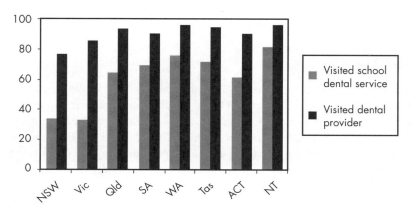

Data source: Spencer 2001

per cent of uninsured non-cardholders avoided or delayed visiting a dentist because of cost, a rate approximately twice that of the insured non-cardholder population. Similar differences occur in the cardholder population with approximately 40 per cent of the uninsured cardholder population reporting delays in dental visits (AIHW Dental Statistics and Research Unit 2002). Following the withdrawal of the Commonwealth dental health program, the states continue to provide services for disadvantaged adults but at a somewhat reduced rate relative to that previously provided with Commonwealth assistance. Dental services therefore remain a significant area of weakness for community-based provision.

Challenges for primary care services

A particular burden placed on community health services is the expectation that these services will 'reorient' the health system away from a curative, secondary, and tertiary focus, to primary health care. This rhetoric often implies, with little evidence, that such a reorientation is achievable and, moreover, will lead to savings for reinvesting in community-based services. However, the stark reality is that hospitals cost almost ten times as much as community and public health activities. As much as one may endorse the need to develop a focus on primary care, it is a recipe for failure to add reorientation objectives to the existing, quite difficult tasks faced by these services. Further, it is undesirable public policy to assume that the health budget is in some way a zero sum game, and that all expansion in public and community health provision should be at the expense of hospital services.

Although there is scope for reallocation of resources within the health budget, this is a politically and industrially difficult task. As was pointed out in chapter 3, the total amount of money spent on health services is identically related to the incomes generated in the health sector. Significant interests are thus affected by funding policy premised only on redistribution within the sector. If one assesses the need for additional spending in an economic framework, so long as cost-effectiveness ratios for new investments in community and public health show that they are warranted, the funding can come from any other area of society where the cost-effectiveness ratios are not so favourable.

Coordinated care

During the mid 1990s there was increasing recognition by governments that services for people with complex care needs were deficient in terms of availability, the complexity of funding arrangements, and the organisation of those services that were available. The government response was to experiment with a new form of organisation involving pooling funds from a number of different funding sources. The experiment, known as the Australian Coordinated Care Trials, was planned during a time of considerable state dissatisfaction with Commonwealth–state relations in health. This was most trenchantly expressed by Paterson (1996) who argued that there were 60 separate Commonwealth funding programs with little coordination, resulting in wasted money and unmet needs. Of course, program boundaries can create problems for service delivery even in unitary countries such as the United Kingdom (Pritchard and Hughes 1995).

The political argument was that the rigid Commonwealth program boundaries were leading to waste and were inhibiting effective service coordination at the local level. The Coordinated Care Trials offered the prospect of sweeping away all Commonwealth program boundaries at the local level, including allowing pooling of funds that would otherwise have been expended under the Medicare Benefits Scheme and the Pharmaceutical Benefits Scheme.

The coordinated care intervention was defined as follows: 'Coordinated care is the explicit process of planning and organising the provision of services through the pooling of funds, within current resource levels, and the development of agreed individual care plans for people who have difficulty accessing appropriate services and/or self-managing their care needs over a period of time' (Leigh et al. 1999, p. 8).

It can be seen that the intervention has a number of key elements. First, there is an explicit process of planning the provision of services; second, it involves pooling of funds within current resource levels; and third, there is development of agreed individual care plans. The target group is defined as those people who have difficulty accessing appropriate services and/or self-managing their care needs. There is an expectation that the populations will be chronically ill ('have needs over a long period of time'). (Descriptions of the funded trials may be found in Leigh et al. 1999.)

Care coordination in the trials was achieved with two main strategies: strengthening the role of general practitioners; or adding a new position of care coordinator. The latter strategy had the most impact, partly because the care coordinator knew better the range of services available and had more time to link beneficial services and patients. Patients valued the care coordinator's experience, especially because they knew whom to contact and who could provide assistance in organising disparate services (Commonwealth Department of Health and Aged Care 2001).

However, the addition of the care coordinator role did not clearly lead to measurable improvements in health or well-being compared to the control groups. Further, savings from improved coordination could not fund the care coordinator role: it added to costs without a commensurate improvement in benefit.

Despite these negative results, the Coordinated Care Trials have been valuable. Unlike many public sector reform processes in Australia, the development of coordinated care was specifically designed to provide empirical evidence for evaluation of the new policy. The evaluation of the trials was one of the largest health service research projects undertaken in Australia to date and provided a model for evidence potentially informing the policy process.

The Coordinated Care Trials addressed an important system issue, and they may yet contribute to the design of new forms of organisation and funding to meet the needs of the chronically ill. Certainly, the flexibility shown by the Commonwealth in allowing the pooling of MBS and PBS funding is an encouraging sign that Commonwealth–state barriers to high quality service delivery are being dismantled.

Residential care

Residential aged care facilities (until 1997 distinguished as 'nursing homes' and 'hostels') are designed to meet the needs of frail elderly people who can no longer stay at home, even with access to the community support services described earlier in this chapter. Residential care has been subject to two major waves of reform: in the mid 1980s, which involved major restructure of funding, and in the late 1990s to increase consumer co-payments (Gibson

Figure 8.14 Australia: Per cent distribution of residential aged care places by type of ownership of facility and state, 30 June 2002

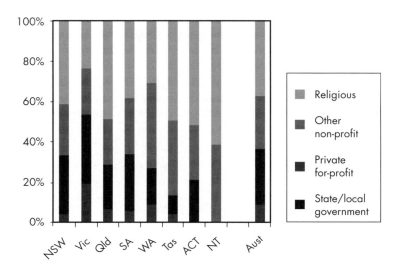

1998; Howe 1998). These changes have also been accompanied by strategies to improve quality of care and strengthen residents' rights (Gibson et al. 1993).

As at 30 June 2002, there were 2961 residential aged care facilities approved by the Commonwealth Department of Health and Ageing providing a total of 144,695 places (an average of 54 places per facility). (The data in this section are drawn from AIHW 2003h.)

Almost three-quarters of all residential aged care places are in government or not-for-profit facilities: facilities operated by religious groups provide 37.5 per cent of all places (see figure 8.14). State and local government provide about 10 per cent of all places.

There is significant difference in the pattern of ownership across the different states. Religious groups provide almost half of all places in Queensland and Tasmania and more than half in the two territories. State and local government provide one-fifth of the places in Victoria, double the provision ratio of any other state.

There are two major sources of funding to support people in residential facilities: a Commonwealth subsidy, which varies with the resident's dependency and need for care, and a patient contribution, the latter in part recognising that residential facilities provide food and shelter that residents would need to pay for wherever they lived.

Government residential care subsidies

The resident's need for care is measured using the Resident Classification Scale (RCS), a continuous scoring system that provides the basis for the eight steps in the differential daily payments to residential care facilities (see table 8.2).

Table 8.2   Basic residential aged care facility subsidy per resident per day (from 1 July 2003)

RCS level	Subsidy per resident per day	Per cent distribution of permanent residents as at 30 June 2002	Per cent distribution of new admissions, 1 July 2001 to 30 June 2002
RCS1*	$115.80–$120.26	18.9	16.9
RCS2*	$105.00–$108.94	25.3	25.8
RCS3*	$90.46–$93.96	14.8	15.8
RCS4*	$63.94–$66.86	4.6	4.4
RCS5	$38.95	10.5	10.8
RCS6	$32.27	10.8	11.4
RCS7	$24.77	13.8	13.8
RCS8	0	1.4	1.1

*Note for 'high care' levels 1-4, the rate depends on state/territory: Queensland, South Australia, Western Australia, and the ACT are on the lowest rate, Tasmania the highest.

The scale value is determined by a scoring system of 20 questions that take into account the resident's communication, mobility, personal hygiene, toileting, bowel management, whether they are physically aggressive, and medication requirements. Specific points are allocated to each type of answer, and a resident with more than 81.0 points is assigned to classification level 1, 69.61 to 81.0 points classification level 2, and so on. Residents with less than 10.6 points are assigned to classification level 8; these residents are not eligible for a care subsidy from the Commonwealth. Categories 1–4 represent high care (formerly restricted to nursing homes) and categories 5–8 represent low care (hostels). There are a number of weaknesses with the RCS, most notably that transformation of a continuous scale into a set of discrete payment rates creates strong incentives for up-coding at the margins. A further weakness is that scale weights are no longer seen as having face validity. The RCS is being reviewed (September 2003) and should be replaced by a new categorisation system in the medium term (Aged Care Evaluation and Management Advisors 2003).

Table 8.2 shows the distribution of residents across the RCS categories both in terms of permanent residents as at 30 June 2002 and admissions in the previous year. In both the 'high care' and 'low care' ranges there is a tendency for the admissions to be marginally lower dependency than permanent residents. This would be consistent with residents deteriorating over time.

Supplements are paid to facilities where 'concessional' residents are up to 40 per cent of bed days (A$7.87 per day) or over 40 per cent of bed days (A$13.49 per day). Resident-related supplements are also paid for oxygen treatment (A$8.21 per day), and enteral feeding. Facility-related supplements are also paid (for example, for facilities in isolated or remote areas).

Residential care subsidies are indexed but it appears that the indexation factor applied is not appropriate for the costs faced in residential care provision and funding levels are becoming inadequate (McCallum and Mundy 2002).

Residents' payments

The resident's payment consists of two major components: a basic daily care charge and a contribution to the capital costs of the facility. Maximum resident payments are specified by the Commonwealth and depend on the resident's income (for daily charges) and assets (for capital-related payments). Although a limited number of facilities that provide a higher level of amenity are exempt from the specification of maximum resident contributions, most places in residential care facilities are subject to Commonwealth-specified fee maxima. These maximum fees differentiate between:

- full pensioners, who as from 1 July 2003 face a maximum daily care fee of A$25.73

- part pensioners, who face an ordinary daily care fee of A$25.73 and a further income-tested fee of up to A$19.91 per day
- nonpensioners ('self-funded retirees'), who face an ordinary daily care fee of up to A$32.12 and an income-tested fee of up to A$45.07 per day.

There are some transitional provisions for people who were receiving hostel level care (RCS levels 5–7) prior to 1 October 1997.

In addition to the contribution to the day-to-day costs of a residential facility, residents may also be required, subject to an assets test, to contribute an accommodation charge (for high level care, RCS 1–4) or 'bond' (lower level care). The accommodation charge or bond effectively provides additional working capital to the residential facility proprietor and is thus analogous to a contribution to the capital costs of the facility. Residents of residential care facilities who require high level care with assets in excess of an indexed threshold (A$27,500 at 1 July 2003) may be asked to pay a capital-related accommodation charge. The maximum accommodation charge is set on a sliding scale and for residents with assets in excess of A$52,886 is A$13.91 per day. The accommodation charge can be levied for a maximum of five years.

Residents in low-level care with assets in excess of the threshold can be asked to pay an accommodation bond, the balance of which is refunded if the resident dies in a residential facility. The provider can take a maximum of A$254.50 monthly for the first five years out of this capital amount but may also retain the interest earned on the full amount for the full period of care.

The limits for asset tests are based on the basic age pension (for example the minimum permissible asset value that a resident may maintain after paying an accommodation bond is set at 2.5 times the basic annual pension per annum). A resident's home is not included in the asset test if the resident's spouse or dependent child is living there or in other special circumstances (for example, another close relative lives there).

Assessment

All proposed residents of aged care facilities need to be approved by an Aged Care Assessment Service (ACAS), a multidisciplinary team funded by the Commonwealth Department of Health and Ageing that assesses applicants. The assessment process takes into account whether the person could be maintained in his or her own home with other forms of support.

Even though ACASs have been set up with funding from the Commonwealth to undertake similar tasks, there is considerable variation in the pattern of decision making of the services. In particular, ACASs in different states have different rates of assessment (in terms of the percentage of the elderly population assessed) and place of assessment (assessing clients in their home versus in residential care). There are also significant differences in the rates of recommendations for residential care versus community services (Kung 1996). To some extent these differences may reflect differences in the environment. For example, Victorian ACASs have significantly higher rates of referral to community services than New South Wales ACASs, which may be a result of better availability of services and Victoria's stronger culture of community-based aged care services.

Commonwealth policy has been to discourage residents with low care needs being accommodated in funded facilities and there has been a decline in residents classified as category 8 and equivalent in recent years: a decline from 16 per cent in 1994 to 1.4 per cent in 2002.

Because all residents in residential care facilities attract a Commonwealth benefit, the Commonwealth has established planning guidelines for approving new facilities. The guidelines are designed to limit the number of funded places to no more than 100 places per 1000 population over 70 (as indicated earlier, these ratios include provision of Community Aged Care Packages). The extent to which Community Aged Care Packages and residential aged care places are indeed substitutes is a moot point, but they are probably not substitutes to meet the needs of more dependent persons requiring access to high level residential aged care; as shown in table 8.2, 42 per cent of those entering high level residential care are in the two highest dependency groups.

The mix of places and packages has changed significantly over the last decade, with packages meeting 15 per cent of the available provision. Concomitantly, the availability of residential aged care places has declined significantly (see figure 8.15; these data are on operational aged care places

Figure 8.15 Australia: Operational residential aged care places and Community Aged Care Packages per 1000 persons 70 and over, 1995–2002

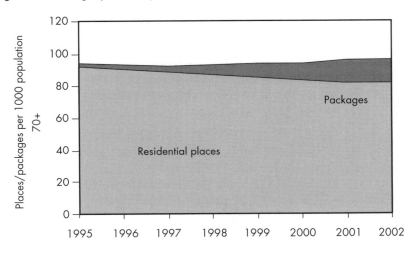

Table 8.3 Australia: Residential aged care places and Community Aged Care Packages per 1000 persons aged 70 years and over, state/territory by geographical area, 30 June 2002

	Major cities	Inner regional	Outer regional	Remote	Very remote	Total (70+)	Total (70+ and Indigenous population aged 50–69)
Places							
NSW	80.0	89.5	68.9	47.5	2.1	81.0	79.4
VIC	75.9	85.8	81.5	68.8		78.5	78.0
Qld	81.0	96.3	86.0	65.4	62.8	85.9	83.1
WA	80.9	95.1	84.6	63.1	94.8	82.8	79.9
SA	85.4	80.5	76.6	71.1	145.8	83.7	82.6
Tas		111.4	22.6	69.0		82.3	79.8
ACT	76.1					76.1	75.2
NT			78.3	163.3	109.4	103.3	51.0
Australia	*79.6*	*91.6*	*73.7*	*69.2*	*78.5*	*81.6*	*79.9*
Packages							
NSW	13.9	17.4	13.5	13.0	10.3	14.7	14.4
VIC	14.8	15.1	5.9	18.2		14.3	14.2
Qld	12.2	13.3	17.4	37.6	42.8	14.0	13.5
WA	12.6	22.1	14.9	34.6	29.2	14.8	14.3
SA	13.9	25.1	10.0	15.3	36.8	14.9	14.7
Tas		21.0	3.0	26.2	1	5.3	14.8
ACT	18.4					18.4	18.2
NT			39.1	98.3	282.5	95.9	47.3
Australia	*13.9*	*16.7*	*12.5*	*30.0*	*65.6*	*14.7*	*14.4*
Total							
NSW	93.9	106.9	82.3	60.6	12.3	95.7	93.8
VIC	90.6	100.9	87.4	86.9	92.7	92.2	96.7
Qld	93.1	109.6	103.3	103.1	105.7	99.9	94.2
WA	93.4	117.2	99.5	97.7	124.0	97.6	97.3
SA	99.3	105.6	86.6	86.4	182.5	98.6	94.6
Tas		132.3	25.7	95.2		97.7	93.4
ACT	94.6					94.5	
NT	117.4	261.6	391.9	199.2	98.4		
Australia	**93.4**	**108.4**	**86.2**	**99.2**	**144.1**	**96.4**	**94.3**

Source: AIHW 2003h

and packages and thus provide the best guide of the experience of families and carers in trying to gain access to a residential care place or a community aged care package compared to data on funded places/packages). At 30 June 2002, there were 81.6 places per 1000 aged 70 and over, almost 10 per cent below the provision ratio of 89.2 five years earlier, suggesting consumers are facing greater difficulties in gaining access to needed residential care (Gibson and Liu 1995). Although the time period between assessment and entry into a residential care facility is more than a month shorter for those assessed in hospitals, the median entry lag for in-hospital assessed residents is 20 days (AIHW 2002b), creating substantial opportunity costs for hospitals and leading to political conflict between the Commonwealth government with funding responsibility for residential care and state governments with direct responsibility for hospitals.

Although the Commonwealth planning guidelines aim to ensure a relatively even distribution of provision across states and by geographic area, the residential aged care places provision ratio varies from 91.6 per 1000 people aged 70 and over in major regional cities to 69.2 in remote areas (see table 8.3). There is also a variation between states with Victoria having 78.5 places per 1000 aged 70 and over, relative to the Queensland ratio of 83.1. The residential care planning process was reviewed by the Commonwealth Auditor-General (1998) who recommended a number of changes to the contemporary process, including stronger links with nonresidential (HACC) provision for aged care.

As would be expected, the likelihood of being accommodated in a residential aged care facility increases with age.

Figure 8.16 Australia: Age- and sex-specific utilisation rates (per 1000 population) for residential aged care by English-speaking status, 2001/02

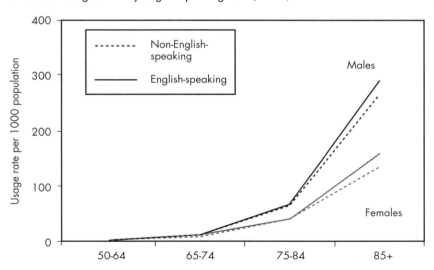

There is substantial variability in the average availability rate of 80 places per 1000 population (see figure 8.16). Males have higher rates of residence than females, English-speaking people have higher rates than people from a non-English speaking background, and there is a threefold difference in residence rates between the 85 and older population compared to the 75- to 84-year-old group. However, even for 90-year-olds, most people in this age group are living in the community. The increasing rates with age have important consequences for planning ratios. The current ratios use the population 70 and over as a denominator, but the 85 and over group are increasing as a proportion of this population and their rate of use is markedly above the younger group in the denominator population. As shown in figure 8.15, total package plus CACP provision per 1000 population has been constant over the last decade. However, the ageing of the population may have effectively reduced access relative to need, and access will reduce further given relative growth in the older-old versus younger-old over the next few decades (Giles et al. 2003).

The average length of stay in a nursing home is between one and two years. Figure 8.17 shows the number of residents by the period spent in a residential facility.

The figure also shows the disposition of residents. It can be seen that for short stays about one-tenth of residents return to the community, but for the majority of residents, the reason for 'leaving' a residential care facility is death (about three in four residents who stay less than four weeks die in the residential facility, rising to nine out of 10 residents who have a stay of more than five years).

Figure 8.17 Australia: Duration of stay of permanent residents in nursing homes, by mode of separation, 1 July 2001 to 30 June 2002

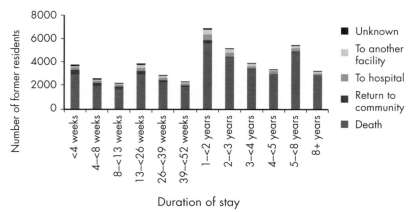

Source: AIHW 2000b

Quality of residential aged care

The quality of residential aged care facilities is supervised by the Aged Care Standards and Accreditation Agency (established under the Aged Care Act 1997) which has responsibility for managing accreditation for all Commonwealth-funded residential aged care services, including monitoring of standards of care for services that are not accredited. The accreditation process in aged care is somewhat similar to that in hospitals (see chapter 6) and includes a self-assessment program together with a visit by assessors appointed by the agency.

The current accreditation framework includes four main elements:
* accreditation standards
* certification of the quality of buildings
* concessional and assistant resident ratios
* prudential arrangements.

The four accreditation standards as specified by the government include:
1 management systems, staffing and organisational development
2 health and personal care
3 residential lifestyle
4 physical environment and safe systems.

In all, there are 44 'expected standards' for these areas (nine outcomes in management, 17 in health, 10 in lifestyle, eight in environment) with explicit criteria specified for each outcome. A four-level rating system is applied (commendable, satisfactory, unacceptable, and critical) with a set of decision rules being published to identify the criteria for awarding each level.

Contemporary policy issues in aged and residential care

In 1996 the Commonwealth embarked on an 'Aged Care Reform' program, in part designed to increase capital funding for residential facilities through increased consumer co-payments, using accommodation bonds. The policy was vehemently opposed by consumers and was largely reversed by late 1997 (Howe 1999) but key elements, including accommodation bonds in a more electorally palatable form, were retained and have since been favourably evaluated (Gray 2001). The underlying purpose of the program was to increase the poor capital stock of nursing homes. The likely cause of this problem was a 'capital strike' by proprietors rather than government underfunding as had been argued by the industry and implicitly assumed by government as the basis of its policy. (Transfer prices for nursing home licences were high before and after the reforms, belying arguments about underfunding; see also Howe 1998.) Given the strong public reaction against the 1996 changes, government is unlikely to attempt a similar strategy for some time.

The current policy provides incentives on residential care facilities to have at least 40 per cent of the places occupied by financially disadvantaged people. The incentive payment appears to be inadequate and some adjustment to funding levels and policy to ensure equitable access for people on low incomes is now necessary.

Australia's long-term care policy has been relatively stable since the early 1980s: an emphasis on expanding HACC and reining in growth of residential care. This policy has been remarkably successful and Australia is not facing an unsustainable increase in its institutionalised elderly population (see Howe 1999). However, cracks are appearing in the system and there are increasing calls for system reform (Kendig and Duckett 2001). One of the most systematic calls for reform has come from the independent Myer Foundation (no date) which has proposed reforms to community care (increasing funding; improving equity; improving efficiency by developing comprehensive care providers), housing (improving funding arrangements for home modification/home maintenance; developing new community housing options for frail older people), and in administration, funding, and planning.

Informal care

Informal caring is an important aspect of communities and a particularly important but often unrecognised and undervalued part of the structure of community services. Formal structures of care do not provide all of the health and personal care that is required to maintain people in the community: a significant proportion of care is provided by families, and friends of carers. Figure 8.18 shows data from the Disability, Ageing and Carers survey (ABS 1999b) on the extent to which assistance is being provided to people with disabilities.

It can be seen that people with lower levels of core activity limitations do not receive assistance at the same level as people with higher levels of core limitation. For example, 82 per cent of people with a profound or severe disability were reported as requiring assistance, relative to 30 per cent of people with a mild core activity limitation. Importantly, for all levels of activity limitation, there is a very high proportion of people who receive informal assistance. Ninety-seven per cent of all those with a profound or severe core activity limitation receive some kind of informal assistance. About 40 per cent of all carers are partners of the person being cared for, about 25 per cent a child, and about 20 per cent a parent.

In every disability category, the number of people receiving informal assistance is greater than those receiving formal assistance, that is, the informal network in communities, including the family and friends of disabled people, is assisting more people in the community than the formal

Figure 8.18 Australia: Assistance provided to people with disabilities, by nature of activity limitation and type of provider, 1998

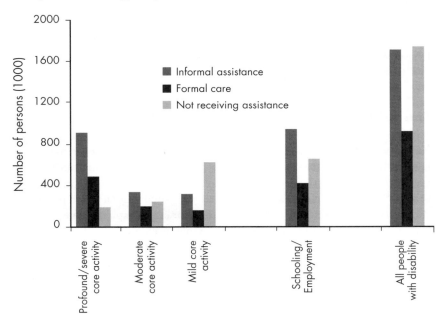

Type of activity limitation

structures. The nature of the assistance provided may be different, but for many people a significant number of hours of care is provided. Almost half of the primary carers of people with a profound disability spent more than 40 hours per week in providing care.

It is important to stress that this voluntary and informal care is a significant and important contribution to the overall assistance being provided to people with disabilities. There is an economic cost to this care provision, especially in terms of the opportunity cost of lost wages or salaries. To some extent, informal care is a replacement for, rather than a complement to, more formal caring arrangements.

In recognition of these opportunity costs, an income and asset tested carer payment equivalent to the age pension has been introduced. The carer payment is paid in circumstances, for example where a carer provides full-time care to an adult with a long-term and severe disability who would otherwise need full-time professional care, or, for example where a carer looks after a dependent child with a profound disability or medical condition. Carers are also assisted by the availability of respite programs in residential care facilities (see Department of Human Services and Health, Aged

Care and Community Care Division 1996 for papers discussing several aspects of policy on carers).

There is probably a large amount of care provided for short-term needs after a person is discharged from an acute hospital. Unfortunately, this type of caring is often taken for granted by the health system, even when the person does not have the family and informal network that is assumed by the discharge policies of many hospitals.

The future of primary and community care

As shown earlier in this chapter, most contacts are with the primary care level of the health care system. However, there is no systematic information on how 'acceptable' the care provided is, nor on the quality of care. Despite this, consumers often develop fierce loyalties to their primary care providers. Providers who make their careers in this sector stay (despite problems in the system) out of a commitment to their patients or clients.

The structural arrangements for care provision vary dramatically across the primary care sector: general practice and specialist medical care involves autonomous private providers with a substantial public subsidy. Aged care provision is dominated by not-for-profit or government agencies. The different structures have different effects on equity. Consumer co-payments are regulated in the aged care sector, but medical practitioners make independent decisions about the level of out-of-pocket costs that their patients will face.

Policy makers lament the paucity of nationally comparable data on this sector, which is localised and varies from state to state and, sometimes, even municipality to municipality. In part, this variability arises from policy-driven issues such as open-ended funding for particular forms of care, and underprovision of some services in some areas. But in part it arises from the nature of the task.

Each patient with a chronic health problem will differ in terms of how much the problem restricts their enjoyment of life, how much family and social support they can count on, what other health problems they suffer, and what sorts of care matter most to them. The more individualised the set of services a patient requires, the less likely it is that a single agency or program can provide all the components. Both comprehensiveness and specialisation are valuable aspects of a health service, but to an extent they are incompatible: a single provider or agency will maximise the coherence of care for an individual, but may sacrifice a degree of specialisation. Conversely, having multiple professional perspectives on a health care problem (nursing, medical, and occupational therapist, for example) will have benefits for patients, but may result in gaps and overlaps in care, or at the very least, higher time-costs to ensure coordination, and information loss and potential loss of alignment of goals as weaknesses in care continuity (Scott 2000; Donaldson 2001).

Policy prescriptions rarely take these intrinsic characteristics of community-based health care into account, seeking single, tidy solutions. Figure 8.19 attempts to distinguish how features of this sector have led to the current complex set of programs, how they interact, and which are amenable to policy intervention.

Figure 8.19 Reasons for underdevelopment of primary and community care

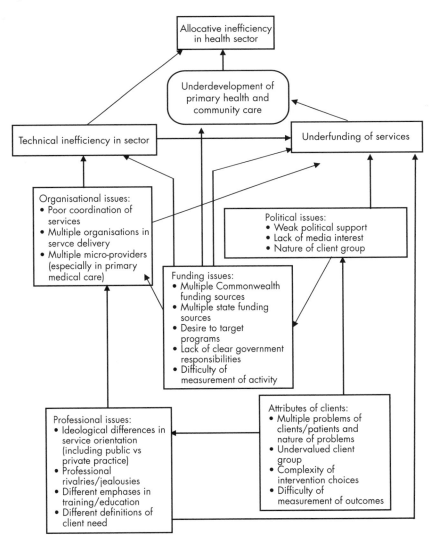

It is important to stress that one of the factors contributing to the weakness of this sector is the nature of the sector itself. Even though primary and community care services are the most frequently used in the health system, they are not glamorous, rarely attract media attention, and thus there is little pressure for political action to improve these services. The most frequent users of primary and community care include the most devalued members of society, including the elderly and people with chronic illnesses and disabilities. Many of the problems being addressed by primary care providers are complex, leading to difficulties in measuring the work of the sector.

A second cluster of causes relate to funding issues: there are multiple Commonwealth and state funding sources, which almost inevitably means there are multiple agencies involved in service provision. Multiple agencies may create problems of coordination (Fine 1995), although as discussed earlier in this chapter, almost two-thirds of clients of the Home and Community Care program deal with only one agency. Other aspects of the structure of provision also create service delivery problems. Because of the multiple nature of the problems of clients, there are a range of professionals involved in the sector with different training, different orientations, and different emphases in treatment. These provider differences are often accompanied by professional rivalries and jealousies about the relative worth of their skills and training, rivalries that may be overlaid by ideological differences between those involved in the private sector (including private practice) and those in public or not-for-profit organisations (Swerissen et al. 2001). The poor coordination of services leads to technical inefficiency in the sector and this further reduces the likelihood that governments will make additional funding available (the argument being that the sector should improve its efficiency before additional funding is granted). However, even if the sector were to become perfectly efficient, it is likely that additional investment in primary and community care services would still be warranted.

Tackling the underfunding requires addressing all of the causative factors and the links between them. Addressing only one causative factor (such as poor coordination) and leaving unaddressed the need to improve the working relationships between professionals and the multiple Commonwealth and state funding sources will not lead to long-term improvement as financial and personal incentives will continue to reduce the effectiveness of the coordination strategies. This is not to say that it is not worthwhile addressing coordination (or indeed any other aspect of the primary and community care sector), rather what is being argued is that addressing the chronic underdevelopment of the sector requires a series of interventions addressing each of these causative elements.

A number of contemporary policies for strengthening primary health and community care focus on addressing multiple funding sources through Commonwealth–state funds pooling (and associated capitated payments) or consolidating multiple funding sources at Commonwealth or state levels. These strategies by themselves will not improve coordination or redress the underdevelopment of the sector. Funds pooling and other macro strategies are often proposed as magic wands that will fix local coordination problems. However, as experience with the Coordinated Care Trials has shown, it is extremely difficult to design new local service delivery structures that lead to measurably improved outcomes for clients.

In the absence of 'magic solutions', underdevelopment in the sector will continue. The quixotic quest for a perfectly coordinated system obviously ignores service reality: strengthening some interrelationships necessarily weakens others. Strong coordination of community and inpatient mental health services inevitably implies weaker links between community mental health and generalist community services and between inpatient psychiatry and other inpatient services. As Leutz (1999, p. 83) paraphrases Abraham Lincoln: 'You can integrate some services for all of the people or all services for some of the people but you can't integrate all services for all of the people.'

In the long term, a well-functioning primary and community care sector is necessary to provide a solid base for the other structures of care provision (secondary and tertiary care), and to facilitate systematic localised public health services. A well-structured primary and community care platform could facilitate the national delivery of health promotion programs, ensure a more efficient skill mix in service delivery, provide for coordinated policy development so that problems of key groups are addressed rather than falling through responsibility gaps (Howe 1997), and hopefully lead to prevention of unnecessary secondary and tertiary care.

A critical issue to be faced in redesign of the sector is the relative role of various professions. It was argued in chapter 4 that critical issues for the future of both the medical and nursing profession relate to the role of the professional. The debate on relative roles is likely to be played out most vigorously in the primary and community care sector. There are obviously some generic roles that are involved in any care provision, as discussed earlier with respect to the future of the medical profession. Addressing issues about relative roles will be facilitated by a restructure of the primary and community care sector. This would provide opportunities to create a broader role for nurses in the sector, and would facilitate nurses working closely with medical practitioners in multiprofessional teams. This, in turn, can only effectively take place if the concept of the sole general practitioner as the foundation stone for medical practice is replaced by a larger multiprofessional group practice (Brand 1996).

There are clearly many questions about restructuring primary and community care. To what extent would the restructure be the same in rural and urban areas? To what extent can financial incentives be used to overcome some of the professional rivalry factors? To what extent is joint Commonwealth–state action necessary to facilitate restructure? In the longer term, a restructure is inevitable. What needs to be debated is the nature, staging, and phasing of such a restructure.

Overall, weaknesses in the primary and community care sector can create problems for the health sector as a whole. A weak primary care sector can mean that health problems are not detected early with resultant increased costs for secondary and tertiary care (Bindman et al. 1995). This results in allocative inefficiency in the health care system as a whole.

9

Pharmaceuticals

Taking a prescription or nonprescription medication is the most common health care activity undertaken by Australians. Australian Health Survey data show that almost 70 per cent of the Australian population used some form of medication in the two weeks prior to interview. (These data are from the 1995 survey; unfortunately the later 2001 survey did not include a question on medication use in the population.) The most common form of medication use was vitamins or minerals (see figure 9.1).

Just over a quarter of the population (258 persons per 1000) used vitamins or minerals in the two weeks prior to interview. The second most common form of medication used was pain relievers (236.2 persons per 1000) followed by medications for heart problems or blood pressure (105.8

Figure 9.1 Australia: Use of medication during previous two weeks by type of medication, 1995 (rate per 1000 population)

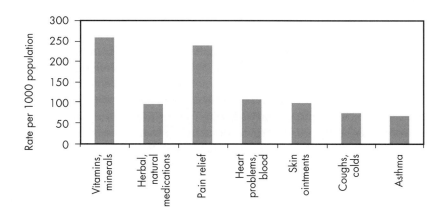

persons per 1000). Use of these medications is not necessarily preceded by any form of medical or other health professional advice and many of these medications (for example, vitamins and herbal medications) do not attract any form of government rebate.

Over two-thirds of encounters with general practitioners involve recommendations about medication, most of these involving prescription medication (Britt et al. 2001); 38.7 per cent of encounters involved one prescription, 13.6 per cent involved two, and 7.5 per cent more than two (40.2 per cent of encounters involved no prescription).

Australia has adopted a National Medicines Policy to guide policy development with respect to pharmaceuticals (Harvey and Murray 1995). Key planks of the policy are:

• timely access to the medicines that Australians need, at a cost to individuals and that the community can afford
• medicines meeting appropriate standards of quality, safety, and efficacy
• quality use of medicines
• maintaining a responsible and viable medicine industry (Commonwealth Department of Health and Aged Care 1999c).

Principal responsibility for the National Medicines Policy rests with the Commonwealth government. The main mechanism for ensuring access to medicines is the Commonwealth's Pharmaceutical Benefits Scheme (PBS). Quality, safety, and efficacy of medicines are regulated through the Therapeutic Goods Administration (TGA). Quality use of medicines involves a range of policies in terms of educational programs, provision of consumer information, and so on. The responsible and viable medicines industry component is achieved through the pharmaceutical industry support program.

Assuring quality, safety, and efficacy: regulatory control

The path from invention to sale of a medication in Australia involves a number of separate regulatory steps (see table 9.1). The regulatory process is a contentious one with manufacturers and others claiming that it has too many barriers and is inefficient, although this view is not confirmed in independent reviews (for example, see Auditor-General 1996, 1997). Regulatory style varies across countries (Wiktorowicz 2003) but tighter regulation may, paradoxically encourage a domestic pharmaceutical industry and strengthen its ability to compete internationally (Scherer 2000, p. 1313).

The TGA, a division of the Commonwealth Department of Health and Aged Care, has principal responsibility for assuring the quality, safety, and efficacy of all products that make therapeutic claims. The evaluation process by the TGA includes premarket assessment (evaluation for quality, safety,

Table 9.1   Issues/roles of approval processes for new drugs in Australia

Issue	Regulatory Body	Regulatory Outcome
Is this a new drug?	Patent and Design Office; part of IP Australia	Patent protection for 20 years
Is the drug safe and efficacious?	Therapeutic Goods Administration (TGA); part of Commonwealth Department of Health and Aged Care	Approval for sale in Australia
Are there untoward outcomes of use of the drug?	Adverse Drug Reactions Advisory Committee	Possible withdrawal from sale
Is the drug cost-effective?	Pharmaceutical Benefits Advisory Committee	Approval for listing/subsidy under Pharmaceutical Benefits Scheme
What should government pay for a drug when first listed under the Pharmaceutical Benefits Scheme?	Pharmaceutical Benefits Pricing Authority (payment to manufacturer)	Recommendation on price to be paid for drug and fee for dispensing by pharmacist
	Pharmaceutical Benefits Remuneration Tribunal (dispensing fee to pharmacists)	
Is the price appropriate given use	Department of Health and Aged Care	Possible renegotiation of price

and efficacy); licensing of manufacturers; and postmarket vigilance. Some life-saving products for individual or experimental use can bypass this regulation under a 'Clinical Trials Notification' scheme.

The premarket assessment takes into account factors such as the strength of the product, possible side effects, potential harm through prolonged use, toxicity, and the seriousness of the medical condition for which the product is intended to be used. The Australian Drug Evaluation Committee advises the TGA in this process. Following premarket assessment, the TGA registers the product on the Australian Therapeutic Goods Register. There are about 7000 to 9000 applications for registration each year. The Therapeutic Goods Act 1989 has adopted a wide definition of therapeutic goods covering those products that are used for humans in:

- preventing, diagnosing, curing, or alleviating a disease
- influencing, inhibiting, or modifying a physiological process
- testing the susceptibility of persons to a disease
- influencing, controlling, or preventing conception
- testing for pregnancy, and/or
- as a replacement or modification of parts of the anatomy.

Therapeutic goods thus not only include medications but also prostheses and tests.

The TGA regulates the advertising and labelling of all registered therapeutic goods. Its regulatory approaches are complemented by state controls over who may prescribe or dispense therapeutic goods. The state legislation specifies, for example, which products can only be sold after a prescription is issued by a medical practitioner or other approved health professional, which products can only be sold in pharmacies, and so on.

The licensing of manufacturers is designed to ensure that the manufacturing process will produce products that vary only minimally from the composition approved by the TGA. The Therapeutic Goods Committee advises the TGA on principles to be observed in the manufacture of therapeutic goods. That committee also oversees development of standards for therapeutic goods, including labelling and packaging.

Timely and affordable access: the Pharmaceutical Benefits Scheme

The Australian Pharmaceutical Benefits Scheme (PBS) was introduced on 1 July 1948 but relatively few prescriptions were provided under this scheme because of opposition from the medical profession. The Liberal Government elected in 1949 altered the scheme (with effect from 4 September 1950), introducing a list of 139 'life saving and disease preventing drugs' that were provided free of charge to the whole community (Sloan 1995). Since then, the range of drugs covered by the PBS has increased dramatically and by August 2003, the PBS covered 601 generic products, available in 1469 forms or strengths and marketed as 2602 different brands. Some of these items are restricted, that is, they require some form of authority to prescribe them (over and above medical registration). Obtaining authority requires contact with the administering agency of the PBS, the Health Insurance Commission and may, for example, require the medical practitioner to certify that specific indications for use of the medication are present. The authority scheme is not well received by doctors and is seen as bureaucratic and not evidence-based (Liaw et al. 2003).

Table 9.2 shows data about the major types of drugs prescribed under the PBS. Drugs are grouped into 'therapeutic groups' using the Anatomical Therapeutics Chemical Code (ATC). (There are five levels to the code: anatomical main group, therapeutic main group, therapeutic subgroup, chemical/therapeutic subgroup, and generic drug name.)

It can be seen that the most frequently prescribed group of drugs are those acting on the cardiovascular system, accounting for just over 30 per cent of all prescriptions and a similar per cent of costs. A further 20 per cent of both prescriptions and costs are for drugs acting on the nervous system. Antineoplastic

Table 9.2 Australia: Number, total cost, and average price of prescriptions issued under Pharmaceutical Benefits Scheme, 1 July 2001 to 30 June 2002 and per cent change since prior year, by Anatomical Therapeutics Chemical Code

	Year ended 30 June 2002			Per cent change 2001 to 2002		
	Number of prescriptions	Total cost ($million)	Average price ($)	Number of prescriptions	Total cost	Average price
Alimentary tract and metabolism	19,082,701	692.4	36.28	6.4%	7.4%	0.9%
Blood and blood forming organs	4,023,864	111.9	27.80	12.3%	38.5%	23.3%
Cardiovascular system	46,587,011	1556.9	33.42	5.3%	8.7%	3.2%
Dermatologicals	2,934,367	81.2	27.68	-2.7%	1.1%	3.9%
Genito-urinary system and sex hormones	6,323,714	159.8	25.27	2.7%	20.4%	17.3%
Systemic hormonal preparations, excl sex hormones	2,304,729	30.2	13.09	3.9%	8.1%	4.0%
General anti-infectives for systemic use	12,550,089	273.1	21.76	-1.1%	2.9%	4.0%
Antineoplastic and immunomodulating agents	961,818	317.7	330.35	8.0%	17.2%	8.5%
Musculo-skeletal system	10,709,738	340.1	31.75	27.2%	14.4%	10.0%
Nervous system	30,564,051	906.5	29.66	3.4%	8.6%	5.1%
Antiparasitic products, insecticides, and repellents	910,580	8.9	9.81	0.4%	2.4%	2.0%
Respiratory system	10,341,286	374.0	36.16	-6.5%	7.3%	14.8%
Sensory organs	6,779,904	104.0	15.33	4.4%	8.1%	3.6%
Various	602,127	43.6	72.41	5.7%	5.4%	-0.3%
Not otherwise classified	294,283	3.1	10.58	-6.5%	0.0%	6.9%
Total	154,970,262	5003.3	32.29	4.7%	9.6%	4.7%

Source: Author's estimates derived from <http://www.hic.gov.au/statistics/dyn_pbs/forms/pbsgtab1.shml>

and immunomodulating agents, although accounting for less than 1 per cent of prescriptions, account for 6 per cent of costs. These drugs cost, on average, ten times as much as the average drug dispensed under the PBS.

Patient moieties or co-payments (officially called 'patient contributions') are structured separately for the general population and concession card-holders. There are three main classes of concession cardholders: Common-wealth Seniors Health Card, Health Care Card, and the Pensioners Concession Card. About eight million concession cards were on issue in 2003 (just over one-third of the total population), about 25 per cent to age pensioners, about 25 per cent to recipients of the Parenting Payment, with the balance spread across about 60 different income support payments. Initially the PBS involved no patient co-payment, but a 50 cent co-payment was introduced for general beneficiaries on 1 March 1960. A co-payment for concession cardholders of A$2.50 per prescription was introduced on 1 November 1990. The co-payment amounts are indexed for inflation and by 2003, the co-payment for concessional beneficiaries had increased to A$3.70 per prescription and for general beneficiaries to A$23.10. The PBS provides some protection from the cumulative impact of these co-payments through a 'safety net threshold' which is set for cardholders at 52 times the co-payment: if concession cardholders require more than 52 prescriptions in any one year, they can obtain a safety net card which entitles them to further prescriptions without any co-payment. The safety net threshold for general beneficiaries applies after they (or their immediate family) purchase PBS items that involve a total co-payment of at least A$708.40 in any calendar year after which prescriptions are supplied for the concessional co-payment.

Where a pharmaceutical is listed on the PBS under more than one brand name, pharmacists may dispense 'generically' identical forms of the drug unless specifically directed not to do so by the prescribing medical practitioner on the prescription form. If generic equivalents are available, the PBS will only pay for the least costly product and the consumer meets any additional costs for a specific brand name alternative in addition to the co-payments described above. This brand name 'moiety' is not counted as part of the safety net arrangements. An additional moiety is also payable if other pharmaceuticals in the same therapeutic class are deemed to be equivalent, and an exemption on clinical grounds has not been granted for that patient. This policy (known as 'Thera-peutic Group Premiums') applies only to items in three therapeutic groups: H2-receptor antagonists, calcium channel blockers, and ACE inhibitors.

The generic substitution policy is facilitated by a government require-ment that, where computer software used by medical practitioners to gener-ate prescriptions for the PBS has a default preferred drug, it defaults automatically to the generic form of a drug rather than a proprietary form of the drug. As at May 2002, 293 products had a brand premium, with the premium ranging from one cent to A$79.48. Over 30 million prescriptions

Figure 9.2 Australia: Trend in expenditure on Pharmaceutical Benefits Scheme, 1948/49 to 2001/02

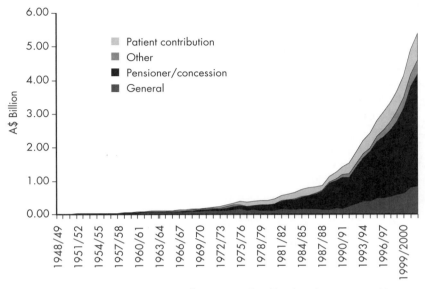

Data source: Commonwealth Department of Health and Aged Care 1999a and later years

had been dispensed with a brand premium, being about 50 per cent of all prescriptions covered by the brand premium policy. (For a fuller discussion of generic drug policy see Löfgren 2002.)

Expenditure on pharmaceutical benefits has increased exponentially

Figure 9.3 Australia: Age–gender specific prescription rates per 100 encounters with general practitioners, Australia, 2000/01

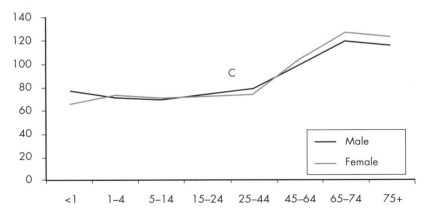

Data source: Britt, Miller, Knox et al 2001

since the commencement of the program, with particularly rapid growth in expenditure on drugs used by pensioners and concession cardholders (see figure 9.2). Importantly, 73 per cent of government pharmaceutical benefits prescription expenditure is for concession cardholders, and therefore shifting costs to consumers can have deleterious equity effects, especially since an increased co-payment will have an impact on both 'essential' and 'discretionary' drugs (McManus et al. 1996). Figure 9.3 shows that people over 65 have a 50 per cent higher prescription rate than people under 45.

This high percentage of use for pensioners should not be surprising because the elderly generally have poorer health status than younger persons and have higher hospital utilisation rates. Expenditure on pharmaceuticals has been growing faster than the economy as a whole in recent years. Since the late 1970s, pharmaceutical expenditure has grown from 0.6 per cent of GDP to 1.1 per cent in 2000/01.

Figure 9.4 shows annual real growth rates in government expenditure and patient contributions.

For most of the last decade patient contributions, which account for 15 per cent of PBS expenditure, have been increasing at around 5 to 8 per cent per annum in real terms. When introduced in 1960, patient contributions represented about 15 per cent of total PBS expenditure. This share rose to around 30 per cent in the mid 1970s to 1980s but since then has declined to the historic level of around 15 per cent. Government expenditure has been increasing faster than patient contributions: at around 7 to 14 per cent per annum. This growth in expenditure is partly driven by increased utilisation and partly by increased prices for dispensed medications. Similar trends are evident in most OECD countries (Jacobzone 2000).

Expenditure on the PBS is the fastest-growing component of health expenditure, growing at 15 to 20 per cent per annum. If the current rates of

Figure 9.4 Australia: Per cent growth in government expenditure and patient contribution, 1991/92 to 2001/02 (real terms)

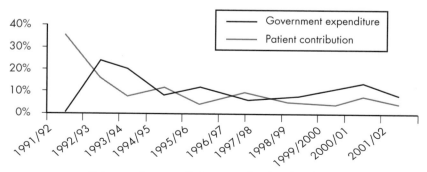

Data source: Commonwealth Department of Health and Aged Care 1999a and later years

Figure 9.5 Annual cost increases in Pharmaceutical Benefits Scheme, 1992/93 to 2000/01, by reason for cost increase

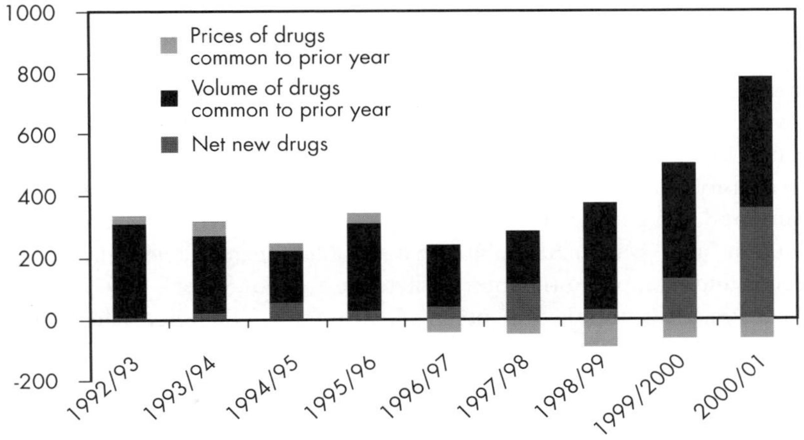

Data source: Sweeny 2002

growth continue, expenditure on the PBS will exceed that on public hospitals by 2007/08 and on all hospitals by 2010/11 (see Walker et al. 1998 for the impact of different growth scenarios on PBS expenditure).

Growth in expenditure is obviously distributed unevenly across the PBS with use of newer drugs increasing faster than older drugs. The average price of a new drug listed on the PBS is about twice that of all drugs on the scheme (Sweeny 2002).

For most of the last decade, the growth in PBS expenditure has primarily been driven by increases in volume of drugs that had been listed on the schedule for at least 12 months rather than by the cost of new drug listings (Sweeny 2002). For the last five years price effects of drugs that have been listed for more than 12 months have acted to moderate growth in expenditure rather than contribute to it (see figure 9.5). The decision to list an item on the PBS can lead to commitment of significant government expenditure, and since 1993 has involved a decision not only about whether the drug is an effective complement to existing items on the PBS, but also an assessment of whether the drug is cost-effective. The legislation that requires cost-effectiveness analysis was passed in 1987; draft guidelines on how listing submissions were to incorporate cost-effectiveness analysis were published in 1990, with definitive guidelines in 1992. These are updated regularly; see www.health.gov.au/pbs/general/pubs/guidelines for the latest guidelines.

The guidelines provide that a drug will be listed on the PBS if:

• it is needed for the prevention or treatment of significant medical conditions not already covered, or inadequately covered, by drugs in the existing list and is of acceptable cost-effectiveness

- it is more effective, less toxic (or both) than a drug already listed for the same indications, and is of acceptable cost-effectiveness, or
- it is at least as effective and safe as a drug already listed for the same indications and is of similar or better cost-effectiveness.

Under the cost-effectiveness arrangements, the pharmaceutical manufacturer needs to present cost-effectiveness data to the Pharmaceutical Benefits Advisory Committee (PBAC: Henry 1992; Harris 1994; Mitchell 1996; Hailey 1997; Hill et. al 1997a; Salkeld et al. 1999). A retrospective study of the decision-making process showed that new pharmaceuticals costing more than A\$68,913 per life year saved are generally not listed on the PBS, while those costing less than A\$36,450 are listed. No apparent decision rules have been found to apply to the intermediate zone (George et al. 1997).

Australia was the first country to incorporate economic evaluation formally in decision-making processes about subsidising drugs, and is still at the forefront of policy in this area (Dickson et al. 2003). However, the operation of PBAC and the economic evaluation policies of the PBS have not been without controversy. Early in 2001, for example, in a controversial move, the government restructured the membership of PBAC to include a person with strong industry links. This initiative was believed to be in response to industry pressure to water down the strong emphasis on economic evaluation followed by PBAC and was seen in the public debate as weakening PBAC (Goddard et al. 2001). These fears do not appear to have translated into reality and economic evaluation still appears to be a central component of the listing recommendations (Aroni et al. 2003). Government need not accept PBAC recommendations and there is also evidence to suggest that it might have been more generous in price negotiations than economic considerations may have warranted (Richardson 2003).

The PBS is principally aimed at supporting supply of pharmaceuticals in the community. There is a special parallel program, known as the Highly Specialised Drugs Program, that provides Commonwealth funding for a limited range of drugs that are to be supplied only through specialist hospitals. The medications covered by this program are approved for specific clinical conditions for community-based patients (that is, not inpatients). The program is a distinct subset of the PBS with the Commonwealth authority to fund medications resting on a separate section of the National Health Act (section 100), rather than through the general PBS arrangements. Drugs are recommended for inclusion in the program only if they meet the following criteria:

- ongoing specialised medical supervision is required
- the drug is for the treatment of long-term medical conditions
- the drug is highly specialised and for an identifiable patient group
- the drug has been approved by the TGA for the specific therapeutic indications proposed
- the drug has a high unit cost.

In 2001/02, there were 46 drugs covered by the Highly Specialised Drug Program at a total cost of A$306m. Over A$70m of total expenditure was for HIV/AIDS anti-retroviral agents and other related drugs (28 separate drugs), A$60m was spent on haemopoietics (two drugs), A$60m on immuno-stimulating agents (six drugs), and A$50m on three immuno-suppressing agents.

As part of the listing decision, the government establishes a price for the drug after advice from the Pharmaceutical Benefits Pricing Authority. In determining the price, the authority takes into account:

• the PBAC comments on clinical and cost-effectiveness
• prices of alternative brands of a drug
• comparative prices of drugs in the same therapeutic group
• cost information, whether provided by the supplier or estimated by the authority
• prescription volumes, economies of scale, and other factors such as expiry dating, storage requirements, product stability, and special manufacturing requirements
• prices of the drug in relevant overseas countries.

The purchasing arrangements for pharmaceuticals covered under the PBS involve a government-agreed price (90 per cent of which is for the supplier, 10 per cent for the wholesaler). The government also undertakes post-marketing surveillance to ensure that the volumes of listed drugs are close to those predicted in the cost-effectiveness analyses and other submissions on which the pricing negotiations were based. This postmarket surveillance does not always appear to be effective (Richardson 2003).

Historically, the government has been able to use its monopsonistic purchasing strength to achieve lower prices relative to those paid in international markets. The ability to do this appears to be weakening as other countries establish schemes similar to the PBS and monitor international pricing negotiations (Löfgren 1998). However, Bessell et al. (1999) have documented an example where the market price rose when the product was deleted from the PBS.

Pricing decisions of the PBS have significant implications for profit that pharmaceutical manufacturers obtain from selling their products in Australia. The major costs of bringing a drug on to the market are in the research and development that can occur over a long period of time. Of course, research and development costs associated with failed research or research that does not lead to a drug that comes on to the market need to be spread over the costs of pharmaceuticals that do come on to the market. In many cases the drug research is subsidised by national research organisations (such as NH&MRC).

Because of pharmaceutical industry pressure to increase the prices paid for drugs under the Pharmaceutical Benefits Scheme, the Commonwealth

Figure 9.6 Ratio of prevailing prices for pharmaceuticals in selected countries compared with PBS prices (Australian PBS=1.0), 2000

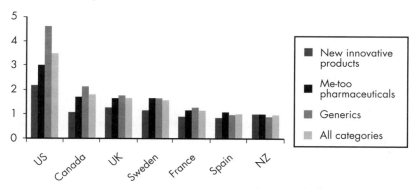

Data source: Productivity Commission 2001

government referred the question of comparative prices to the Productivity Commission. International comparison of pricing is difficult, in part because of the existence of discounting arrangements in several countries: list prices may not reflect prices actually paid in the marketplace. Accordingly, in its major study of comparative prices of drugs, the Productivity Commission reported high and low estimates of the difference between costs in other countries and costs in Australia (see figure 9.6). The high estimate is the greatest difference likely to be found.

There are a number of broad general conclusions that can be drawn from figure 9.6. Prices in Australia are certainly substantially less than prices in the USA. On the other hand, prices in Australia are similar to prices in other countries. The success of the PBS in restraining prices has attracted the ire of the US pharmaceutical manufacturing industry (Lokuge and Denniss 2003).

There are significant differences in price relativities for different types of drugs. The differences between new and innovative pharmaceuticals are much lower than for all pharmaceuticals, suggesting that the Australian purchasers (particularly those involved in setting prices under the PBS) are not able to extract the same price discounts for newer drugs relative to older preparations.

Because listing under the PBS provides a significant marketing boost (by reducing the effective price faced by consumers to the co-payment), government is in a strong position to negotiate over price. However, where a pharmaceutical company has a new medication significantly superior to others, or which is unique, it can threaten to rely on consumers paying the full price for the drug rather than accept a lower price from government. In these circumstances, consumers are likely to place significant pressure on government to list the product.

A viable medicines industry

Government has a mixed set of objectives with respect to pricing of pharmaceuticals under the PBS. On the one hand the higher the price, the greater will be the government's expenditure on the PBS. On the other hand, government also has the objective of encouraging development of the pharmaceutical industry in Australia. In pursuit of this latter objective, government aims to ensure that a pharmaceutical industry based in Australia receives adequate returns on its investment. These two objectives have bureaucratic advocates from the Department of Health and Aged Care, who are responsible for the PBS, and from the Department of Industry, Science and Resources, who are responsible for the development of Australian industry (Löfgren 1998).

A number of industry development schemes have operated over the years to support the pharmaceutical industry, and to provide partial compensation for the pharmaceutical industry for the impact of government exercising its monopsony purchasing power under the PBS. Effectively, these schemes provided a higher price for nominated products supplied by participating companies in return for those companies undertaking manufacturing, research, and development in Australia (for a review of these earlier schemes see Bureau of Industry Economics 1991; Industry Commission 1996). The current industry support scheme breaks the nexus between price suppression and industry support: it is explicitly cast as an industry development scheme designed to increase pharmaceutical research and development in Australia. The scheme, known as the Pharmaceuticals Partnerships Program (P^3), which was planned to commence on 1 July 2004, has a five-year life. The program provides A\$150 million over its life in the form of subsidies of 30 cents for each dollar of increased research and development activity. The maximum grant to a company is A\$10 million. The program encourages partnerships between local and multinational companies and so, to some extent, recognises the continuing agglomeration of the global pharmaceutical industry (Rasmussen 2002).

The high rate of growth in the cost of pharmaceuticals has led governments in Australia (and around the world) to develop a number of strategies to limit this expenditure. Table 9.3 shows some of the strategies that have been utilised (Saltman and Figueras 1997; Maynard and Bloor 2003).

In broad general terms, the government can shape pharmaceutical policy by intervening at any point of the drug distribution chain with initiatives targeted at manufacturers, medical practitioners who prescribe drugs, pharmacists who dispense drugs, and consumers.

Different policy initiatives will have different equity effects and will have different impacts. Policies to reduce consumption of pharmaceuticals could

Table 9.3 Targets for control of government pharmaceutical expenditure

	Demand	Supply
Price	Patient co-payments*	Ceilings on promotion expenditure
	Encourage prescription of 'generic' (non-brand name) drugs*	Pay pharmacists a flat rate rather than a percentage
	Encourage prescription of alternative medication in same therapeutic class*	Negotiate prices based on lowest in other countries*
Volume	Patient education programs*	Fixed PBS budgets for individual medical practitioners
	Managed care arrangements	Incentives on medical profession as a whole to limit prescribing*
		Practice guidelines
		Limit inclusion on the approval list (including through use of cost-effectiveness analysis)*
		Provide education program to pharmacists, doctors*

*This strategy used in Australia

involve a mix of price strategies on the demand side, increasing consumer co-payments or, alternatively, acting on supply by attempting to change the behaviour of manufacturers by reducing the incentives to manufacturers to promote increased use of pharmaceuticals. One of the most powerful supply-side strategies is using price volume contracts to reduce the price paid under the PBS as volume increases. The two different strategies have different equity impacts and different effectiveness. Organisational and system-wide change by changing incentives on the manufacturers will have a far more pervasive effect than educational strategies on medical practitioners and minimise the adverse equity impacts of consumer co-payment strategies.

Quality use of medicines

Figure 9.1 shows the extensive use of medication in the community whether or not it is subsidised by government. Inappropriate use of medicines in the community can have serious consequences including admission to hospital. About 3 per cent of all hospital admissions are drug related (Roughead et al. 1998b). Adherence to evidence-based prescribing protocols is also cost-effective (Nelson et al. 2001).

The fourth arm of the National Medicines Policy is to promote the quality use of medicines: ensuring that the right drug is provided to the right patient, and taken the right way (Stuart and Briesacher 2002). Although such a policy could involve a mix of strategies, the emphasis in Australia has been on sporadic educational programs rather than systematic use of incentives on manufacturers or medical practitioners. Such campaigns encourage consumers to be more judicious in their use of medication and/or attempt to educate medical practitioners to reduce their prescribing. Consumers have the least power in the chain of supply and are also the least well placed to judge what medication is necessary and efficacious.

Despite the regulation of claims made by pharmaceutical manufacturers in their advertising to medical practitioners, manufacturers advertising to medical practitioners do not promote the scientific basis of their products (Loke et al. 2002). Because there are few price volume agreements in place under the PBS, manufacturers have a very strong incentive to increase sales when the marginal cost production of the additional drugs is well below the revenue from the PBS. These incentives on manufacturing companies overwhelm the educational campaigns on medical practitioners. Pharmaceutical marketing budgets are large and this results in 'entanglement' between doctors and the manufacturing companies as the manufacturers encourage medical practitioners to prescribe their products through enticements (Moynihan 2003). Manufacturing companies also support consumer organisations to lobby for inclusion of relevant drugs on the PBS and use the consumer organisations to advocate use of the manufacturer's product (Herxheimer 2003).

The primary interest of the pharmaceutical industry is in maximising sales, and this usually translates into maximising government expenditure. Australia uses a range of strategies to rein in pharmaceutical benefits expenditure, for example by providing feedback to general practitioners on costs (Beilby and Silagy 1997; see also National Health Strategy 1992; Harvey and Murray 1995; Hill et al. 1997b). Despite government programs to promote evidence-based prescribing and improve consumer information (Shenfield and Tasker 1997), the pharmaceutical industry has been remarkably successful in creating 'needs' (Moynihan et al. 2002), persuading medical practitioners to prescribe the latest drug even if benefits to the consumer are marginal (Moulds 1992; Day 1998; Roughead et al. 1998c, but see Roughead et al. 1999 for a positive evaluation of the 'Quality Use of Medicines' policy).

Supply arrangements and the pharmacy workforce

Payments to pharmacists for dispensing prescriptions under the PBS are set following negotiations between the Commonwealth government and the Pharmacy Guild of Australia. The contemporary arrangements are incorporated in the Third Community Pharmacy Agreement that is for the five-year period 1 July 2000 to 30 June 2005. The agreement provides for differential base dispensing fees for dispensing 'ready prepared' items (A\$4.40 fee in 2000/01) and 'extemporaneously prepared' items (A\$6.28). In either case the pharmacist also receives a mark-up of 10 per cent on the agreed price if that price is less than A\$180, A\$18 if the price is between A\$180 and A\$450, and 4 per cent if the price is above A\$450. The base fees are indexed annually. The agreement also provides for upward or downward adjustment of payments if the average mark-up increases by more than 4 per cent over that projected in the agreement or if prescriptions increase faster or slower than projected. The operation of these claw-back and supplementation arrangements both protect government from additional expenditure on pharmacists simply because of increases in average prescription prices and protect pharmacists from the impact on total remuneration if prescription volume declines. The agreement also provides that pharmacists can receive a range of other miscellaneous fees and allowances.

In 1999 there were 14,747 employed pharmacists, an increase of 6.6 per cent from 1996 (AIHW 2003g). The number of pharmacies however, remains unchanged at just under 5000 (4926 in 1999 compared to 4953 in 1996). The Commonwealth government has pursued a policy of limiting the number of pharmacies as the dispensing fee incorporated in the PBS payment arrangements is in part based on the number of prescriptions dispensed per pharmacy. The Commonwealth believes that if it can increase the number of prescriptions dispensed per pharmacy it might be able to reduce the dispensing fee per prescription, thus achieving some benefits of economies of scale. The Australian Community Pharmacy Authority is the body that oversees the process of relocating existing, and approving new, pharmacies.

The number of employed pharmacists per 100,000 population increased by 12.5 per cent over the period 1994–99. Over a longer time frame (from the 1961 to the 1996 Census) there was a reduction in the number of practising pharmacists per 100,000 population of 13.8 per cent. This is in contrast with the increase in practising pharmacists that occurred over the same period in the USA (24 per cent increase).

There is a shortage of pharmacists (AIHW 2003g), but whether this will continue into the medium term is a moot point as the number of commencing pharmacy students increased by 57 per cent between 1992 and 2000.

Across Australia there were 77.7 pharmacists per 100,000 population in 1999. As with other health professions there is variation in the supply of pharmacists by geographic location (see figure 9.7). Community pharmacists are fairly evenly distributed across metropolitan and regional areas (with around 60 to 70 pharmacists per 100,000 population). There are fewer community pharmacists in smaller rural areas and in remote areas as community pharmacies may not be financially viable with a smaller population base/market. Hospital pharmacists are unevenly distributed, with higher levels of employment in metropolitan areas and large rural centres and low levels of employment elsewhere. Pharmacy services in small rural towns would normally be supplied

Figure 9.7 Australia: Employed pharmacists per 100,000 population by type of practice and geographic area, 1999

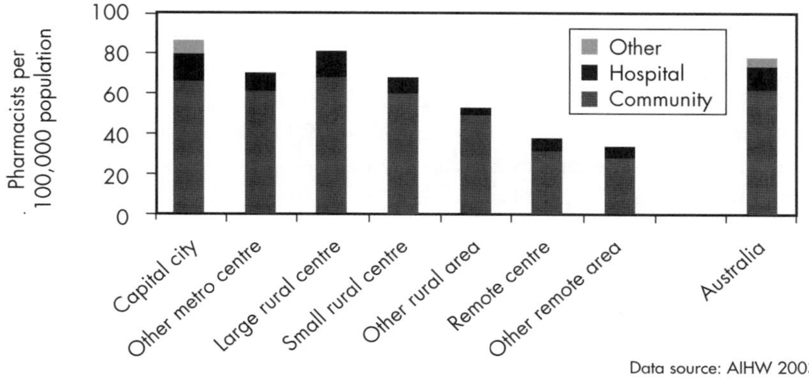

Data source: AIHW 2003g

by the local community pharmacy rather than by the hospital employing its own pharmacist.

Evaluation

Australia's arrangements for the supply of pharmaceuticals are the envy of many other developed countries. The Pharmaceutical Benefits Scheme performs well in terms of our criteria of equity, efficiency, quality, and acceptability. In terms of equity, the structure of the PBS minimises the financial barriers to access to pharmaceuticals. The safety net arrangements also ensure that the cumulative impact of the co-payment also protects the chronically ill, whether or not they have access to a concession card. The low co-payment for concession cardholders ensures that they have access to the medication prescribed for them: only 2 per cent of people over 65 have reported that they did not fill a prescription because of cost (Schoen 2003). However, co-payments for the general population are much higher than for concession cardholders and may create a barrier, especially for people on low incomes. Blendon et al. (2002) have reported that 23 per cent of Australians did not fill a prescription because of cost. In terms of efficiency the Pharmaceutical Benefits Scheme again performs well in the sense that all new drugs are subject to economic evaluation prior to listing on the scheme.

Because new drugs listed on the PBS have been evaluated for their cost-effectiveness, it could be argued that any increased expenditure on the PBS is worthwhile in terms of savings in other sectors of the health industry (for example, hospitals), in increased productivity (reduced time off work), or in terms of improved quality of life generally. Thus even where there is increased expenditure on these drugs, this may be efficient and cost-effective when viewed in a wider economic context.

The success of the cost-effectiveness strategy relies on rigorous standardised cost-effectiveness analyses undertaken in accordance with published guidelines (Morgan et al. 2000). It also relies on ensuring that pre-listing estimates of demand (based on the indications tested in the cost-effectiveness analyses) hold true once the drug is marketed. However, pharmaceutical companies are normally the sponsors of cost-effectiveness analyses submitted for review. Friedberg et al. (1999) and Neumann et al. (2000) have shown that drug-company funded cost-effectiveness analyses are more likely than studies funded from other sources to report favourable cost-effectiveness results. There is also a tendency for drug-company sponsored studies to overstate qualitative conclusions (that is, a favourable qualitative conclusion in the face of neutral or negative quantitative results). Studies sponsored by pharmaceutical manufacturers are also more likely to report outcomes favouring the sponsor than research funded from other sources (Lexchin 2003). Although the Department of Health and Aged Care undertakes 'postmarketing surveillance' of new PBS listings, renegotiation of prices in the face of unexpected increased sales volumes is relatively unusual. A weakness of the PBS in terms of efficiency lies in this area of postmarket surveillance: the economic evaluation is based on a particular range of conditions and evidence from particular research studies and the prescription use of the drug in practice, and its promotion by the manufacturers, may not be in accordance with the research and the basis of the listing decision. Efficiency of the scheme would be promoted if there were stronger incentives on manufacturers to restrain use in line with the research evidence, possibly by expanded use of pricing arrangements.

Although the PBS incorporates incentives for the quality use of medicines, the incentives are primarily directed at the weakest points of the supply chain in terms of the effectiveness of policy instruments. Educational strategies aimed at consumers and medical practitioners should be supplemented by stronger incentives on manufacturers to encourage quality use of medicines. Evidence of overprescription can be seen in the rate of admissions to hospitals for drug related adverse events.

Finally, the PBS appears to be popular and so would rate highly in terms of the criterion of acceptability.

As noted above, almost 80 per cent of pharmaceutical benefits expenditure is for pensioners and concessional beneficiaries, that is, the program is already highly targeted. As a corollary, in 1989/90, 26 per cent of persons in the lowest income decile benefited from the PBS subsidy for pharmaceuticals compared with 5 per cent of persons in the highest income decile (Schofield 1998). Further use of demand side strategies, such as patient co-payments, would thus have an adverse impact on equity, but this effect has not precluded advocacy of this policy option, especially by pharmaceutical manufacturers (Löfgren 1998). It should therefore be anticipated that expenditure on the PBS will continue to rise as new therapeutic agents are developed and replace older, cheaper products.

10

Policy Challenges for the Australian Health Care System

The previous chapters of this book have discussed the inputs and institutions of the health care system and contemporary policy issues. In this concluding chapter, discussion will focus on critical policy challenges for the Australian health care system. The criteria used here for evaluating health care systems were outlined in the Introduction: equity, efficiency, quality, and acceptability. There are challenges for the Australian health care system in each of these areas. The stance adopted here is that the Australian health care system has a large number of strengths and that only minor structural change is necessary. This position is in contrast with that often adopted in public debates on the health sector where advocates for particular positions claim the existence of a 'crisis' in the sector to facilitate adoption of their favoured nostrum.

Equity

The quest for equity has been a major issue in the Australian health care system since the 1960s. There are two elements of equity to be addressed: equity of access and equity of outcomes.

Equity of access

The most significant development in terms of equity of access was obviously Scotton and Deeble's work underpinning the introduction of universal health insurance to address financial barriers to access (see Scotton and Macdonald 1993 for an account of the processes involved in this) and to ensure equity in financing (Lairson et al. 1995). Their work led to the introduction of Medibank in 1975 and its reinstatement as Medicare in 1984. Australia was a relative latecomer in addressing mutualisation of funding for hospital and medical care. The introduction of Medibank was fiercely contested (De Voe and Short 2003), and the policy direction was then progressively reversed by the Fraser Government over the period 1975 to 1981 (Duckett 1984). Prior to the 1996 election, the then Leader of the Opposition John Howard promised that 'Medicare would be retained in its entirety'. Actions in the first term of the Howard Government were consistent with that promise. However, in its second term the commitment appears to be weakening with a retreat from support for universality. This is most obvious in the government response to the decline in bulk billing which is predicated on bulk billing being a service for 'the poor' rather than all Australians. The decline in bulk billing suggests that equity of access may be under threat through creation of financial barriers to access in the primary medical care system. Access to public hospitals without financial barriers continues to be available. The absence of financial barriers does not, however, guarantee equity: consultation times for consumers with lower socioeconomic status are shorter than high status consumers (Martin et al. 1997; Wiggers and Sanson-Fisher 1997; Furler et al. 2002). There are also still financial barriers to access to specialist services (Scott 1997).

An important aspect of financial barriers is the differential access to timely care. Baume (1995) has demonstrated that there are significant waiting times in gaining access to private surgeons but the most publicly debated issue in this area remains waiting times for elective surgery in public hospitals. This is despite a significant reduction in waiting times for the most urgent surgery in Victoria and other states (Street and Duckett 1996).

In terms of other dimensions of equity, Australia's record is poor. There are significant differences between urban and rural areas in access to primary and hospital health care. Identification of the nature of the problem here is complex, as geographic equity is usually described relatively; for example, there are fewer doctors per 1000 population in rural Australia relative to urban areas. Figure 4.13 shows trends in general practitioner:population ratios in urban and rural areas in Australia. There has been a significant increase in general practitioner provision in both metropolitan and rural areas but there is still a higher ratio in capital cities relative to rural and remote areas. What is noteworthy, however, is that the contemporary level of rural access is above the metropolitan level in 1984/85.

Figure 4.13 does not show the distribution of medical practitioners within a single category such as small rural centres. In the past, most towns may have had one or two doctors, but some now have three and others none. Towns with only one doctor are vulnerable to that doctor retiring or otherwise relocating, especially as community expectations of 24-hour access to the practitioner may conflict with the lifestyle expectations of doctors and their families.

Access to hospital services in rural communities is also perceived to be a problem, in part because of the need to travel significant distances to gain access to specialist services. In a sense, this is almost inevitable, as super-specialist services need to be concentrated to achieve economies of scale and expertise and are available in only a limited number of tertiary hospitals. Infrastructure requirements even for more generalist hospital services are increasing, leading to the concentration of hospitals in the larger rural centres and closure of smaller rural hospitals. However, small rural communities value their local hospital highly, largely because of the hospital's perceived role as a source of emergency care, and so rural hospital closures are hotly contested politically.

The third element of equity of access is the issue of racial barriers to access. Access issues here are complex. Deeble et al. (1998) have shown that health expenditure for Indigenous populations is not too dissimilar from that for the non–Indigenous population. But given the differences in health outcomes for Aboriginal people discussed below and in chapter 2, there is a strong case for greater levels of expenditure.

Equity of outcomes

The picture in terms of equity of outcomes of care is much less clear, in part because there are few regularly collected measures of outcomes, in part because outcomes are affected not only by the quality of care that is provided but also by environmental factors (as discussed in chapter 2). What we do know about equity of outcomes is that the health status of our Aboriginal and Torres Strait Islander populations is appalling, and should be a major focus of policy attention. Clearly, the factors affecting the health status of the Aboriginal and Torres Strait Islander population are not going to be remedied only by actions in the health sector, as broader issues of dignity, identity, and justice need to be taken into account as part of any strategy to improve the health status of Indigenous peoples. One element of this is undoubtedly the need for further progress on reconciliation (Jackson and Ward 1999).

There is also significant difference in health status between people with low incomes and those with high incomes, and between the employed and the unemployed. Similar differences have been found in a number of countries including the USA and the United Kingdom. These problems should not be seen as intractable. A recent report in the United Kingdom identified a number of strategies for addressing this problem of inequity of outcomes (Acheson 1998; but see Williams 1999b for a critique). Many European countries have also adopted policies to reduce inequalities (Mackenbach and Bakker 2000).

Quality

Unfortunately, methods for measuring quality have not been subject to the same methodological advances as has occurred in measurement of efficiency. As was discussed in chapter 6, the evidence from Australian studies of quality of hospital care suggests that an adverse event, with serious consequences, occurs in a significant proportion of hospital admissions. Almost one-quarter of 'sicker Australians' believe that there have been errors in their treatment in the last two years (Blendon et al. 2003); although Australian results for perceived quality of care are similar to the other countries (see table 10.1).

Another element of quality of care relates to system design issues and here, poor quality arises because of weaknesses in continuity of care. About one-quarter of Australian respondents saw five or more doctors. Half the respondents had to repeat information and many respondents had problems with lost or delayed records. There are two main proposals for enhancing continuity: integration of acute and primary care services and changing Commonwealth–state financial responsibilities.

Table 10.1   Medical practitioner interactions and care coordination among sicker adults in five countries, 2002

	Aus %	Can %	NZ %	UK %	US %
Number of different doctors and other health professionals seen in past two years:					
One	13	18	13	16	13
Two	25	23	23	18	19
Three	19	17	19	19	22
Four	14	13	10	12	14
Five or more	26	27	30	30	29
Care coordination experience in past two years:					
Had to tell same story to multiple health professionals	49	50	47	49	57
Records/results did not reach doctors office in time for appointment	14	19	16	23	25
Sent for duplicate tests/procedures by different health professionals	13	20	17	13	22
Received conflicting information from different doctors or health professionals.	23	23	24	19	26
Mistake made in past two years:					
Believed a medical mistake was made in treatment or care	19	20	18	13	23
Given the wrong medication or wrong dose by a doctor, hospital, or pharmacist	11	11	13	10	12
Either type or error was made.	23	25	23	18	28

Source: Blendon et al. 2003

Continuity or coordination of care might be inhibited by our existing Commonwealth–state division of responsibility that can create incentives for care to be provided in inappropriate settings. Additional expenditure in tightly constrained state programs would, in many instances, lead to improved efficiency for the same, or better, health outcomes from the whole system, compared with additional expenditure on Commonwealth entitlement programs such as the Medicare Benefits Schedule. There is significant anecdotal evidence of poor coordination of acute and primary care services, principally described as poor discharge planning. Although poor discharge planning has recently been attributed to the introduction of casemix funding, anecdotes about poor discharge planning have circulated for decades.

It is naive to imagine that elimination of Commonwealth–state discontinuities or casemix funding, however, will eradicate coordination problems. There are many anecdotes of poor coordination within institutions (especially large institutions such as teaching hospitals) and even unitary health systems, such as the United Kingdom National Health Service, have coordination problems (see Pritchard and Hughes 1995).

A further example of poor coordination is within the primary health and community services sector, where multiple agencies provide services to consumers who have multiple health care needs. The reasons for poor coordination in this sector were discussed in chapter 8. The Coordinated Care Trials (also discussed in chapter 8) represent one attempt to address such service integration issues in the context of Australia's complex Commonwealth–state health funding arrangements.

Efficiency

Efficiency, broadly defined, is the second of the key criteria for evaluating health care systems. From an economic perspective, a focus on efficiency requires attention to two main elements: allocative efficiency and dynamic efficiency.

Allocative efficiency

Allocative efficiency is concerned with ensuring the best allocation of resources in the health care system, so that the inputs allocated to the health care system yield the best possible outcomes. As discussed in chapter 1, this involves addressing technical efficiency, effectiveness, and appropriate priority setting.

Technical efficiency

There has been significant improvement in technical efficiency in the health care sector over the last 20 years and remarkable efficiency improvements have been achieved through the introduction of casemix funding, which commenced in Victoria in 1993 (Duckett 1995b).

The complexity of Commonwealth–state relations in health is said to lead to technical inefficiency, because of multiple reporting requirements. A more important aspect of Commonwealth–state relations relates to cost shifting: existing Commonwealth–state divisions of responsibility and other aspects of program design almost inevitably lead to cost-shifting as managers seek to address budget problems by transferring programs to readily accessible Commonwealth entitlement programs such as Medicare or the Pharmaceutical Benefits Scheme. This allows managers' attention to be diverted from directly improving efficiency, with a possible overall loss of system efficiency.

There are also real problems of Commonwealth–state relations in terms of the political process and accountability. This dissipation of responsibility in the health sector means that whenever state or Commonwealth politicians are under pressure, they almost inevitably attempt to shift blame to politicians at the other level (the so-called 'blame game'). Dissipation of responsibility undermines the functioning of political accountability for government actions.

Effectiveness

The second key element of allocative efficiency relates to effectiveness. It is about ensuring that the ratio of outputs to outcomes is optimised. There are a number of elements to this, one of which is 'efficacy', the extent to which the outputs of the health care service lead to the ideal outcome under the best possible conditions (using a definition from Cochrane 1971). One of the key objectives of policy is to ensure that actual effectiveness (in terms of the ratio of outputs to actual outcomes) moves closer to this ideal. It is also an object of policy to move the outcome frontier, that is, to improve the best possible (ideal) outcome. This latter task is the focus of medical and health services research.

Many factors affect the actual outcome ('effectiveness') of an intervention or system, including the design of the care system, the environment into which a patient is discharged, the safety of the manufacturing devices and pharmaceuticals used (part of the role of the Therapeutic Goods Administration as discussed in chapter 9), and the quality of care provided (discussed above).

Priority setting

The third element of allocative efficiency relates to priority setting: deciding on the appropriate division of resources between diseases (for example the appropriate relative emphasis on orthopaedic services versus cardiac services) and also within disease such as in terms of preventive versus curative investments. Segal and Richardson (1994) have provided a framework for addressing within-disease choices. However, attempts to use economic analysis to assist between-disease choices, most notably Oregon's priority setting experiment, have generally failed—in Oregon's case because community and economic priorities were not coincident (Tengs et al. 1996). This does not augur well for those who advocate a simple application of cost-effectiveness analysis.

Spending on prevention accounts for a relatively small proportion of health expenditure in Australia, although, as was shown in chapter 7, some public health expenditure is recorded as 'environmental protection'. This by itself does not imply that preventive services should be expanded. The cost-effectiveness of preventive services has been subject to considerable academic debate (see Russell 1986, 1987). Before advocating any increase in expenditure (or increased relative expenditure) on prevention, we need to demonstrate that such expenditure will be cost-effective.

Another aspect of priority setting relates to the balance of services, for example, funding of allied health care and natural therapies vis-à-vis medical services. When Scotton and Deeble were developing their policy on universal health insurance, the main focus of the health care system was doctors and hospitals. The health care system in Australia in the twenty-first century is significantly different to that of the 1960s. There has been a notable expansion in the role of allied health personnel, partly associated with the increased chronicity of the health problems of the Australian population associated with ageing. The important role that allied health personnel play in rehabilitation services, and the change in the allied health workforce in terms of supply and skill levels, have also contributed to the increased importance of these disciplines in the health care system. The Australian population is embracing natural therapies for similar reasons.

Financing arrangements have not kept pace with these changes and so it may be that there is an overinvestment in services for which there is a Medicare rebate and underinvesting in other more effective or cost-effective services. Certainly, there is evidence that poorer people have less access to some allied health services relative to those on higher incomes (Schofield 1999). To some extent the Coordinated Care Trials are trying to address this in the case of allied health, but there is no systematic investigation of policy on natural therapies.

The final aspect of priority setting is whether all hospitalisations are necessary. Stamp et al. (1998) have shown that many Aboriginal people are admitted to hospitals for conditions where admissions could be prevented (or at least the incidence reduced) with good primary care. There is now also abundant evidence that there is considerable variation in utilisation across Australia and separation rates for many conditions vary considerably between local government areas (Richardson 1998b), variations that cannot be explained in terms of demography or other clinical factors. The lack of utilisation review and analysis of the appropriateness of care allows this variability to continue. The high level of variation of hospital separation rates is one of the underlying factors that provides supporting evidence for those who advocate moving to managed care in Australia. Although managed care is not the only policy response to variation in utilisation rates, variation in utilisation patterns is clearly a contemporary problem in the Australian health care system.

Dynamic efficiency

Dynamic efficiency refers to the extent to which the health care system as a whole, and its constituent elements, adapt to change and innovation.

The Australian health care system is relatively open to adopting new technologies (drugs, surgical, and diagnostic) soon after their development. Australia has a strong and dynamic medical research system with publications and citations increasing over recent decades (Butler 2001). Spending on medical research in 1990/91 equated to about 2 per cent of national health expenditure, and Australia's medical research is of high quality, measured in terms of citations (Butler et al. 1998). In 1990/91, the largest single source of research expenditure was funding from business enterprises (such as the pharmaceutical industry), although almost 40 per cent of the person-years spent on research was in universities (Nichol et al. 1994). A recent Federal government report (Health and Medical Research Strategic Review 1999) proposed a substantial increase in government funding of medical research through the main government granting body, the NH&MRC. A substantial increase in research funding was announced in the 1999/2000 budget.

Industry (and some consumer) groups criticise the processes of our regulatory bodies that monitor safety and efficacy (for example, the TGA) and cost-effectiveness (Pharmaceutical Benefits Advisory Committee and the Medical Service Advisory Committee). This is an inherent side effect of attempting to slow the introduction of ineffective (or cost-ineffective) technologies, that is, striking the balance between allocative and dynamic efficiency objectives. Overall, there is relatively speedy introduction of new technologies at the clinical level.

Our track record on system level change is not so good. There are relatively powerful interest groups in the health system (such as health insurers and the medical profession) who for many years combined to delay the introduction of universal health insurance. Australia was one of the last countries in the Western developed world to adopt a system of universal financing for health care, following a long and bitter struggle to introduce

Medibank (Scotton and Macdonald 1993). It may be that the struggle over universal health insurance distracted policy makers' attention from other needed reforms.

It is still extraordinary, for example, that Australia does not have a comprehensive platform on which to build community-based health services. The brief flirtation with a national policy in this area, through the community health program initiated in the Whitlam years, was soon undone in the Fraser years. This is still a major gap in the Australian health care system. Dynamic efficiency then at the system level leaves much to be desired. Unlike the USA, Australian health policy culture does not emphasise systematic trials and experimentation in health policy innovation, the Coordinated Care Trials being the most notable counter-example.

Acceptability

Along with equity and efficiency, a key criterion for evaluating health care systems is acceptability of the system from the perspective of patients, communities, and providers.

Patient acceptability

In recent years there has been a burgeoning interest in understanding the factors that affect patient satisfaction, how to measure it, and how to improve it (Draper and Hill 1996). However, there are no nationally accepted measures of patient satisfaction, and policy use of patient satisfaction questionnaires is still subject to significant political overlays. Governments usually trumpet very high levels of overall patient satisfaction with hospital care, but the results mask significant differences between hospitals and very poor performance on some specific questions evaluating patient experience with the system.

A major development in the health system since the early 1980s has been the strengthening of the consumer movement (see Bastian 1998 for an argument that the antecedents of the health consumer movement date back to the nineteenth century). Although a fledgling Medical Consumers Association was formed in the 1970s (Bates 1983), systematic funding of health consumer organisations did not occur until the mid 1980s. By the early 1990s, a number of organisations were funded by the Commonwealth to serve as a voice for consumers' interests (House of Representatives Standing Committee on Community Affairs 1991). The largest of these at the national level is the Consumers Health Forum but the Victorian-based Health Issues Centre is also nationally active. There is now also a broad range of groups working in the interest of consumers with chronic illnesses. These organisations are able to challenge the provider-based disease specialty organisations that had previously dominated discourse in this area (Short 1998). A network of self-help groups has also assisted in exchanging information between and advocacy for people with chronic illness.

The emergence of consumer organisations was in response to an increasing dissatisfaction with the way in which consumers were treated in the health care system. This dissatisfaction was in part the stimulus for the women's health movement (Broom 1991; Gray 1998) and also for groups of people with chronic illnesses and those from a non-English speaking background (Reid and Boyce 1995). People with chronic illness have, by definition, a long-term relationship with the health system and are thus better able to evaluate the quality of their interactions with the system because they are able to compare their care across time (and providers).

The dissatisfaction with the health system is also evident among other socially devalued groups. Although people from non-English speaking backgrounds, for example, generally have better health than their Australian-born counterparts (Donovan et al. 1992; Mathers 1998), they face problems of communication through language and a lack of cultural sensitivity in the health care system (Dollis et al. 1993). Aboriginal and Torres Strait Islander peoples also encounter lack of cultural sensitivity in interacting with the health care system.

The hand of consumers has been strengthened by the development of government organisations to assist in the resolution of consumer complaints. These organisations were introduced from the late 1980s onwards, and were specifically mandated in the 1993–98 Medicare Agreement. The title and legislative bases of health complaints bodies vary (Health Care Complaints Commission in New South Wales, Health Services Commissioner in Victoria), as do their statutory powers. However, their basic function is to receive consumer complaints about any aspect of the health system (including public and private hospitals, medical practice, naturopaths) and to attempt to mediate between the complainant and the provider. The complaints are often about the way in which consumers are treated in terms of dignity and communication when they interact with the health care system. A key role of the complaints organisation is to increase the likelihood that providers will listen to complainants (because of the external support provided by the complaints organisation), and to ensure providers address the individual situation of the complainant and change their structures so that the same complaint is not likely to recur.

The powers of complaints organisations vary between states, in particular as to whether the organisation has the ability to mandate redress by the relevant provider. All complaints organisations provide annual reports that detail the nature of the complaints that have been received and the way in which they have been resolved. Public shaming is often a powerful tool in encouraging resolution of complaints. A similar organisation (the Private Health Insurance Ombudsman) has been established by the Commonwealth specifically to deal with complaints against private health insurance organisations.

Community acceptability

Blendon et al. (2003) report the latest in a series of cross-national studies of peoples' views of health care systems.

The most recent study focused on the attitudes of 'sicker' respondents, people who had experience with the health system. The results show that almost two-thirds of sicker Australians were very satisfied or fairly satisfied with the health system (see table 10.2). These figures are similar to those of the other countries studied with the exception of New Zealand and the USA where there are significantly lower levels of satisfaction.

The nature of the problems with the health system differed across countries, with Australia and most other countries reporting different priorities for the biggest problems compared to the USA. In Australia, the two biggest problems, shortages of health professionals or hospital beds and the consequence of that in terms of waiting times, could be seen as being

Table 10.2 Health system views among sicker adults in five countries, 2002

	Aus %	Can %	NZ %	UK %	US %
Satisfaction with health system:					
Very satisfied	15	21	14	25	18
Fairly satisfied	48	41	36	41	36
Not very satisfied	21	23	32	21	25
Not at all satisfied	14	13	16	10	19
Two biggest problems with health care system:					
High cost of health care	19	13	21	6	48
Inadequate coverage of services	9	8	6	8	25
Shortages of health professionals/hospital beds	31	54	20	33	5
Waiting times	31	27	41	39	3
Inadequate government funding	20	16	23	24	1
Single most important thing government can do to improve health care:					
Spend more money	30	32	34	30	4
Reduce waste/reduce fraud/allocate resources better	7	6	10	17	8
Increase number of health professionals/hospitals	14	19	6	17	2
Reduce costs	5	1	5	3	16
Improve coverage of services/people	4	3	5	1	21
Reduce waiting times	6	3	9	9	-

Source: Blendon et al. 2003

attributable to funding constraints. The high cost of health care was seen by about one-fifth of Australians as one of the two biggest problems with the health care system. This could reflect the high co-payments for non-cardholders for pharmaceuticals and the consequences of the recent decline in bulk billing of medical services. Interestingly, the solution to the problems was seen as principally a government requirement, namely, to spend more money.

Overall, in international terms, Australian respondents have a somewhat similar perception of the problems with the health care system and also report similar levels of satisfaction to their overseas counterparts.

A key element of the Australian health care system is consumer choice, and this undoubtedly contributes to the historically high level of acceptability. Australians have almost no constraints on choice with respect to primary care provider and, in the case of primary medical care, this is heavily subsidised. In the United Kingdom, consumers must sign up to a general practitioners list and there are formalised procedures that must be observed for transferring from one list to another. Similarly, in the USA, most managed care plans restrict consumer choice to a designated panel of providers from whom consumers are allowed to seek (reimbursed) care.

Some policy analysts have suggested adoption of managed care in Australia (Scotton 1995, 1999). It is easy to understand the attraction of managed care in the USA (where it might provide the way around political obstacles to increased access) and in developing countries (where managed care might provide increased access at relatively low cost). However, the Australian situation is quite different, as Medicare has so far managed to provide high levels of access at a moderate cost. Thus the driving force for managed care in Australia is not increasing access but, principally, reducing cost. The trade-off thus entails reduced choice for reduced social cost, and it is unlikely that this trade-off will be politically acceptable to consumers and voters. It is sometimes argued that managed care can be seen to increase 'quality', but given the very poor measurement of quality in Australia, it is difficult to see how this will be demonstrated to consumers. The social contract to maintain universal coverage is fragile. The loss of widespread public support by implementing a managed care strategy could result in a taxpayer revolt and/or reversion to less equitable, predominantly private financing of health care.

Provider acceptability

The Medicare system of high quality, low cost universal access is vulnerable if providers can persuade the public and political parties that it is failing. The most notable instance of this was the campaign by the medical profession (and the health insurance funds) to destabilise Medibank and facilitate its dismantling under the Fraser Government in the late 1970s. The interests of providers are not always coincident with the interests of consumers (Duckett 1984), and it is important that policy not be driven solely by provider acceptability. However, provider acceptability affects the system and, to a degree, affects the extent to which it is able to achieve dynamic efficiency.

Some elements of the medical profession still rail against universal health insurance. However, these criticisms should not be dismissed, as health professionals often have a high level of personal commitment to provision of high quality care and a clear understanding of the effects of various reforms. What is important, however, is that we disentangle the financial and professional interest of the providers from the interests of consumers and the system as a whole.

Overseas alternatives

This chapter has reviewed a number of outstanding problems of the Australian health care system in addressing equity, efficiency, and accepta-bility. These issues are often used to support the adoption of an alternative structure for the health system, with the United Kingdom, New Zealand and, occasionally, the USA hailed as providing guidance. Health systems in these countries have been the subject of major restructure in recent years. Indeed, the 1990s could be characterised as a decade of major health reform in a number of countries. A hallmark of these reforms has been the attempt to introduce competition into previously integrated and controlled national health services and to distance government from health sector activities. They are underpinned by a belief that market-type incentives can be used to improve both the efficiency and consumer responsiveness of the systems. They also rely on the contemporary theory that government is better at 'steering' than actually 'rowing' (the metaphor derives from Osborne and Gaebler 1992), and that the appropriate role of government is to decide policy direction, but leave program delivery to nongovernment agencies. This view, particularly popular in the USA, results in 'smaller government' (fewer direct employees) and in less direct political accountability for the quality, range, and accessibility of services funded by government.

Although the reforms have differed in some important aspects (see Saltman and von Otter 1989 for a characterisation of the reform directions and Saltman and Figueras 1998 for a review of the reforms), there have been two common underlying threads of the reform processes. First has been the identification of separate roles for the funder, purchaser, provider, and owner. Policy directions have, in particular, emphasised the split of the purchaser and provider roles, with the purchaser being responsible for ensuring that the 'required services in the right volume (are) delivered at the right quality and at the right price' (unpublished paper prepared in 1992 for senior health officials). The provider function has also been strengthened by corporatising providers and encouraging them to function in a more market-oriented manner. A second strand of the policy has been a strengthening of the role of the purchaser in priority setting. The two most widely known examples of these reforms are the Thatcher reforms of the National Health Service from 1989–91 and the New Zealand reforms of 1990. Strengthening of the purchaser function in the USA has occurred through the growth of managed care.

The reforms to the United Kingdom National Health Service

Prior to the Thatcher reforms in the United Kingdom, the National Health Service (NHS) was highly centralised with an integrated care delivery structure. A key element of the 1989–91 reforms was the separation of the roles of provider and purchaser. In their ultimate form, the providers were organised as separate units (known as NHS Trusts). The NHS Trust, which was either a hospital or a community service provider (or in some cases mixtures of hospitals and community services), negotiated contracts for delivery of services from a range of purchasers.

The NHS reforms brought in two distinct types of purchasers. One type was area-based purchasers (area health authorities) which had responsibility for identifying the health needs of their population and purchasing relevant services. The second type of purchaser was 'general practice (GP) fundholders'. General practices were given responsibility for purchasing health care (for example, outpatient care) from providers for the patients on their list. GP fundholders were funded on a per capita basis and would then negotiate with providers for services. While GP fundholding was relatively popular with general practitioners (over 50 per cent of all services were purchased by GP fundholding), there was conflict between the role of the GP fundholders and the roles of area health authorities. There was also considerable disquiet that patients of GP fundholders (who were quite generously funded) would have preferential access to services over patients covered by the less well-funded area health authorities.

Provider contracts with both sets of purchasers were relatively crude. Theoretically, contracts were specified in price, volume, and quality terms, but because of the very poor development of quality measures and the slow development of casemix in the United Kingdom, most were in the form of 'block contracts'. These did not standardise for casemix differences within a broad category of services and provided no quality measures.

The implementation of the Thatcher reforms was bitterly opposed by health professionals, including the medical and nursing professions. The New Labour Government elected in 1997 has begun to dismantle the

Thatcher reforms and has introduced a further round of significant changes to the NHS. In particular, the language of competition and purchasing has been replaced by a language of cooperation and trust (Goddard and Mannion 1998). The evaluations of the NHS internal market changes have produced mixed results (Klein 1998; Le Grand et al. 1998), perhaps not surprisingly given differences in management skills and the contexts in which reforms were implemented. Wyke et al. (2003) concluded 'budgetary incentives are not "magic potions" which have similar effects on behaviour wherever they are introduced'. Whether the language of trust and co-operation will be sustained and provide a sound basis for the NHS is still an open question (Malin et al. 2002).

New Zealand

New Zealand also implemented a purchaser/provider split for its health service in early 1990. Six purchasing authorities were established for New Zealand's population, four of which were population based. The other two were a Public Health Commission to purchase public health services and a Clinical Training Agency to purchase training and development services. The four population-based purchasing agencies were called Regional Health Authorities. Providers were organised into Crown Health Enterprises (CHEs). The purchasing strategies of the four Regional Health Authorities diverged, some adopting sophisticated casemix contracts whereas others pursued strategies similar to the block contracts under the NHS.

There was considerable criticism of the New Zealand reforms, which were electorally unpopular. Then Prime Minister Jim Bolger specifically identified the government's health policy as a major reason for its substantial loss of support in the 1993 election (Easton 1997). Following the 1996 election and the formation of a Coalition Government, the New Zealand reforms have been significantly changed. The four Regional Health Authorities were abolished and a single national health funding authority was created. Moves have been made to replace the language of commercialisation and business with language based on partnership and cooperation. Gauld (2001) summarised the past few decades of reform: 'there is little to suggest that any of the health sector reforms implemented in New Zealand over the last ten years performed significantly better than any prior structure'.

The USA

Health reform in the USA has been substantially different from the directions pursued in countries that started from a unified national health service. In particular, with a very large national share of privately funded insurance, the major reforms have been led by market pressures rather than changes in government policy. With the collapse of the Clinton proposals for universal health care coverage in 1994, there has been substantial restructuring of the health care market in the USA, with a dramatic increase in the proportion of the insured covered by managed care organisations. This marked a profound transformation from a system where most people were insured through 'indemnity' plans similar to Australian private health insurance. About 17 per cent of the US population remains uninsured.

The term 'managed care' immediately connotes a positive (who can support the opposite, 'unmanaged care'?), but it has no precise meaning. In practice, US managed care organisations can be structured quite differently along the critical dimensions of system choice outlined in the Introduction. Hacker and Marmor (1999) have outlined the different options for managed care organisations in terms of constraints on consumer and provider choice and risk pooling of physicians. All are designed to reduce costs to the insurer, with the aim of offering lower premiums to consumers.

The tools and techniques used by managed care organisations, and the relative emphasis on each of these tools, varies between organisations. The key tool, however, is selective provider contracting, that is, the managed care organisation only contracts with a limited number of providers. It thus has the potential to achieve three benefits:

- economies of scale, by concentrating consumers on fewer providers
- stronger market power with respect to the limited number of providers contracted, reflected in potentially lower unit prices
- ability to influence treatment behaviour of the selected providers.

Managed care in Australia

Managed care or health funding based on capitation is an increasingly common response to key problems facing health systems throughout the world. Not surprisingly, the introduction of managed care has been proposed for Australia. There are some benefits of managed care but there are also attendant risks. To a very large extent, the balance of risks and benefits will depend on the design of a managed care policy. Jackson (1996) has identified a number of the features of an ethically sound, practical managed care development for Australia; this involves voluntary enrolment, a focus on a limited number of chronic conditions, payment based on validated risk-assessment tools, and safeguards to assure standards of care. Each departure from these core elements increases the likelihood that the risk of managed care will outweigh the benefits to the Australian health care system.

It is important that policy makers clarify several aspects of any proposed Australian managed care initiative. First, a clear articulation of the policy goal is required. As noted above, managed care advocates emphasise either the cost-saving potential of managed care or its ability to provide a more appropriate mix of services (and, only occasionally, both). Managed care policies designed to meet the cost-saving objective would look quite different from those designed to provide a more comprehensive and responsive service mix.

Second, it is important to clarify whether managed care is to be a voluntary supplement for defined populations or a compulsory and universal approach. Advocates of the cost-saving goal typically propose a wider net for managed care, at least for Medicare or public patients.

Third, strategies to ensure public accountability of any managed care organisation need to be developed before any form of third party care management is implemented. There are real risks with the introduction of managed care including the ethical considerations flagged above and the potential erosion of trust in the health care system (Mechanic 1996; Mechanic and Schlesinger 1996). Despite the development of sophisticated methods of 'risk adjustment' and premium setting (Duckett and Agius 2002), managed care organisations will still have significant incentives and scope to avoid poor 'risks' ('cream skimming', that is, the selection of healthier than average enrolees to be covered by a plan while receiving payment on the basis of an average health profile for their care) rather than accept risks and engage in health promotion and other long-term strategies. This raises issues of adequate financial accountability for plans. Traditionally, the way of dealing with such uncertainty in terms of design was to require that the managed care organisation be not-for-profit, thus allaying at least some concerns about profit-making incentives on owners of the organisation. Such solutions are no longer in vogue and so other forms of accountability need to be developed. This will require clear specification of what is to be expected from managed care organisations, sanctions for poor performance and some form of public scrutiny (Duckett and Swerissen 1996).

Fourth, some account will have to be taken of the persistent opposition to managed care by the medical profession. Organised medicine opposed the 1995 health insurance reforms because it saw these as presaging the introduction of 'US style managed care' in Australia. Managed care is not popular among US physicians (White 1995) and the medical profession in Australia is able to trade on 'horror stories' emanating from the USA where professional autonomy has been or might be infringed in undesirable ways. These US horror stories are further reinforced by stories of the adverse impact of managed care on the demand for medical services, thus affecting US clinicians' incomes.

The medical profession in Australia has traditionally been opposed to any moves to increase accountability to third parties, arguing that they undermine the 'doctor–patient relationship'. This argument may simply be for presentational purposes, as increased accountability of doctors to their peers or government has not diminished accountability to patients, but rather supplemented or reinforced it. The underlying issue for the medical profession remains, however, that third party intervention may place the medical practitioner in a conflict between the interest of the third party payer and that of the patient (Clancy and Brody 1995; Emanuel and Dubler 1995; Kassirer 1995; Rodwin 1995).

But it is not only medical practitioners who are sceptical of the benefits of managed care. Under current arrangements in Australia, patients feel they have extensive freedom of choice for medical care, especially in ambulatory care. This range of choice would inevitably be reduced under managed care, although for some consumers better access to a range of nonmedical services may offset these limitations to some extent.

The Australian 1995 health insurance reforms provide for health insurance organisations to be engaged in selective provider contracting with both hospitals and doctors. This is without a doubt the fundamental basis for introduction of any of the managed care components into Australia.

Managed care or managed competition should not be seen as a panacea. A recent evaluation of the USA's experience provides a salutary warning for Australian policy advocates, as Steiner and Robinson (1998) point out: 'There is some strong evidence in relation to the overall performance of managed care in terms of changes in utilisation, quality and patterns of treatment. Applying this evidence directly to (another country), however, is complicated'.

The US health system is more expensive than the Australian system at the same time as exhibiting significant access problems. Strategies to rein in health expenditure when it stands at 16 per cent of GDP may not be productive in the context of health expenditure at less than 10 per cent of GDP. Similarly, improvements in preventive activities (one of the success stories of managed care in the USA) have been achieved in Australia through organised public health programs. However, this does not mean that there are no lessons for Australia.

In considering the potential application of managed care in Australia it is worthwhile unpacking the concept of managed care into two key components: influencing the behaviour of providers through incentive tools, and through information and education strategies.

The incentive approaches to controlling provider behaviour are the aspects of managed care that give rise to most opposition from providers and are simultaneously of most concern to consumers. Because they directly oppose doctors' interests with those of their patients, these approaches are likely to face overwhelming opposition to their use in Australia. Private sector capitation and/or strong utilisation management processes of managed care are unlikely to be implemented in this country.

However, there is more scope for introduction of information/education strategies developed for the US managed care industry. A number of managed care organisations are developing new approaches to quality measurement (Bernstein et al. 1993) and combining databases about the experience of their enrolees with information from other research efforts from the USA (such as the Patient Outcome Research Teams). These approaches could well be used to improve the quality of care in Australia. A useful step for government (or private health insurance funds) would be to consider purchasing advisory services from managed care or like organisations to assist in providing information to providers to help inform and influence their practice patterns.

The Health Insurance Commission has developed state-of-the-art approaches to analysing its vast data holdings to assist in the identification of possible fraud and overservicing. It would be a logical step for the Health Insurance Commission to develop its data handling capacities to provide better feedback to medical practitioners (and possibly hospitals) about ways of improving practice based on the results of the analysis occurring in the more advanced US managed care organisations. Similarly, the Health Insurance Commission could begin to use techniques developed by US managed care organisations to reward quality of care rather than volume of care (Hanchak et al. 1996; Murray et al. 1996).

An ideal system?

An ideal health system should be designed to maximise achievement of the three broad health system goals described in the Introduction: equity, efficiency, and acceptability. First and foremost, an ideal health system is one that is patient-centred and ensures that high quality care is available to all people in a timely fashion. The vignette in the case study below illustrates a number of attributes of an ideal system: it is well integrated, accessible, dynamic, and respectful of patient autonomy.

Case study

A woman with dizziness is concerned about her health. She rings the state Call Centre, which advises her to visit her local health team. She is able to see the general practitioner quickly. The practitioner asks her a series of questions from the relevant research-based protocol and undertakes a clinical examination. The general practitioner emails the results to a local specialist and books an appointment with the specialist who orders some further investigations consistent with the state research-based care path.

The specialist is able to schedule these from her office. On the basis of the test results and clinical examination, the specialist thinks hospitalisation is necessary and schedules admission to the local hospital. Advice of this impending admission is automatically conveyed electronically to the general practitioner and the social worker in the referring health team. The social worker contacts the hospital to discuss discharge planning issues before the patient is admitted. The patient is discovered to have a brain tumour.

The specialist advises against an operation but suggests a number of sources for information about the patient's condition. The patient contacts the Call Centre for further information about alternatives and discusses these with the specialist. The patient (and her family) accept the specialist's advice and she is discharged to the local palliative care team. The patient does not need to make any out-of-pocket payment at any point in this chain.

This case is randomly selected by the hospital audit committee for quality review. The committee suggests slight changes to the protocol for handling dizzy patients in the community. The statewide protocol committee funds a small-scale randomised controlled trial to assess the cost-effectiveness of the change before it is definitively implemented.

The case is not subject to utilisation review because there are no significant deviations from the care path and resource use (reported from the hospital's clinical costing system) is within normal bounds for that condition.

Emphases in the ideal health system

Emphasis on equity of outcomes

Ill health is unevenly distributed in Australia (rich versus poor, Aboriginal versus non–Aboriginal) and, in an ideal health system, these disparities would be eliminated. This would require cross–sectoral strategies and positive discrimination in health promotion and community development programs.

Emphasis on community-based programs

The disability field has adopted a concept of advocating the 'least restrictive alternative' as the goal for housing for the disabled: that people with a disability should be accommodated in the type of housing that involves the least possible restrictions on their autonomy. A similar concept should be practised in health care: that services should be provided in the home or community settings where feasible and that hospitalisation or centralisation should only occur where there were demonstrable benefits in a more distant site of care.

Emphasis on quality of care

The desire for high quality health care is something that unites providers and consumers. In order to promote high quality care, quality should be measured both in the clinical sense (the best possible outcome, given the patient's condition) and from a patient perspective (that they are treated with dignity, that they are provided with appropriate information). Feedback should be given to hospitals and other health agencies on their performance against quality measures and, in the medium term, performance should also be reported publicly.

Emphasis on real consumer choice and accountability

Consumers should have choices (not constrained by their financial means) about alternative sites of care (that is, what hospital or health team is most convenient for them), and should be involved in treatment decision making. Assessments of relative benefits of treatments and trade-offs in terms of surgery or medical interventions should involve the fully informed consumer. Consumer choice is facilitated by allowing consumers choice of any hospital or agency for their care and by providing information to assist choice.

Emphasis on efficiency

The ideal health system needs to be financially sustainable. This in turn means that decision-making processes (and care delivery) must be organised to maximise efficiency, broadly defined to include technical, allocative, and dynamic efficiency. Payment systems to agencies should reward efficiency and penalise inefficiency. Substitutable services should be subsidised so that consumers (and referring providers) are agnostic as to which service is used.

The ideal system

What would an ideal health system look like? First, it would start with strategies to assist consumers to make informed choices. This would require a telephone (and Internet) call centre that would be able to provide health advice (according to evidence-based protocols), and advice about sources of care including costs, waiting times, and quality.

Second, an ideal health system would be based on locally accessible multidisciplinary health teams. The teams should include general practitioners, nurses, pharmacists, physiotherapists, and so on. The teams should have links to locally based specialists. In rural areas especially, the teams may include a number of nurses with rights to prescribe commonly needed medications ('nurse practitioners'), to ensure accessible primary care.

Third, there needs to be a network of hospitals and day procedure centres. Hospitals would not be the centre of the new system, even though they are the most expensive part of any health care system. Hospitalisation is a rare event; only about 1 per cent of the population is hospitalised in any one year. What is critical is ensuring good links between hospitals and primary care and local specialists. This is a communication rather than a management task.

The ideal system would need to be supported by a sophisticated information technology infrastructure, facilitating transmission of information between the various providers of care, when authorised by the patient.

Funding of this system should be on an equitable basis, through general taxation. Individual providers should have incentives for efficiency: hospitals should be funded on a casemix basis, primary care teams on a mix of activity (fee-for-service) and program payments. Although capitation payments are often suggested as the preferred method of payment in primary care and for patients with chronic conditions, capitation has a number of weaknesses. First, it requires consumers to elect to be treated by a single primary care team (in order to identify the capitated population). Some consumers may want to identify with a single provider, but others may want to exercise choice as to the provider or provider group they wish to have treat a particular problem. Second, the technology for capitation payment is still in its infancy and, although theoretically capitation gives providers an incentive to 'keep people healthy', in fact capitation payments provide a far greater incentive for providers to avoid taking on 'bad risks' (Newhouse 1996, 1998), resulting in efficiency losses in the system and reduced access for those who probably need it most.

From theory to practice

Specifying ideal systems is relatively easy. The difficult task is managing the transition from the current system to this nirvana. Some aspects of the transition are straightforward: we know how to ensure technical efficiency of inpatient care; we fund on the basis of casemix-adjusted activity. Other aspects are not so clear because the technologies are not so well developed or there may not be consensus on either the desirability of the change or how to achieve it. Improving consumer choice and accountability, for example may be seen to conflict with the desire of some professionals for autonomy and respect for their judgment. Measuring effectiveness of health interventions is a complex task, and the research to do this is expensive. Jurisdictional barriers between governments, departments, and other agencies will be defended.

There is no perfect policy which, when implemented, will allow the health system to operate in equilibrium without intervention. The health system is dynamic, and the system needs to be capable of incorporating worthwhile innovations. Some policy instruments that are necessary to achieve one goal (for example output-based funding for technical efficiency) will need to be accompanied by strategies to ensure that they do not compromise achievement of other goals (for example output-based funding might lead to unnecessary admissions and hence increased expenditure and reduced allocative efficiency).

The basis for any change must be good, publicly accessible information. The more information in the public domain about equity, efficiency, and acceptability of the current system, the less will be the power of those who seek to frustrate progress towards the ideal for self-interested or other reasons. Second, the expectations of the health system need to be explicit. This should involve a clear linkage between funding provided and output expectations, with accompanying accountability systems. For inpatient care, a range of goals might be set relating to activity levels, quality, timeliness, consumer acceptability, and so on. In primary care a similar range of goals might be set but supplemented by goals relating to prevention, including prevention of hospital admissions. At the least this involves transparency in the relationships between the myriad providers and funders.

Getting the ideal system to work will require a mix of strategies. There are three broad sets of instruments that societies have available to promote the achievement of health policy goals: financial incentives, hierarchical structures and regulation, and professional norms and cultures. The mix of these used to achieve social goals varies across social policy sectors, countries, and over time (Tuohy 1999). Government action tends to concentrate on use of the first two strategies. The late 1990s probably marked the apogee of the use of financial incentives in most areas of policy, and there is now a substantial literature on when financial incentives rather than hierarchical strategies are appropriate in system design (for example, Williamson 1975, 1986; Ashton 1997). Government can exercise considerable influence over the health system through using financial incentives to influence provider behaviour, establishing the structures and agencies for achieving health system goals, and setting the rules within which organisations and professions work. However, government has relatively less influence over control of professional cultures and norms, as these are primarily the preserve of the professions themselves.

Systems theory has adopted a concept of equifinality; that there are a number of ways systems can be organised to achieve the same ends. In that light, the organisational arrangements of the health care system (networks versus areas versus individual hospitals) are seen to be less important. What does become critical is how these organisations operate, what goals they are pursuing, and what they are achieving. Although financial incentives have an important role in defining goals and so on, so, too, do hierarchical relationships and professional norms and cultures. Strategies to move towards the ideal must therefore attempt to use all three instruments of change, and particularly the last, given the influential role played by professional norms and cultures in health.

Conclusion

There are a number of significant challenges that face the Australian health care system over the next decade. These are not the ones traditionally lamented, of an ageing population driving health expenditure out of control. As was discussed in earlier chapters, the cost of the health system is relatively stable. Rather, the key problems facing the system are internal ones: choices about the roles of doctors and nurses, addressing the glaring inequities in health outcomes, ensuring quality, and addressing technical and allocative efficiency. In the medium term, information technology may substantially change the role of practitioners; consumers may benefit from improved access to information through the Internet.

However, one cannot be sure that these positive moves will conspire to ensure the onward steady march of progress. The health system remains a contested terrain and the interest of purchasers, providers, and consumers do not always coincide. The interests of funders and consumers may also diverge. Increasing globalisation of the economy may lead to pressures for further reshaping of the health care system.

It is the thesis of this book, though, that debates about the future of the health care system should involve consumers and health professionals of all kinds, and that these debates should sort fact from fiction, evaluating policy proposals against available evidence. The stronger the information base about what is happening in the health care system, the more likely that the strong gains we have made in Australia in terms of equity, efficiency, and acceptability of the system can be consolidated, and gains in quality can be achieved.

Appendices

Appendix 1 Australia: Preliminary estimates of total health service expenditure, current prices, by area of expenditure and source of fund, 2001/02 (A$ million)

| | Government Sector | | | | | Nongovernment sector | | | | | | |
| | Commonwealth | | | State & local | Total government | Health insurance funds | | | Individuals | Other | Total non-government | Total |
	Direct expenditure	Health insurance rebates	Total			Gross	Rebates	Net				
Hospitals	8649	1048	9697	8092	17,789	3783	1048	2735	561	1151	4447	22,236
Public (nonpsychiatric)	7889	104	7993	7707	15,700	375	104	271	236	471	978	16,678
Public (psychiatric)	-1	-1	385	385		0	18	7	24	409		
Private	761	944	1704	0	1704	3407	944	2464	308	673	3444	5149
High-level residential aged care	3093		3093	213	3306				831	0	831	4137
Ambulance	74	52	126	517	643	189	52	137	256	50	443	1086
Total institutional	11,816	1100	12,916	8822	21,738	3972	1100	2872	1648	1201	5721	27,459
Medical services	8,879	166	9045	0	9045	598	166	432	1195	515	2142	11,187
Other health professionals	453	116	569	0	569	420	116	304	1415	234	1952	2521
Pharmaceuticals	4813	18	4830	0	4830	64	18	46	4030	83	4159	8989
Benefit paid items	4746	0	4746	0	4746	0	0	0	841	0	841	5586
All other items	67	18	85	0	85	64	18	46	3189	83	3318	3403
Aids and appliances	99	88	187	0	187	318	88	230	1932	54	2216	2403

Appendix 1 Australia: Preliminary estimates of total health service expenditure, current prices, by area of expenditure and source of fund, 2001/02 (A$ million) (cont.)

| | Government Sector | | | | | Nongovernment sector | | | | | | |
| | Commonwealth | | | State & local | Total government | Health insurance funds | | | Individuals | Other | Total non-government | Total |
	Direct expenditure	Health insurance rebates	Total			Gross	Rebates	Net				
Other noninstitutional	1552	463	2015	3382	5397	1665	463	1203	2293	15	3511	8908
Community/public health	644	1	645	2671	3316	1	1	0	-1	6	5	3321
Dental services	75	262	337	365	702	946	262	684	2293	10	2987	3689
Health administration	832	200	1032	347	1379	718	200	518	0	0	518	1897
Other noninstitutional (nec)	1	0	1	0	1	0	0	0	0	0	0	1
Research	834	0	834	166	1000	0	0	0	0	226	226	1226
Total noninstitutional	*16,630*	*850*	*17,480*	*3548*	*21,028*	*3065*	*850*	*2215*	*10,864*	*1128*	*14,206*	*35,235*
Total recurrent	**28,445**	**1950**	**30,396**	**12,370**	**42,766**	**7037**	**1950**	**5087**	**12,512**	**2329**	**19,927**	**62,693**
Capital outlays	90	0	90	1462	1552	0	0	0	0	1305	1305	2856
Capital consumption	27	0	27	1005	1033	0	0	0	0	0	0	1033
Total capital	**118**	**0**	**118**	**2467**	**2584**	**0**	**0**	**0**	**0**	**1305**	**1305**	**3889**
Direct health expenditure	**28,563**	**1950**	**30,513**	**14,837**	**45,350**	**7037**	**1950**	**5087**	**12,512**	**3633**	**21,232**	**66,582**
Nonspecific tax expenditure	150		150		150			0	-150		-150	0
Total health expenditure	**28,713**	**1950**	**30,663**	**14,837**	**45,500**	**7037**	**1950**	**5087**	**12,362**	**3633**	**21,082**	**66,582**

Source: AIHW (2003) Health expenditure Australia 2001–02, Canberra

Appendix 2 Australia: Funding flows for hospital and medical services

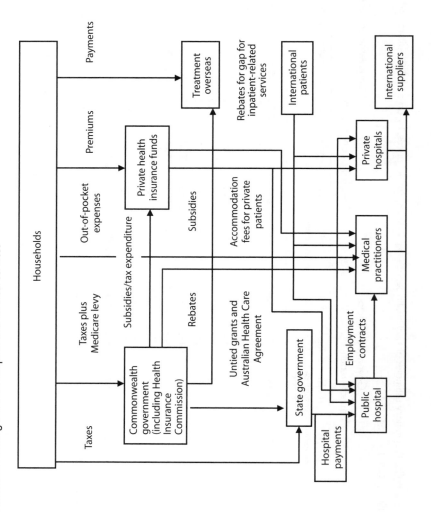

Appendix 3 Evolution of Medicare/health insurance arrangements

	Medical rebates	Hospital access	Levy/Private health insurance
Medibank July 1975	• Universal rebate at 85% of schedule fee with maximum gap between fee and rebate of $5 (85%/$5) • Bulk billing available	• Universal access to public hospitals without charge for treatment by hospital nominated doctor ('hospital patient')	• No levy
October 1976 (Medibank Mark II)			• Levy: 2.5% of taxable income • Levy opt-out provision for people with private insurance
May 1978	• General population 75%/$10 • Bulk billing restricted to pensioners (85%/$5) and socially disadvantaged (75%/-)		
November 1978	• General population: 40%/$20 (paid through health insurance funds whether member of not) • Pensioners, socially disadvantaged unchanged		• Levy abolished
May 1979	• General population: rebate only for that part of schedule fee in excess of $20 (0%/$20) • Pensioner: unchanged		
September 1981	• Rebates restricted to those with medical insurance, paid at 30% of schedule fee (30%/-)	• 'Free' public hospital care abolished	
Medicare, February 1984 (Hawke Labor Government)	• Universal 85%/$10 • Universal bulk billing available	• 'Free' public hospital care restored	• Levy: 1%
November 1986	• Out of hospital: 85%/$20 but subject to total gap not to exceed $150 p.a. • In hospital 75%/-but basic private hospital insurance to cover remaining 25%		• Levy: 1.25%
July 1993			• Levy: 1.4%

Appendix 3 Evolution of Medicare/health insurance arrangements (cont.)

	Medical rebates	Hospital access	Levy/Private health insurance
July 1995			• Levy: 1.5%
July 1996			• Levy: 1.5% (From 1 July 1996 to 30 June 1997 there was a 0.2% surcharge on the Medicare levy to pay for a guns buy-back scheme introduced following the Port Arthur massacre.)
July 1997 (Howard Coalition Government)			• Levy surcharge of 1% introduced for those with household income over $100,000 p.a. who do not have private health insurance • Capped means-tested rebate for hospital and ancillary insurance
January 1999			• Uncapped 30% rebate payable for health insurance (both hospital and ancillary) without means test
July 2000			• Regulation of private health insurance premiums changed to allow differential premiums based on age at which contributor first took out health insurance ('life-time community rating').

Bibliography

Abbott, P. D. and L. O. Goldsmith 1952, 'History and functions of the Commonwealth Health Department, 1921–1952', Public Administration XI:119–28, 146.

Abelson, P. 2002, 'Economic evaluation of public health programs in Australia from 1970 to 2000', *2001 Proceedings of Twenty-third Australian Conference of Health Economists*, pp. 285–310.

Acheson, D. 1998, Report of the independent inquiry into inequalities in health (Acheson Report), London: Stationery Office.

Aday, L. A., C. E. Begley, D. R. Lairson and C. H. Slater 1998, *Evaluating the healthcare system*, Chicago: Health Administration Press.

Aged Care Evaluation and Management Advisors 2003, *Resident Classification Scale Review*, Commonwealth Department of Health and Ageing, Aged and Community Care Service Development and Evaluation Report No. 43, Canberra: Australian Government Publishing Service.

Aiken, L. H., S. P. Clarke and D. M. Sloane 2002, 'Hospital staffing, organization, and quality of care: Cross-national findings', *International Society for Quality in Health Care*, 14(1):5–13.

Aiken, L. H., S. P. Clarke, D. M. Sloan, J. Sochalski and J. H. Silber 2002, 'Hospital nurse staffing and patient mortality, nurse burnout, and job dissatisfaction', *American Medical Association*, 288(16):1987–93.

Alexander, J. 2000, 'The changing role of clinicians: Their role in health reform in Australia and New Zealand,' in A.L. Bloom (ed.) *Health reform in Australia and New Zealand*, Melbourne: Oxford University Press, pp. 161–77.

Allison, G. and P. Zelikow 1999, *Essence of decision: Explaining the Cuban missile crisis*, New York: Longman.

Alt Statis and Associates 1994, 'Service provision targets: A report for the Home and Community Care Program', Aged and Community Care Service Development and Evaluation Report No. 15, Canberra: Australian Government Publishing Service.

Andersen, T. F. and G. Mooney (eds) 1990, *The challenges of medical practice variations*, London: Macmillan Press.

Anderson, L. M., S. C. Scrimshaw, M. T. Fullilove, J. E. Fielding and Task Force on Community Preventive Services 2003, 'The Community Guide's model for linking the social environment of health', *American Journal of Preventive Medicine*, 24(3S):12–20.

Ansari, M. Z., M. J. Ackland, D. J. Jolley, N. Carson and I. G. McDonald 1999, 'Inter-hospital comparison of mortality rates', *International Journal for Quality in Health Care*, 11(1):29–35.

Antonazzo, E., A. Scott, D. Skatun and R. F. Elliott 2003, 'The labour market for nursing: A review of the labour supply literature', *Health Economics*, 12:465–78.

Antonovsky, A. 1993, 'Complexity, conflict, chaos, coherence, coercion and civility', *Social Science & Medicine*, 37:968–81.

Applied Economics 2003, *Returns on investment in public health: An epidemiological and economic analysis prepared for the Department of Health and Ageing*, Canberra: Commonwealth Department of Health and Ageing.

Arblaster, L., M. Lambert, V. Entwistle, M. Forster, D. Fullerton, T. Sheldon and I. Watt 1996, 'A systematic review of the effectiveness of health service interventions aimed at reducing inequalities in health', *Journal of Health Services Research and Policy*, 1:93–103.

Aroni, R., R. de Boer and K. Harvey 2003, 'The Viagra affair: Evidence as the terrain for competing "partners"', in V. Lin and B. Gibson (eds) *Evidence-based health policy*, Melbourne: Oxford University Press, pp. 97–109.

Arrow, K. J. 1963, 'Uncertainty and the welfare economics of medical care', *American Economic Review* 53:941–73.

Ashton, T. 1997, 'Contracting for health services in New Zealand: A transaction cost analysis', *Social Science & Medicine* 46:357–67.

Auditor-General 1996, *Drug evaluation by the Therapeutic Goods Administration*, Canberra: Australian National Audit Office.

Auditor-General 1997, *Pharmaceutical Benefits Scheme*, Canberra: Australian National Audit Office.

Auditor-General 2000, *Home and Community Care*, Audit Report No. 36 1999–2000, Canberra: Australian National Audit Office.

Auditor-General 2002, *Home and Community Care follow up audit*, Audit Report No. 32 2001–02, Canberra: Australian National Audit Office.

Auditor-General of Victoria 1998, *Acute health services under casemix: A case of mixed priorities*, Special Report No. 56, Melbourne: Victorian Government Printer.

Australian Bureau of Statistics 1994, *Apparent determinants of private health insurance*, Canberra: ABS.

Australian Bureau of Statistics 1996a, *Australians and the environment*, ABS Cat. No. 4601.0, Canberra: ABS.

Australian Bureau of Statistics 1996b, *Causes of death, Australia*, Cat. No. 3303.0, Canberra: ABS.

Australian Bureau of Statistics 1996c, *Detailed expenditure items: 1993–94 household expenditure survey, Australia*, Cat. No. 6535.0, Canberra: ABS.

Australian Bureau of Statistics 1997a, *Australian social trends*, Cat. No. 4102.0, Canberra: ABS.

Australian Bureau of Statistics 1997b, *National health survey: SF-36 population norms*, Cat. No. 4399.0, Canberra: ABS.

Australian Bureau of Statistics 1997c, *1995 National health survey: Summary of results, Australia*, Cat. No. 4364.0, Canberra: ABS.

Australian Bureau of Statistics 1998a, *Community Services 1995–96, Australia*, Cat. No. 8696.0, Canberra: ABS.

Australian Bureau of Statistics 1998b, *How Australians use their time*, Cat. No. 4153, Canberra: ABS.

Australian Bureau of Statistics 1999a, *Government finance statistics 1996/97*, Cat. No. 5512.0, Canberra: ABS.

Australian Bureau of Statistics 1999b, *Disability, ageing and carers, Australia: Summary of findings*, Cat. No. 4430.0, Canberra: ABS.

Australian Bureau of Statistics 1999c, *Environment protection expenditure, Australia*, Cat. No. 4603.0, Canberra: ABS.

Australian Bureau of Statistics 1999d, *Population by age and sex, Australian states and territories.* Cat. No. 3201.0, Canberra: ABS.

Australian Bureau of Statistics 1999e, *Deaths*, Cat. No. 3302.0, Canberra: ABS.

Australian Bureau of Statistics 1999f, *Optometry and optical dispensing services*, Cat. No. 8553.0, Canberra: ABS.

Australian Bureau of Statistics 2000, *Household expenditure survey: Detailed expenditure items, Australia*, Cat. No. 6535.0, Canberra, ABS.

Australian Bureau of Statistics 2001, *The health and welfare of Australia's Aboriginal and Torres Strait Island peoples* ABS Cat. No. 4704.0, AIHW Cat. No. IHW6, Canberra: ABS.

Australian Bureau of Statistics 2002, *National Health Survey. Summary of Results*, Cat. No. 4364.0, Canberra: ABS.

Australian Bureau of Statistics and Australian Institute of Health and Welfare 2002, *Hospital statistics. Aboriginal and Torres Strait Islander Australians, 1999–2000*, ABS, Cat. No. 4711.0, Canberra: ABS & AIHW.

Australian Council on Healthcare Standards 1998, *Measurement of care in Australian hospitals*, Sydney: ACHS.

Australian Council on Healthcare Standards 2002a, *Determining the potential to improve quality of care (3rd edn). ACHS clinical indicator results for Australia and New Zealand 1998–2001*, Sydney: ACHS.

Australian Council on Healthcare Standards 2002b, *The EQuIP Guide. A framework to improve quality and safety of health care (3rd edn)*, Sydney: ACHS.

Australian Health Workforce Advisory Committee 2002a, *The midwifery workforce in Australia*, Sydney: AHWAC.

Australian Health Workforce Advisory Committee 2002b, *The critical care nursing workforce in Australia*, Sydney: AHWAC.

Australian Institute of Health and Welfare 1998a, *Medical labour force 1996*, Cat. No. HWL 10, Canberra: Ausinfo.

Australian Institute of Health and Welfare 1998b, *Nursing labour force 1995*, Cat. No. HWL 8, Canberra: Ausinfo.

Australian Institute of Health and Welfare 1998c, *Breast and cervical cancer screening in Australia 1996–97*, Cat. No. CAN 3, Canberra: AIHW.

Australian Institute of Health and Welfare and Commonwealth Department of Health and Aged Care 1999, *Residential aged care facilities in Australia 1998: A statistical overview*, AIHW Cat. No. AGE 14, Canberra: AIHW.

Australian Institute of Health and Welfare 1999a, *Australian hospital statistics 1997/98*, Cat. No. HSE 6, Canberra: Ausinfo.

Australian Institute of Health and Welfare 1999b, *BreastScreen Australia Achievement Report 1997 and 1998*, Canberra: AIHW, p. 9.

Australian Institute of Health and Welfare 1999c, *Health Expenditure Bulletin No. 15: Australia's health services expenditure 1997–98*, Cat. No. HWE 13, Canberra: AIHW.

Australian Institute of Health and Welfare 2000a, *Optometrist Labour Force 1999*, (National Labour Force Series No. 18), Cat No. HWL17, Canberra: AIHW.

Australian Institute of Health and Welfare 2000b, *Residential aged care facilities in Australia 1998–99*, (Aged Care Statistics Series), Cat. No. AGE 16, Canberra: AIHW.

Australian Institute of Health and Welfare 2001a, *Occupational therapy labour force 1998*, HWL 21, Canberra: AIHW.

Australian Institute of Health and Welfare 2001b, *Physiotherapy labour force 1998*, HWL 22, Canberra: AIHW.

Australian Institute of Health and Welfare 2002a, *Alcohol and other drug treatment services in Australia 2000–01: First report on the National Minimum Data Set*, Drug Treatment Series No. 1, Cat. No. HSE 22, Canberra: AIHW.

Australian Institute of Health and Welfare 2002b, *Entry period for residential aged care*, AIHW Cat. No. AGE 24, Canberra: AIHW.

Australian Institute of Health and Welfare 2002c, *National public health expenditure report 1999–00*, AIHW, Health and Welfare Expenditure Series, Canberra: AIHW.

Australian Institute of Health and Welfare 2002d, *Podiatry labour force 1999*, AIHW Cat. No. HWL 23, Canberra: AIHW.

Australian Institute of Health and Welfare 2002e, *Waiting times for elective surgery in Australia 1999–00*, Cat. No. HSE 18, Canberra: AIHW.

Australian Institute of Health and Welfare 2003a, *Australian hospital statistics 2001–02*, AIHW Cat. No. HSE 25, Canberra: AIHW.

Australian Institute of Health and Welfare 2003b, *Community Aged Care Packages in Australia 2001–02: A statistical overview*, AIHW Aged Care Statistics Series No. 14, Cat. No. AGE 30, Canberra: AIHW.

Australian Institute of Health and Welfare 2003c, *Medical labour force 1999*, Cat. No. HWL 24, Canberra: AIHW.

Australian Institute of Health and Welfare 2003d, *Medical labour force 2000*, Bulletin No. 5, Canberra: AIHW.

Australian Institute of Health and Welfare 2003e, *Mental health services in Australia 2000–01*, Mental Health Series No. 4, Canberra: AIHW.

Australian Institute of Health and Welfare 2003f, *Nursing labour force 2001*, AIHW National Health Labour Force Series No. 26, Cat. No. HWL 26, Canberra: AIHW.

Australian Institute of Health and Welfare 2003g, *Pharmacy labour force to 2001*, AIHW Cat. No. HWL 25, Canberra: AIHW.

Australian Institute of Health and Welfare 2003h, *Residential aged care in Australia 2000–01: A statistical overview*, AIHW Aged Care Series No. 11, Cat. No. AGE 22, Canberra: AIHW.

Australian Institute of Health and Welfare Dental Statistics and Research Unit 2002, 'Dental insurance and access to dental care', DSRU, Research Report No. 5, Adelaide: DSRU.

Australian Institute of Health, Law and Ethics 1998, *Public health law in Australia: New perspectives*, Canberra: The Institute.

Australian Medical Workforce Advisory Committee 1998a, *Influences on participation in the Australian Medical Workforce: AMWAC 1998.4*, Sydney: AMWAC.

Australian Medical Workforce Advisory Committee 1998b, *Sustainable specialist services, AMWAC 1998.7*, Sydney: AMWAC.

Australian Medical Workforce Advisory Committee 1999, *Temporary resident doctors in Australia. Distribution, characteristics and role, AMWAC 1999.3*, Canberra: AMWAC.

Australian Medical Workforce Advisory Committee and Australian Institute of Health and Welfare 1996, *Female participation in the Australian medical workforce,* AMWAC 1996.7, Sydney: AMWAC.

Australian Medical Workforce Advisory Committee and Australian Institute of Health and Welfare 1998, *Medical workforce supply and demand in Australia: A discussion paper*, AMWAC Report 1998.8, AIHW Cat. No. HWL 12, Sydney: AIHW.

Ayanian, J. Z. and J. S. Weissman 2002, 'Teaching hospitals and quality of care: A review of the literature', *The Milbank Quarterly*, 80(3):569–93.

Baldock, J. and A. Evers 1992, 'Innovations and care of the elderly: The cutting-edge of change for social welfare systems. Examples from Sweden, the Netherlands and the United Kingdom', *Ageing and Society*, 12:289–312.

Baldwin, R. and C. Walker 1995, 'The separation of policy and operations in organisation: A New South Wales case study', *Australian Journal of Public Administration*, 54:185–95.

Ballard, J. 1998, 'The constitution of AIDS in Australia: Taking "government at a distance" seriously', in M. Dean and B. Hindess (eds) *Governing Australia: Studies in contemporary rationalities of government*, Cambridge, UK: Cambridge University Press, pp. 125-38.

Ballard, J. 1999, 'HIV-contaminated blood and Australian policy: The limits of success', in E.A. Feldman and R. Bayer (eds) in *Blood feuds: AIDS, blood and the politics of medical disaster*, New York: Oxford University Press, pp. 243–70.

Banta, D. 2003, 'The development of health technology assessment', *Health Policy* 63:121–32.

Barer, M., M. Nicoll, M. Diesendorf and R. Harvey 1990, *Australian private medical care costs and use, 1976 and 1986*, Canberra: Australian Government Publishing Service.

Barer, M. L., V. Bhatla, R. G. Evans and G. L. Stoddard 1993, 'Who are the Zombie masters and what do they want?', University of British Columbia Health Policy Research Unit, HPRU 93:13D.

Barraclough, S. 1997, 'Australia's international health relations', in H. Gardner (ed) *Health Policy in Australia*, Melbourne: Oxford University Press, pp. 227–42.

Barraclough, S. and J. Smith 1994, 'Change of government and health services policy in Victoria, 1992/93', *Australian Health Review*, 17:7–21.

Barros, P. P. 1998, 'The black box of health care expenditure growth determinants', *Health Economics*, 7:533–44.

Bartlett, B. and D. Legge 1994, *Beyond the maze: Proposals for more effective administration of Aboriginal health programs*, Working Paper No. 34, Alice Springs: National Centre for Epidemiology and Population Health.

Bastian, H. 1998, 'Speaking up for ourselves: The evolution of consumer advocacy in health care', *International Journal of Technology Assessment and Health Care*, 14:3–23.

Bates, D. V. 1994, *Environmental health risks and public policy: Decision making in free societies*, Vancouver: UBC Press.

Bates, D. W. and A. A. Gawande 2003, 'Improving safety with information technology', *New England Journal of Medicine*, 348(25):2526–34.

Bates, D. W., R. S. Evans, H. Murff, P. D. Stetson, L. Pizziferri and G. Hripcsak 2003, 'Detecting adverse events using information technology', *Journal of the American Medical Informatics Association*, 10(2):115–28.

Bates, E. M. 1983, *Health systems and public scrutiny: Australia, Britain and the United States*, Beckenham: Croom Helm.

Baum, F. 1998, *The new public health: An Australian perspective*, Melbourne: Oxford University Press.

Baume, P. 1994, *A cutting edge: Australia's surgical workforce 1994: Report of the inquiry into the supply of, and requirements for, medical specialist services in Australia*, Melbourne: Australian Government Publishing Service.

Baume, P. E. 1995, 'Waiting times for non-urgent specialist appointments', *Medical Journal of Australia*, 162:648–9.

Beaglehole, R. and M. R. Dal Poz 2003, 'Public health workforce: Challenges and policy issues', *Human Resources for Health*, 1(4):1–10.

Beaglehole, R. and R. Bonita 1997, *Public health at the crossroads: Achievements and prospects*, Cambridge, New York: Cambridge University Press.

Beauchamp, T. L. and J. F. Childress 2001, *Principles of biomedical ethics*, New York: Oxford University Press.

Beaver, C. 1999, 'Health priority setting in the Northern Territory: Principles and models in operation', in *Strategic health care investment seminar: Summary of proceedings*, Sydney: Department of Health & Aged Care and Territory Health Services.

Beckmann, U., I. Baldwin, M. Durie, A. Morrison and L. Shaw 1998, 'Problems associated with nursing staff shortage: An analysis of the first 3600 reports submitted to the Australian incident monitoring study (AIMS-ICU)', *Anaesthesia and Intensive Care*, 26(4):396–400.

Beilby, J. J. and C. A. Silagy 1997, 'Trials of providing costing information to general practitioners: a systematic review', *Medical Journal of Australia*, 167:89–92.

Bellomo, R., D. Goldsmith, S. Russell and S. Uchino 2002, 'Postoperative serious adverse events in a teaching hospital: A prospective study', *Medical Journal of Australia*, 176(4 March):216–18.

Benn, S. 1997, 'The EHCA 1985 (NSW): A historical perspective on issues arising in the control of toxic chemicals', *Australian Journal of Political Science*, 32:49–64.

Bernstein, A. B. and A. K. Gauthier 1999, 'Choices in health care: What are they and what are they worth?', *Medical Care Research and Review* 56(Suppl. 1):5–23.

Bernstein, S. J., E. A. McGlynn, A. L. Siu, C. P. Roth, M. J. Sherwood, J. W. Keesey, J. Kosecoff, N. R. Hicks and R. H. Brook 1993, 'The appropriateness of hysterectomy: A comparison of care in seven health plans', *Journal of the American Medical Association*, 269:2398–402.

Bessell, T. L., J. E. Hiller and L. N. Sansom 1999, '"Pharmacist only" medicines', *Australian and New Zealand Journal of Public Health*, 23:661–2.

Bickerdyke, I., R. Dolamore, I. Monday and R. Preston 2002, *Supplier-induced demand for medical services*, Productivity Commission Staff Working Paper, Canberra, November.

Bidmeade, I. and C. Reynolds 1997, *Public health law in Australia: Its current state and future directions*, Canberra: Australian Government Publishing Service.

Bigg, I., S. Azmi and C. Maskell-Knight 1998, 'The Commonwealth's proposal for the 1998–2003 Health Care Agreements', *Australian Health Review*, 21:8–18.

Bindman, A. B., K. Grumbach, D. Osmond, M. Komaromy, K. Vranizan, N. Lurie, J. Billings and A. Stewart 1995, 'Preventable hospitalisations and access to health care', *Journal of the American Medical Association*, 274:305–11.

Birch, S. L. 1999, 'The 39 steps: The mystery of health inequalities in the UK', *Health Economics*, 8:301–8.

Blakeman, T. M., M. F. Harris, E.J. Comino and N.A. Zwar 2001, 'Evaluating general practitioners' views about the implementation of the Enhanced Primary Care Medicare items', *Medical Journal of Australia* 175(16 July):95–8.

Blendon, R. J., C. Schoen, C. M. DesRoches, R. Osborn and K. Zapert 2003, 'Common concerns amid diverse systems: Health care experiences in five countries', *Health Affairs*, 22(3):106–21.

Blendon, R. J., C. Schoen, C. M. DesRoches, R. Osborn, K. L. Scoles and K. Zapert 2002, 'Inequities in health care: A five-country survey', *Health Affairs* 21(3):182–91.

Blendon, R. J., R. Leitman, I. Morrison and K. Donelan 1990, 'Satisfaction with health systems in ten nations', *Health Affairs Summer*, pp. 185–92.

Bloom, A. L. (ed.) 2000, *Health reform in Australia and New Zealand*, Melbourne: Oxford University Press.

Bloor, K. and A. Maynard 2003, *Planning human resources in health care: Towards an economic approach. An international comparative review*, Ottawa: Canadian Health Services Research Foundation.

Bolman, L. G. and T. E. Deal 1991, *Reframing organizations: Artistry, choice and leadership*, San Francisco: Jossey-Bass Inc.

Bond, L., T. Nolan, P. Pattison and J. Carlin 1998, 'Vaccine preventable diseases and immunisations: A qualitative study of mothers' perceptions of severity, susceptibility, benefits and barriers', *Australian and New Zealand Journal of Public Health*, 22:441–6.

Booth, J. L. and B. T. Collopy 1997, 'A national clinical indicator database: Issues of reliability and validity', *Australian Health Review*, 20:84–95.

Borland, R., M. Borland and R. Mullins 1997, 'Prevalence of workplace smoking bans in Victoria', *Australian and New Zealand Journal of Public Health*, 21:694–8.

Boulding, K. E. 1967, 'The boundaries of social policy', *Social Work*, 12:3–11.

Boyce, N., J. McNeill, D. Graves and D. Dunt 1997, *Quality and outcome indicators for acute healthcare services*, Canberra: Australian Government Publishing Service.

Braithwaite, J. 1997, 'The 21st-century hospital', *Medical Journal of Australia*, 166(1): 6.

Braithwaite, J., L. Lazarus, R. F. Vining and J. Soar 1995, 'Hospitals: To the next millennium', *International Journal of Health Planning and Management*, 10:87–98.

Braithwaite, J., R. F. Vining and L. Lazarus 1994, 'The boundaryless hospital,' *Australian and New Zealand Journal of Medicine*, 24:565–71.

Brand, D. J. 1996, 'General practice reform: The shared management model', *Medical Journal of Australia*, 164:221–3.

Brasure, M., S. C. Stearns, E. C. Norton and T. Ricketts III 1999, 'Competitive behavior in local physician markets', *Medical Care Research and Review*, 56:395–414.

Braybrooke, D. 1987, *Meeting needs*, Princeton: Princeton University Press.

Brayley, N. and J. Marrow 1996, 'Health care resource groups in accident and emergency medicine', *Journal of Accident and Emergency Medicine*, 13:143–4.

Breen, K., V. Plueckhahn and S. Cordner 1997, *Ethics, law and medical practice*, Sydney: Allen & Unwin.

Brennan, D. S. and A. J. Spencer 2002a, 'Practice activity trends among Australian private general dental practitioners: 1983–84 to 1998–99', *International Dental Journal* 52(2):61–6.

Brennan, D. S. and Spencer, A. J. 2002b, *Dentists' practice activity in Australia: 1983–84 to 1998–99*, Australian Institute of Health and Welfare, Cat. No. DEN 101, Canberra: AIHW.

Britt, H., G. Sayer, G. Miller, J. Charles, S. Scahill, F. Horn and A. Bhasale 1999, *Bettering the evaluation and care of health: A study of general practice activity*, AIHW Cat. No. GEP-1, Canberra: Ausinfo.

Britt, H., G. Miller, S. Knox, J. Charles, L. Valenti, J. Henderson and Y. Pan 2001, *General practice activity in Australia 2000–01*, Australian Institute of Health and Welfare (General Practice Series No. 8), Cat. No. GEP 8, Canberra: AIHW.

Britt, H., G. C. Miller and S. Knox 2001, *Imaging orders by general practitioners in Australia 1999–00*, A joint report by the University of Sydney and the Australian Institute for Health and Welfare, Cat. No. GEP 7, Canberra: AIHW.

Britt, H., G. C. Miller, S. Knox, J. Charles, L. Valenti, J. P. Henderson, C. Sutton and C. Harrison 2002, *General practice activity in Australia 2001–02*, Australian Institute of Health and Welfare, Cat. No. GEP 10, Canberra: AIHW.

Britt, H., L. Valenti and G. Miller 2002, 'Time for care. Length of general practice consultations in Australia', *Australian Family Physician*, 31(9):876–80.

Broadhead, P. 1985, 'Social status and morbidity in Australia', *Community Health Studies*, 9:87–98.

Broadhead, P. 1987, 'Surveying health: A sociological perspective', *Australian and New Zealand Journal of Sociology*, 23:104–13.

Brodie, P. and L. Barclay 2001, 'Contemporary issues in Australian midwifery regulation', *Australian Health Review*, 24(4):103–18.

Brooks, P. M. 2003, 'The impact of chronic illness: Partnerships with other healthcare professionals', *Medical Journal of Australia*, 179:260–2.

Brooks, P. M., H. M. Lapsley and D. B. Butt 2003, 'Medical workforce issues in Australia: "Tomorrow's doctors—too few, too far"', *Medical Journal of Australia*, 179(18 August):206–8.

Broom, D. H. 1991, *Damned if we do: Contradictions of women's health*, Sydney: Allen & Unwin.

Brown, W. J. and S. Redman 1995, 'Setting targets: A three-stage model for determining priorities for health promotion', *Australian Journal of Public Health*, 19:263–9.

Bryant, R. 2001, 'The regulation of nursing in Australia: A comparative analysis', *Journal of Law and Medicine*, 9(1):41–57.

Bryce, M. 2000, 'APHA shores up "fragmenting industry" for joint campaign to push private health care', *Healthcover*, 10:46–51.

Bureau of Industry Economics 1991, *The pharmaceutical Industry: Impediments and opportunities. Program Evaluation No. 11*, Canberra: Australian Government Publishing Service.

Burnley, I. H. 1997, 'Disadvantage and male cancer incidence and mortality in New South Wales 1985–1993', *Social Science & Medicine*, 45:465–76.

Burrows, C., K. Brown and A. Gruskin 1993, 'Who buys health insurance? A survey of two large organisations', *Australian Journal of Social Issues*, 28:106–23.

Butler, J. R. G. 1993, 'Commonwealth/state financial relations in health: An update', in C. Selby-Smith (ed.) *Economics and Health: 1993 Proceedings of the Fifteenth Australian Conference of Health Economists*, Canberra: Faculty of Business and Economics and National Centre for Health Program Evaluation, pp. 256–77.

Butler, J. R. G. 1995, *Hospital cost analysis*, Dordrecht: Kluwer Academic.

Butler, J. R. G. 1999, 'Is the economic burden of illness worth measuring?', in A. H. Harris (ed.) *Economics and health 1998: Proceedings of the twentieth Australian conference of health economists*, Sydney: School of Health Services Management, University of New South Wales, pp. 256–77.

Butler, J. R. G. 2001, *Policy change and private health insurance: Did the cheapest policy do the trick?*, Canberra: National Centre for Epidemiology and Population Health, ANU.

Butler, J. R. G. 2002, 'Policy change and private health insurance: Did the cheapest policy do the trick?', *Australian Health Review*, 25(6):33–41.

Butler, J. R. G. and J. P. Smith 1992, 'Tax expenditures on health in Australia: 1960/61 to 1988/89', *The Australian Economic Review*, 3rd Quarter:43–58.

Butler, L., N. Biglia and P. Bourke 1998, *Australian biomedical research: Funding acknowledgements and performance*, Canberra: National Health & Medical Research Council.

Cameron, A. C. and J. McCallum 1996, 'Private health insurance choice in health: The role of long-term utilisation of health services', in *Economics and Health: 1995*, Sydney: School of Health Services Management, UNSW, pp. 143–57.

Cameron, A. C. and P. K. Trivedi 1991, 'The role of income and health risk in the choice of health insurance: Evidence from Australia', *Journal of Public Economics* 45:1–28.

Cameron, A. C., P. K. Trivedi, F. Milne and J. Piggott 1988, 'Microeconometric model of the demand for health care and health insurance in Australia', *Review of Economic Studies* 55:85–106.

Cameron, P. A., M. P. Kennedy and J. J. McNeil 1999, 'The effects of bonus payments on emergency service performance in Victoria', *Medical Journal of Australia* 171:243–6.

Caplan, G. A., J. A. Ward, N. J. Brennan, J. Coconis, N. Board and A. Brown 1999, 'Hospital in the home: A randomised controlled trial', *Medical Journal of Australia* 170:156–60.

Carrin, G. and P. Hanvoravongchai 2003, 'Provider payments and patient charges as policy tools for cost-containment: How successful are they in high-income countries?', *Human Resources for Health* 1(6).

Carter, M. 2000, 'Integrated electronic health records and patient privacy: Possible benefits but real dangers', *Medical Journal of Australia* 172:28–30.

Cass, A., J. Cunningham, P. Snelling, Z. Wang and W. Hoy 2003, 'Urban disadvantage and delayed nephrology referral in Australia', *Health and Place* 9:175–82.

Catchlove, B. R. 2001, 'The why and the wherefore', *Medical Journal of Australia*, 175:68–70.

Celler, B. G., N. H. Lovell, and J. Basilakis 2003, 'Using information technology to improve the management of chronic disease', *Medical Journal of Australia* 179(5):242–6.

Chanda, R. 2002, 'Trade in health services', *Bulletin of the World Health Organization*, 80(2):158–63.

Chandler, I. R., R. B. Fetter and R. C. Newbold 1991, 'Cost accounting and budgeting', in R. B. Fetter (ed.) *DRGs: Their design and development*, Ann Arbor: Health Administration Press, pp.91–120.

Chapman, S. and S. Wutzke 1997, 'Not in our backyard', *Australian and New Zealand Journal of Public Health* 21:614–20.

Cherkin, D. C., R. A. Deyo, M. Battie, J. Street and W. Barlow 1998, 'A comparison of physical therapy, chiropractic manipulation and provision of an educational booklet for the treatment of patients with low back pain', *New England Journal of Medicine* 339:1021–9.

Chernovsky, D. 1995, 'Health system reforms in industrialized democracies: An emerging paradigm', *The Milbank Quarterly* 73:339–72.

Clancy, C. M. and H. Brody 1995, 'Managed care: Jekyll or Hyde?', *Journal of the American Medical Association* 273:338–9.

Clare, R. and A. Tulpulé 1994, *Australia's ageing society*, Canberra: Economic Planning Advisory Council.

Clark, R. B. 2001, *Australian Patient Survey: Final report to the Commonwealth Department of Health and Aged Care*, Canberra: Commonwealth Department of Health and Aged Care.

Coburn, D. 2003, 'Beyond the income inequality hypothesis: Class, neo-liberalism, and health inequalities', *Social Science & Medicine*, 58(1): 41–56.

Cochrane, A. L. 1971, *Effectiveness and efficiency*, London: The Nuffield Provincial Hospital Trust.

Cohen, D. R. and J. B. Henderson 1988, *Health, prevention and economics*, Oxford: Oxford University Press.

Coile Jr, R. C. 2002, *Futurescan 2002: A forecast of healthcare trends 2002=2006*, Chicago: Health Administration Press, American College of Healthcare Executives.

Collins, D. J. and H. M. Lapsley 1991, *National Campaign Against Drug Abuse: Estimating the economic costs of drug abuse in Australia*, Monograph Series No. 15, Canberra.

Collins, D. J. and H. M. Lapsley 1996, *National Drug Strategy: The social costs of drug abuse in Australia in 1988 and 1992*, No. 30, Canberra: Australian Government Publishing Service.

Collins, F. S. 1999, 'Shattuck Lecture—Medical and societal consequences of the human genome project', *New England Journal of Medicine* 341:28–37.

Collopy, B. T. 1996, 'Report on the introduction of clinical indicators in surgery', *Journal of Quality in Clinical Practice* 16:183–4.

Collopy, B. T., M. Z. Ansari, J. L. Booth and J. A. Brosi 1995, 'The Australian Council on Healthcare Standards care evaluation program', *Medical Journal of Australia* 163:477–80.

Collyer, F. and K. White 1997, 'Enter the market: Competition, regulation and hospital funding in Australia', *Australian and New Zealand Journal of Sociology* 33:344–63.

Committee on Data Standards for Patient Safety 2003, *Key capabilities of an electronic health record system*, Washington D.C.: Institute of Medicine.

Commonwealth Department of Health and Aged Care 1999a, *PBS expenditure and prescriptions 1998 to 1999*, Canberra: Department of Health and Aged Care.

Commonwealth Department of Health and Aged Care 1999b, *Medical Statistics 1984–85 to September 1999*, Canberra: Commonwealth Department of Health and Aged Care.

Commonwealth Department of Health and Aged Care 1999c, *National medicines policy*, Canberra: Production Unit, Parliamentary and Access Branch.

Commonwealth Department of Health and Aged Care 2000, *Medicare Statistics September Quarter 2000*, Canberra: Commonwealth Department of Health & Aged Care, Table D1.

Commonwealth Department of Health and Aged Care 2001, *The Australian Coordinated Care Trials: Final technical national evaluation report on the first round of trials*, Canberra: Commonwealth Department of Health and Aged Care.

Commonwealth Department of Health and Ageing 2002, *HACC Program National Minimum Data Set* 2001–02 Bulletin.

Commonwealth Department of Health and Family Services 1996, 'The final report of the Taskforce on Quality in Australian health care', Canberra: Australian Government Publishing Service.

Commonwealth Department of Health and Family Services 1998, *Report on the national hospital cost data collection 1996/97*, Canberra: Australian Government Publishing Service.

Commonwealth Department of Human Services and Health 1994, *Nursing education in Australian universities: Report of the national review of nurse education in the higher education sector—1994 and beyond*, Canberra: Australian Government Publishing Service.

Commonwealth Department of Human Services and Health 1995, *Health promotion projects: Evaluation of the General Practice Demonstration Practice Grants Program 1992–94 (Report 2)*, Canberra: Australian Government Publishing Service.

Commonwealth Grants Commission 1995, *Equality in diversity: History of Commonwealth Grants Commission*, Canberra: Australian Government Publishing Service.

Commonwealth Grants Commission 1999, *Report on general revenue grant relativities*, vol. 1, Main Report, Canberra: Australian Government Publishing Service.

Connelly, J. 1999, 'Public health policy: Between victim blaming and the nanny state—will the third way work?', *Policy Studies* 20:51–67.

Cooper, G. 1999, 'Hospital in the home in Victoria: Factors influencing allocation decisions', *Australian Journal of Primary Health Interchange* 5:60–9.

Crawford, R. 1977, 'You are dangerous to your health: The ideology and politics of victim blaming', *International Journal of Health Services* 7:663–80.

Crerar, S. K., C. B. Dalton, H. M. Longbottom and E. Kraa 1996, 'Foodborne disease: Current trends and future surveillance needs in Australia,' *Medical Journal of Australia* 165:672–5.

Crichton, A. 1990, *Slowly taking control? Australian governments and health care provision 1788–1988*, Sydney: Allen & Unwin.

Crouch, M. and C. Colton 1983, *The course of community health in New South Wales, 1958–1982*, Sydney: University of New South Wales.

Cullis, J. G. and P. R. Jones 2000, 'Waiting lists and medical treatment: Analysis and policies', in A. J. Culyer and J. P. Newhouse (eds), *Handbook of health economics: Volume 1B*, Amsterdam: Elsevier, pp. 1201–49.

Cumpston, H. J. 1953, 'Public Health Administration', *Public Administration* XII:10.

Cunningham, J. and Y. Paradies 2000, 'Mortality of Aboriginal and Torres Strait Islander Australians 1997', Occasional Paper Cat. No. 3315, Canberra: ABS.

Cutler, D. M. (ed.) 2003, *A framework for evaluating medical care systems. A disease-based comparison of health systems: What is best and at what cost?*, Paris: OECD.

Daly, S., D. A. Campbell and P. A. Cameron 2003, 'Short-stay units and observation medicine: A systematic review', *Medical Journal of Australia*, 178(2 June):559–63.

Daniel, J., L. Johnson, S. Kennedy, K. Tallis and R. Webster 1997, 'Measuring outputs, inputs and productivity for Australian public acute care hospitals', in A.H. Harris (ed.) *Proceedings of the nineteenth Australian conference of health economists*, Sydney: School of Health Services Management, University of New South Wales, pp. 425–58.

Davidson, L., S. Chapman and C. Hull 1979, *Health promotion in Australia 1978/79: A report prepared for the Commonwealth Department of Health*, Canberra: Australian Government Publishing Service.

Davis, P. and T. Ashton (eds) 2001, *Health and public policy in New Zealand,* Auckland: Oxford University Press.

Davis, P., P. Graham and N. Pearce 1999, 'Health expectancy in New Zealand 1981–1991: Social variation and trends in a period of social and economic change.' *Journal of Epidemiological and Community Health* 53:519–27.

Davis, P., R. Lay-Yee, J. Fitzjohn, P. Hider, R. Briant and S. Schug 2002, 'Compensation for medical injury in New Zealand: Does "no-fault" increase the level of claims making and reduce social and clinical selectivity?', *Journal of Health Politics, Policy and Law*, 27(5):833–54.

Day, R. 1998, 'Pharmaceutical company promotion: striking a balance.' *Australian and New Zealand Journal of Medicine* 28:291–3.

Declaration of Alma Ata 1978, Adopted at the International Conference on Primary Health Care, Alma Ata, USSR: World Health Organization.

Deeble, J. 1999, 'Medicare: Where have we been? Where are we going?', *Australian and New Zealand Journal of Public Health* 23:563–70.

Deeble, J. S. 2002, 'Capital investment in public hospitals', *Australian Health Review* 25(5):45–60.

Deeble, J., C. Mathers, L. Smith, J. Goss, R. Webb and V. Smith 1998, *Expenditures on health services for Aboriginal and Torres Strait Islander people*, Cat. No. HWE 6, Canberra: AIHW.

Degeling, P. J. 1994, 'Unrecognised structural implications of casemix management', *Health Services Management* 7:9–21.

Delnoij, D., G. Van Merode, A. Paulus and P. Groenewegen 2000, 'Does general practitioner gatekeeping curb health care expenditure?', *Journal of Health Services Research and Policy* 5:22–6.

Dent, O. F. and K. J. Goulston 1999, 'Trends in the specialist workforce in internal medicine in Australia, 1981–1995', *Medical Journal of Australia* 170:32–5.

Department of Education, Training and Youth Affairs 2000, *Students 1999*, Canberra: DETYA.

Department of Health and Family Services 1996–1997, *Drug evaluation by the Therapeutic Goods Administration*, The Auditor-General Performance Audit Report No. 8, 1996–97, Canberra: Australian National Audit Office.

Department of Health and Family Services 1997, *Pharmaceutical Benefits Scheme*, The Auditor-General Performance Audit Report No. 12, Canberra: Australian National Audit Office.

Department of Human Services and Health, Aged and Community Care Division 1996, *Towards a national agenda for carers: Workshop papers*, No. 22, Canberra: Australian Government Publishing Service.

De Voe, J. 2003, 'A policy transformed by politics: The case of the 1973 Australian Community Health Program', *Journal of Health Politics, Policy and Law*, 28(1):77–108.

De Voe, J. E. and S. D. Short 2003, 'A shift in the historical trajectory of medical dominance: The case of Medibank and the Australian doctors' lobby', *Social Science & Medicine* 57:343–53.

Dickson, M., J. Hurst and S. Jacobzone 2003, *Survey of pharmacoeconomic assessment activity in eleven countries*, OECD Health Working Papers No. 4, Paris: OECD.

DiMaggio, P. J. and W. W. Powell 1991, 'The Iron Cage revisited: Institutional isomorphism and collective rationality in organizational fields', in W. W. Powell and P. J. DiMaggio (eds), *The new institutionalism in organizational analysis*, Chicago: The University of Chicago Press, pp. 63–82.

Doherty, R. L. 1988, *Australian medical education and workforce into the 21st Century: Committee of Inquiry into Medical Education and Medical Workforce*, Canberra: Australian Government Publishing Service.

Dollis, N., S. M. Gifford, C. Henenberg and J. Pirkis 1993, *Removing cultural and language barriers to health*, National Health Strategy Issues Paper No. 6, Melbourne: National Health Strategy.

Donabedian, A. 1973, *Aspects of medical care administration: Specifying requirements for health care*, Cambridge, MA: Harvard University Press.

Donaldson, M. S. 2001, 'Continuity of care. A reconceptualization', *Medical Care Research and Review* 58(3):255–90.

Donelan, K., R. J. Blendon, C. Schoen, K. Davis and K. Binns 1999, 'The cost of health system change: Public discontent in five nations', *Health Affairs* 18:206–16.

Donovan, J., E. d'Espaignet, C. Merton and M. van Ommeren 1992, *Immigrants in Australia: A health profile*, Canberra: AIHW.

Dooland, M. 1992, *Improving dental health in Australia*, National Health Strategy, Background Paper No. 9.

Douglas, R. M. and D. C. Saltman 1991, *W(h)ither Australian general practice?*, NCEPH Discussion Paper No. 1, Canberra: NCEPH.

Dowling, S., S. Barrett and R. West 1995, 'With nurse practitioners, who needs house officers?', *British Medical Journal* 311:309–13.

Dowling, S., R. Martin, P. Skidmore, L. Doyal, A. Cameron and S. Lloyd 1996, 'Nurses taking on junior doctors' work: A confusion of accountability,' *British Medical Journal* 312:1211–14.

Dowsett, G. 1998, 'Pink conspiracies: Australia's gay communities and national HIV/AIDS policies, 1983–96', in A. Yeatman (ed.) *Activism and the policy process*, Sydney: Allen & Unwin.

Draper, M. and S. Hill 1996, 'Feasibility of national benchmarking of patient satisfaction with Australian hospitals', *International Journal for Quality in Health Care* 8:457–66.

Dror, D. M., A. S. Preker, et al. 2002, 'The role of communities in combating social exclusion', in D. M. Dror and A. S. Preker (eds) *Social reinsurance: A new approach to sustainable community health financing*, Washington D.C.: World Bank.

Duckett, S. J. 1979, 'Chopping and changing Medibank part 1: Implementation of a new policy', *Australian Journal of Social Issues* 14:230–43.

Duckett, S. J. 1980, 'Chopping and changing Medibank part 2: An interpretation of the policy making process', *Australian Journal of Social Issues* 15:79–91.

Duckett, S. J. 1984, 'Structural interests and Australian health policy', *Social Science & Medicine* 18:959–66.

Duckett, S. J. 1988, 'Hospital financing reform: The first steps', *The Australian Quarterly* 60:435–47.

Duckett, S. J. 1994a, 'Hospital and departmental management in the era of accountability: Addressing the new management challenges', *Australian Health Review* 17:116–31.

Duckett, S. J. 1994b, *Reform of public hospital funding in Victoria*, Sydney: School of Health Services Management, No. 77, University of New South Wales.

Duckett, S. J. 1995a, 'The Australian health care system: An overview', in G. Lupton and J. M. Najman (eds) *Sociology of health and illness: Australian readings*, Melbourne: Macmillan Education Australia.

Duckett, S. J. 1995b, 'Hospital payment arrangements to encourage efficiency: The case of Victoria, Australia', *Health Policy* 34:113–34.

Duckett, S. J. 1998, 'Casemix funding for acute hospital inpatient services in Australia', *Medical Journal of Australia* 169 (Supplement, 19 October):S17–S21.

Duckett, S. J. 2003, 'Making a difference in health care', in S. Ryan and T. Bramston (eds) *The Hawke government: A critical perspective*, North Melbourne: Pluto Press, pp. 215–24.

Duckett, S. J. and P. Agius 2002, 'Performance of diagnosis-based risk adjustment measures in a population of sick Australians', *Australian and New Zealand Journal of Public Health*, 26(6):500–7.

Duckett, S. J. and T. Jackson 1999, 'Do the elderly cost more? Casemix funding in acute settings', in R. Nay and S. Garrett (eds) *Nursing older people: issues and innovations*, Sydney: Maclennan & Petty, pp. 3–17.

Duckett, S. J. and T. Jackson 2000, 'The new health insurance rebate: An inefficient way of assisting public hospitals', *Medical Journal of Australia* 172(9):439–44.

Duckett, S. J. and T. Jackson 2001, 'Paying for hospital emergency care under a single-payer system', *Annals of Emergency Medicine*, 37(3):309–17.

Duckett, S. J. and T. Jackson 2003, 'Do the elderly cost more? Casemix funding for elderly patients in acute inpatient settings', in R. Nay and S. Garrett (eds) *Nursing older people: Issues and innovations*, 2nd edn, Melbourne: MacLennan and Petty. In press.

Duckett, S. J., C. G. Scarf, A. M. Schmiede and C. J. Weaver 1981, *The organisation of medical staff in Australian hospitals*, Melbourne: Longman Cheshire.

Duckett, S. J. and H. Swerissen 1996, 'Specific purpose programs in human services and health: Moving from an input to an output and outcome focus', *Australian Journal of Public Administration* 55:7–17.

Dunn, C., K. Sadkowsky and P. Jelfs 2002, *Trends in deaths: Australian data, 1987-1998 with updates to 2000*, AIHW, Mortality Surveillance Series No. 3 Cat. No. PHE 40, Canberra.

Easton, B. 1997, *The commercialisation of New Zealand*, Auckland: Auckland University Press.

Easton, D. 1979a, *A framework for political analysis*, Chicago: University of Chicago Press.

Easton, D. 1979b, *A systems analysis of political life*, Chicago: University of Chicago Press.

Eastwood, H. 2000, 'Why are Australian GPs using alternative medicine? Postmodernisation, consumerism and the shift towards holistic health', *Journal of Sociology*, 36(2):133–56.

Eckermann, S. 2002, in J. R. G. Butler and L. B. Connelly (eds) *2001 Proceedings of the Twenty-third Australian Conference of Health Economists*, Sydney: AHES, pp. 433–63.

Economic and Budget Review Committee 1992, *Hospital services in Victoria: Efficiency and effectiveness of health service agreements: the impact of the mix of public and private patients on the funding of the public hospital system*, 35th Report to Parliament of Victoria, Melbourne: Government Printer.

Edwards, D., S. Peacock and R. Carter 1998, 'Beyond the individual: Benefits and community health', in J. C. Baldry (ed.) *Economics and Health: 1998*, Sydney: School of Health Services Management, pp. 93–120.

Edwards, N. 2002, 'The future role of the hospital', *Journal of Health Services Research and Policy* (1):1–2.

Edwards, N. and A. Harrison 1999, 'Planning hospitals with limited evidence: A research and policy problem', *British Medical Journal*, 319(20 November): 1361–3.

Elixhauser, A., C. Steiner and I. Fraser 2003, 'Volume thresholds and hospital characteristics in the United States', *Health Affairs*, 22(2):167–77.

Emanuel, E. J. and N. N. Dubler 1995, 'Preserving the physician–patient relationship in the era of managed care', *Journal of the American Medical Association* 273:323–39.

Evans, R. G. 1990a, 'Tension, compression and shear: Directions, stresses and outcomes of health care cost control', *Journal of Health Politics, Policy and Law* 15:101–28.

Evans, R. G. 1990b, 'The dog in the night-time: Medical practice variations and health policy', in T. F. Anderson and G. Mooney (eds) *The challenges of medical practice variations*, London: Macmillan Press, pp. 117–52.

Evans, R. G. 1995, 'Healthy populations or healthy institutions: The dilemma of health care management', *Journal of Health Administration Education* 13:453–72.

Evans, R. G. 1997, 'Going for the gold: The redistributive agenda behind market-based health care reform', *Journal of Health Politics, Policy and Law* 22:427–65.

Evans, R. G. and G. L. Stoddart 1990, 'Producing health, consuming health care', *Social Science & Medicine* 31:1347–63.

Feder, J., H. L. Komisar and M. Niefeld (in press), 'Long term care in the United States,' *Health Affairs*.

Fells, E. 2003, 'The proliferation of identity politics in Australia: An analysis of ministerial portfolios, 1970-2000', *Australian Journal of Political Science*, 38(1):101–17.

Ferguson, K. 1998, 'The nexus of health reform and health professional practice: Narratives of health professionals in times of change,' EdD thesis, Melbourne: La Trobe University.

Ferlie, E. B. and S. M. Shortell 2001, 'Improving the quality of health care in the United Kingdom and the United States: A framework for Change', *The Milbank Quarterly*, 79(2):281–315.

Fetter, R. B. 1991, 'Diagnosis related groups: Understanding hospital performance', *Interfaces* 21:6–26.

Filmer, D. and L. Pritchett 1999, 'The impact of public spending on health: does money matter?' *Social Science & Medicine* 49:1309–23.

Fine, M. 1995, 'Community-based services and the fragmentation of provision: A case study of home and community care services in a suburban community', *Australian Journal of Social Issues* 30:143–61.

Fitzgerald, P. D. 2001, 'The ethics of doctors and big business', *Medical Journal of Australia*, 175:73–5.

Flynn, K. E. and M. A. Smith 2002, 'From physician to consumer: The effectiveness of strategies to manage health care utilization', *Medical Care Research and Review*, 59(4):455–81.

Food Regulation Review Committee 1998, *Food a growth industry: The report of the Food Regulation Review*, Canberra: Ausinfo.

Frankel, S., S. Ebrahim and G. Davey-Smith 2000, 'The limits to demand for health care', *British Medical Journal* 321(1 July):40–4.

French, J. R. and B. Raven 1959, 'The bases of social power', in D. Cartwright (ed.) *Studies of social power*, Ann Arbor: University of Michigan Press, pp. 118–49.

French, J. R. and B. Raven 1968, 'The bases of social power,' in D. Cartwright and A. Zander (eds) *Group dynamics*, 3rd edn, New York: Harper and Rowe, pp. 259–69.

Friedberg, M., B. Saffran, T. J. Stinson, W. Nelson and C. L. Bennett 1999, 'Evaluation of conflict of interest in economic analyses of new drugs used in oncology', *Journal of the American Medical Association* 282:1453–57.

Furler, J. S., E. Harris, P. Chondros, P. G. Powell Davies, M. F. Havris and D. Y. Young 2002, 'The inverse care law revisited: Impact of disadvantaged location on accessing longer GP consultation times', *Medical Journal of Australia* 177(2):80–3.

Gardner, H. (ed.) 1995, *The politics of health: The Australian experience*, Melbourne: Churchill Livingstone.

Gardner, H. (ed.) 1997, *Health policy in Australia*, Melbourne: Oxford University Press.

Gardner, H. and S. Barraclough (eds) 2002, *Health policy in Australia*, Melbourne: Oxford University Press.

Garg, P. P., K. D. Frick, M. Diener-West and N. R. Powe 1999, 'Effect of the ownership of dialysis facilities on patients' survival and referral for transplantation', *New England Journal of Medicine* 341:1653–60.

Garnick, D. W. and K. Swartz 1999, 'Meeting information needs: Lessons learned from New Jersey's individual health insurance reform program', *Medical Care Research and Review* 56:456–70.

Gauld, R. 2001, *Revolving doors: New Zealand's health reforms*, Wellington, NZ: Institute of Policy Studies & the Health Services Research Centre, Victoria University.

George, B., A. Harris and A. Mitchell 1997, 'Reimbursement decisions and the implied value of life: Cost effectiveness analysis decisions to reimburse pharmaceuticals in Australia 1993–96', in A. Harris (ed.) *Economics and Health: 1997 Proceedings of the nineteenth Australian conference of health economists*, Sydney: University of New South Wales, pp. 1–18.

George, J. 1998, *States of health: Health and illness in Australia*, Melbourne: Addison Wesley Longman.

Gerdtham, U.-G. 1992, 'Pooling international health care expenditure data', *Health Economics* 1:217–31.

Gerdtham, U.-G., J. Sogaard, B. Jönsson and F. Andersson 1992, 'A pooled cross-section analysis of health care expenditures of the OECD countries', *Developments in Economics and Public Policy* 1:287–310.

Germov, J. 1995, 'Medi-fraud, managerialism and the decline of medical autonomy: de-professionalisation and proletarianisation reconsidered', *Australian and New Zealand Journal of Sociology*, 31(3):51–66.

Germov, J. (ed.) 2002, *Second opinion: An introduction to health sociology*, Melbourne: Oxford University Press.

Gibson, D. 1996, 'Reforming aged care in Australia: Change and consequence', *Journal of Social Policy* 25:157–79.

Gibson, D. 1998, *Aged care: Old policies, new problems*, Cambridge: Cambridge University Press.

Gibson, D. and Z. Liu 1995, 'Planning ratios and population growth: Will there be a short-fall in residential aged care by 2021?', *Australian Journal on Ageing* 14:57–62.

Gibson, D., G. Turrell and A. Jenkins 1993, 'Regulation and reform: Promoting residents' rights in Australian nursing homes', *Australian and New Zealand Journal of Sociology*, 29:73–91.

Giles, L. C., I. D. Cameron and M. Crotty 2003, 'Disability in older Australians: Projections for 2006-2031', *Medical Journal of Australia* 179:130–3.

Gillespie, J. A. 1991, *The price of health: Australian governments and medical politics 1910–1960*, Cambridge: Cambridge University Press.

Gleeson, M. 1989, 'Organizational change in Australian Catholic hospitals', PhD thesis, Sydney: University of New South Wales.

Godber, E., R. Robinson and A. Steiner 1997, 'Economic evaluation and the shifting balance towards primary care: Definitions, evidence and methodological issues', *Health Economics* 6:275–94.

Goddard, M. and R. Mannion 1998, 'From competition to co-operation: New economic relationships in the national health service', *Health Economics* 2:105–19.

Goddard, M., D. Henry and D. J. Birkett 2001, 'Securing the future of the Pharmaceutical Benefits Scheme', in G. Mooney and A. Plant (eds) *Daring to dream: The future of Australian health care*, Perth: Black Swan Press, pp. 79–88.

Goldsmith, J. 2000, 'From the field: How will the internet change our health system?', *Health Affairs* 19:148–56.

Gosden, T., F. Forland, I. S. Kristiansen, M. Sutton, B. Leese, A. Giuffrida, M. Sergison and L. Pedersen 2001, 'Impact of payment method on behaviour of primary care physicians: A systematic review', *Journal of Health Services Research and Policy* 6(1):44–55.

Grant, C. 1985, *Australian hospitals: Operation and management*, New York: Churchill Livingstone.

Gray, G. 1996, 'Reform and reaction in Australian health policy', *Journal of Health Politics, Policy and Law* 21:587–615.

Gray, G. 1998, 'How Australia came to have a national women's health policy', *International Journal of Health Services* 28:107–25.

Gray, L. 2001, *Two year review of aged care reforms*, Canberra: Commonwealth Department of Health and Aged Care.

Gupta, N., K. Diallo, P. Zurn and M. R. Dal Poz 2003, 'Assessing human resources for health: What can be learned from labour force surveys?', *Human Resources for Health* 1(5):1–16.

Haas, M. 1993, 'Evaluation of physiotherapy using cost-utility analysis', *Australian Physiotherapy* 39:211–16.

Haas, M., R. L. Rushwork and M. I. Rob 1996, 'Health services and the elderly: An evaluation of utilisation data', *Australian Journal of Ageing* 13:176–80.

Hacker, J. S. and T. Marmor 1999, 'How to think about "Managed Care"', *University of Michigan Journal of Law Reform* 32(4):661–84.

Hadorn, D. and Steering Committee of the Western Canada Waiting List Project 2003, 'Setting priorities on waiting lists: Point-count systems as linear models', *Journal of Health Services Research and Policy* 8(1):48–53.

Hadorn, D. C. and A. C. Holmes 1997a, 'The New Zealand priority criteria project. Part 1: Overview', *British Medical Journal* 314:131–4.

Hadorn, D. C. and A. C. Holmes 1997b, 'The New Zealand priority criteria project. Part 2: Coronary artery bypass graft surgery', *British Medical Journal* 314:135–8.

Hadorn, D. C. and Steering Committee of the Western Canada Waiting List Project 2002, 'Developing priority criteria for magnetic resonance imaging: Results from the Western Canada Waiting List Project', *Health Policy and Practice* 53(4):210–18.

Hailey, D. 1994, 'Health care technology in Australia', *Health Policy* 30:23–72.

Hailey, D. 1997, 'Australian economic evaluation and Government decisions on pharmaceuticals, compared to assessment of other health technologies', *Social Science & Medicine* 45:563–81.

Hailey, D. M. 1993, 'The influence of technology assessments by advisory bodies on health policy and practice', *Health Policy* 25:243–54.

Hall, J., R. De Abreu Lourenco and R. Viney 1999, 'Carrots and sticks—the fall and fall of private health insurance in Australia', *Health Economics* 8:653–60.

Hall, J., R. Viney and M. Haas 1998, 'Taking a count: The evaluation of genetic testing', *Australian and New Zealand Journal of Public Health* 22:754–8.

Hall, P. A. 1999, 'Social capital in Britain', *British Journal of Politics* 29:417–61.

Halligan, J. 1987, 'Reorganising Australian government departments, 1987', *Canberra Bulletin of Public Administration* 52:40–7.

Halligan, J., I. Beckett and P. Earnshaw 1992, 'The Australian Public Service Reform

Program', in J. Halligan and R. Wettenhall (eds) *Hawke's Third Government: Australian Commonwealth Administration 1987–1990*, Canberra: University of Canberra/RIPAA (ACT Division), pp. 7–56.

Hammond, P. B. and R. Coppock (eds) 1990, *Valuing health risks, costs and benefits for environmental decision making: Report of a conference*, Washington DC: National Academy Press.

Hanchak, N. A., N. Schlackman and S. Harmon-Weiss 1996, 'U.S. healthcare's quality-based compensation model', *Health Care Financing Review* 17:143–59.

Hannan, E. L. 1998, 'Measuring hospital outcomes: Don't make perfect the enemy of the good!', *Journal of Health Services Research and Policy* 3:67–9.

Harding, A., R. Percival, D. Schofield and A. Walker 2002, 'The lifetime distributional impact of government health outlays', *Australian Economic Review* 35(4):363–79.

Hardy, B. 1998, *Australian Market Basket Survey 1996*, Canberra: Australia and New Zealand Food Authority.

Harrinvirta, M. and M. Mattila 2001, 'The hard business of balancing budgets: A study of public finances in seventeen OECD countries', *British Journal of Political Science* 31:497–521.

Harris, A. H. 1994, 'Economic appraisal in the regulation of pharmaceuticals in Australia: Its rationale and potential impact', *Australian Economic Review* (2nd quarter):98–105.

Harris, M. F. and P. J. T. Mercer 2001, 'Reactive or preventive: The role of general practice in achieving a healthier Australia', *Medical Journal of Australia*, 175:92–3.

Harvey, K. and M. Murray 1995, 'Medicinal drug policy', in H. Gardner (ed.) *The politics of health: The Australian experience*, Melbourne: Churchill Livingstone, pp. 238–83.

Haycock, J., A. Stanley, N. Edwards and R. Nicholls 1999, 'Changing hospitals', *British Medical Journal* 319(6 November):1262–4.

Hayes, L. J., S. Quine, R. Taylor and G. Berry 2002, 'Socio-economic mortality differentials in Sydney over a quarter of a century, 1970–94', *Australian and New Zealand Journal of Public Health* 26(4):311–17.

Hays, R., G. Miller, B. Booth, B. Harris, M. Harris and J. Stirton 1998, 'The development of general practice standards in Australia', *Medical Education* 32:199–204.

Hays, R. B., D. A. Wallace and T. K. S. Gupta 1997, 'Training for rural family practice in Australia', *Teaching and Learning in Medicine* 9:80–3.

Hazelton, M. 1990, 'Medical discourse on contemporary nurse education: An ideological analysis', *Australian and New Zealand Journal of Sociology* 26:107–25.

Health and Medical Research Strategic Review 1999, *The virtuous cycle, working together for health and medical research*, Canberra: Department of Health and Aged Care.

Health Care Complaints Commission 1999, *The cosmetic surgery report: Report to the NSW Minister for Health*, Sydney: Health Care Complaints Commission.

Health Insurance Commission 1998, *Annual Report 1997/98*, Canberra: HIC.

Health Insurance Commission 2001, *Annual Report 1999–2000*, Canberra: HIC, Table 3.

Health Solutions 1994, *Independent assessment of casemix payment in Victoria: A report to the Casemix Development Program Commonwealth Department of Human Services and Health*, Melbourne: Health Solutions Pty Ltd.

Healy, J. 2002, 'The care of older people: Australia and the United Kingdom', *Social Policy and Administration* 36(1):1–19.

Hede, A. 1993, 'Reforming the policy role of inter-governmental councils', in A. Hede and S. Prasser (eds) *Policy making in volatile times*, Sydney: Hale & Iremonger, pp. 193–210.

Henry, D. 1992, 'Economic analysis as an aid to subsidisation decisions: The development of Australian guidelines for pharmaceuticals', *PharmacoEconomics* 1:54–67.

Hensher, M. and N. Edwards 2002, 'The hospital and the external environment: Experience in the United Kingdom', in M. McKee and J. Healy (eds), *Hospitals in a changing Europe*, Buckingham, UK: Open University Press, pp. 83–99.

Herxheimer, A. 2003, 'Relationships between the pharmaceutical industry and patients' organisations', *British Medical Journal* 326(31 May):1208–10.

Hickham, D. H., S. Severance, A. Feldstein, L. Ray, P. Gorman, P. Schuldheis, W. R. Hersh, K. P. Krages and M. Helfand 2003, *The effect of health care working conditions on patient safety*, Evidence Report/Technology Assessment No. 74, Agency for Healthcare Research and Quality, Rockville, MD.

Hickie, J. B. 1994, 'Success of a new health administration strategy. The patient focused institute with a tripartite management', *Medical Journal of Australia* 161:324–7.

Hicks, N. 1978, *'This sin and scandal': Australia's population debate 1891–1911*, Canberra: Australian National University Press.

Hill, S., D. Henry, B. Pekarsky and A. Mitchell 1997a, 'Economic evaluation of pharmaceuticals: What are reasonable standards for clinical evidence—the Australian experience', *British Journal of Clinical Pharmacology* 44:421–5.

Hill, S. R., D. D. Henry and A. J. Smith 1997b, 'Rising prescription drug costs: Whose responsibility?', *Medical Journal of Australia* 167:6–7.

Holahan, J., A. Weil and J. M. Wiener 2003, 'Which way for federalism and health policy?', *Health Affairs*, W3:317–33.

Holman, C. D. J. 1992, 'Something old, something new: Perspectives on five "new" public health movements', *Health Promotion Journal of Australia* 2:4–11.

Holmes, N. and S. M. Gifford 1997, 'Narratives of risk in occupational health and safety: Why the "good" boss blames his tradesman and the "good" tradesman blames his tools', *Australian and New Zealand Journal of Public Health* 21:11–16.

Hopkins, S. and M. P. Kidd 1996, 'The determinants of the demand for private health insurance under Medicare', *Applied Economics* 28: 1623–32.

Hospitals and Health Services Commission 1974, *Annual report: Hospitals and Health Services Commission*, Canberra: The Commission.

House, J. S. 2001, 'Understanding social factors and inequalities in health: 20th century progress and 21st century prospects', *Health and Social Behavior* 43(June):125–42.

House of Representatives Standing Committee on Community Affairs 1991, *'You have your moments': A report on funding of peak health and community organisations*, Canberra: Australian Government Publishing Service.

Howe, A. 1998, 'The economics of aged care: achieving quality and containing costs', in G. Mooney and R. Scotton (eds) *Economics and Australian health policy*, St Leonards: Allen & Unwin, pp. 137–53.

Howe, A. L. 1997, 'From states of confusion to a national action plan for dementia care: The development of policies for dementia care in Australia', *International Journal of Geriatric Psychiatry* 12:165–71.

Howe, A. L. 1999, 'Extending the pillars of social policy financing to aged care', *Social Policy and Administration* 33(5):534–51.

Humphreys, J. S., S. Mathews-Cowey and H. C. Weinand 1997, 'Factors in accessibility of general practice in rural Australia', *Medical Journal of Australia* 166:577–80.

Hunter, E. 1993, *Aboriginal health and history: Power and prejudice in remote Australia*, Melbourne: Cambridge University Press.

Hurst, J. and L. Siciliani 2003, *Tackling excessive waiting times for elective surgery: a comparison of policies in twelve OECD countries*, Paris: OECD.

Hutton, D. and L. Connors 1999, *A history of the Australian environment movement*, London: Cambridge University Press.

Iezzoni, L. I. (ed.) 1994, *Risk adjustment for measuring health care outcomes*, Ann Arbor: Health Administration Press.

Iezzoni, L. I. 1997, 'Annals of internal medicine', *American College of Physicians* 127:666–74.

Iliffe, S. and S. Shepperd 2002, 'What do we know about hospital at home? Lessons from international experience', *Applied Health Economics and Health Policy* 1(3):141–7.

Industry Commission 1995, *Work health and safety: Inquiry into occupational health and safety*, Report No. 47, Canberra: Industry Commission.

Industry Commission 1996, *The pharmaceutical industry*, Report No. 51, 3 May, Canberra: Australian Government Publishing Service.

Jackson, G. and M. Tobias 2001, 'Potentially avoidable hospitalisations in New Zealand, 1989–98', *Australian and New Zealand Journal of Public Health* 25(3):212–19.

Jackson, L. R. and J. E. Ward 1999, 'Aboriginal health: Why is reconciliation necessary?', *Medical Journal of Australia* 170:437–40.

Jackson, P. M. 1988, 'Public choice and public sector management', *Public Money and Management* 10:13–20.

Jackson, T. 1985, 'On the limitations of health promotion', *Community Health Studies* IX:1–9.

Jackson, T. 1996, 'A proposal for managed care payment options for patients with chronic conditions', *Australian Health Review* 19:27–39.

Jackson, T. 2001, 'Using computerised patient-level costing data for setting DRG weights: The Victorian (Australia) cost weight studies', *Health Policy* 56:149–63.

Jackson, T., S. Mitchell and M. Wright 1989, 'The community development continuum', *Community Health Studies* XIII:66–73.

Jackson, T. and P. Sevil 1996, *The development of relative resource weights for non-admitted patients*, Centre for Health Program Evaluation, Monash University.

Jackson, T. and P. Sevil 1997, 'Problems in counting and paying for multi-disciplinary out-patients clinics', *Australian Health Review* 20:38–54.

Jackson, T., J. Watts, D. Muirhead and P. Sevil 1997, *Non-admitted patient services: A literature review and analysis*, Melbourne: Acute Health Services Division.

Jackson, T., J. Watts, L. Lane and R. Wilson 1999, 'Data comparability in patient level clinical costing systems', *Casemix Quarterly* 1(1):36–45.

Jacobs, R. and D. Dawson, 2003, 'Hospital efficiency targets', *Health Economics*, 12:669–84.

Jacobzone, S. 2000, *Pharmaceutical policies in OECD countries: Reconciling social and industrial goals*, Labour Market and Social Policy Occasional Papers No. 40, Paris: OECD.

James, M. 1999, 'Towards an integrated needs and outcome framework', *Health Policy* 46:165–77.

Jegers, M., K. Kesteloot, D. De Graeve and W. Gilles 2002, 'A typology for provider payment systems in health care', *Health Policy*, 60:255–73.

Jin, R. L., C. P. Shah and T. J. Svoboda 1997, 'The impact of unemployment on health: A review of the evidence', *Journal of Public Health Policy* 18:275–301.

Johnson, T. 1997, *The 1996 course experience questionnaire*, Melbourne: Graduate Careers Council of Australia.

Jönsson, B. and I. Eckerlund 2003, 'Why do different countries spend different amounts on health care?', in OECD (ed.) *A disease-based comparison of health systems. What is best and at what cost?*, Paris: OECD, pp. 107–19.

Judge, K., J. Mulligan and M. Benzeval 1998, 'Income inequality and population health', *Social Science & Medicine* 46:567–79.

Karmel, P. 1973, *Expansion of medical education: Report of the Committee on Medical Schools to the Australian Universities Commission*, Canberra: Australian Government Publishing Service.

Kassirer, J. P. 1995, 'Managed care and the morality of the marketplace', *New England Journal of Medicine* 333:50–2.

Kast, F. E. and J. E. Rosenzweig 1972, 'General systems theory: Applications for organization and management', *Academy of Management Journal* 15:447–65.

Kearney, B. J. 1996, 'Health technology assessment', *Journal of Qualitative Clinical Practice* 16:131–43.

Kelaher, M. and L. Manderson 2000, 'Migration and mainstreaming: Matching health services to immigrants' needs in Australia', *Health Policy* 54:1–11.

Kendig, H. and S. J. Duckett 2001, *Australian directions in aged care: the generation of policies for generations of older people*, Commissioned Paper Series 2001/05, Sydney: Australian Health Policy Institute, University of Sydney.

Kenkel, D. S. 2000, 'Prevention', in A. J. Culyer and J. P. Newhouse (eds) *Handbook of health economics: Volume 1B*, Amsterdam: Elsevier, pp. 1675–1720.

Kewley, T. H. 1973, *Social security in Australia 1900–72*, Sydney: Sydney University Press.

Kidd, M. and F. Braun 1992, *Problems encountered by overseas-trained doctors migrating to Australia*, Canberra: Australian Government Publishing Service.

Kinnear, P. 2001, *Population ageing: Crisis or transition?*, Discussion Paper No. 45, Canberra: The Australia Institute, ANU.

Klein, R. 1998, 'Why Britain is reorganizing its National Health Service—yet again', *Health Affairs* 17:111–25.

Korda, R. J., L. Strazdins, D. H. Broom and L. L.-Y. Lim 2002, 'The health of the Australian workforce: 1998–2001', *Australian and New Zealand Journal of Public Health* 26(4):325–31.

KPMG Peat Marwick 1993, *National costing study: Production of cost weights for AN-DRGs. Version 1: Summary report*, Adelaide: KPMG Peat Marwick.

Kung, F. T. Y. 1996, 'Variation in performance of Aged Care Assessment Teams', *Health Systems Research Reports No. 2*, Melbourne: La Trobe University.

Kunz, E. F. 1975, *The intruder: Refugee doctors in Australia*, Canberra: Australian National University Press.

Lairson, D. R., P. Hindson and A. Hauquitz 1995, 'Equity on health care in Australia', *Social Science & Medicine* 41:475–82.

Lalonde, M. 1974, *A new perspective on the health of Canadians: A working document*, Ottawa: Health and Welfare.

Larson, J. S. 1999, 'The conceptualization of health', *Medical Care Research and Review* 56:123–36.

Laven, G. A., J. J. Beilby, D. Wilkinson and H. J. McElroy 2003, 'Factors associated with rural practice among Australian-trained general practitioners', *Medical Journal of Australia* 179(21 July):75–9.

Lawrence, G. L., C. R. MacIntyre, et al. 2003, 'Measles vaccination coverage among five-year-old children: Implications for disease elimination in Australia', *Australian and New Zealand Journal of Public Health* 27(4):413–19.

Lawson, J. S. and D. Black 1993, 'Socioeconomic status: The prime indicator of premature death in Australia', *Journal of Biosocial Science* 25:539–52.

Leask, J.-A. and S. Chapman 1998, '"An attempt to swindle nature": Press anti-immunisation reportage 1993–1997', *Australian and New Zealand Journal of Public Health* 22:17–26.

Leeder, S. R. 1993, *Pathways to better health*, Canberra: National Health Strategy.

Leeder, S. R. 1995, 'The contribution of epidemiology to the definition of health goals and targets for Australia', *International Journal of Epidemiology* 24:S109–12.

Leeder, S. R. 1999, *Healthy medicine: Challenges facing Australia's health services*, Sydney: Allen & Unwin.

Leeder, S. R. and A. Dominello 1999, 'Social capital and its relevance to health and family policy', *Australian and New Zealand Journal of Public Health* 234:424–9.

Legge, D. 1983, 'Quality assurance in US hospitals: A view from Australia', *Australian Clinical Review* September:34–43.

Le Grand, J., N. Mays and J.-A. Mulligan (eds) 1998, *Learning from the NHS internal market. A review of the evidence*, London: Kings Fund.

Leigh, J., D. Tyson, B. Pekarsky and C. Silagy 1999, 'The Australian Coordinated Care Trials and their evaluation—an introduction', in Commonwealth Department of Health and Aged Care (ed.) *The Australian Coordinated Care Trials: Background and trial descriptions*, Canberra: Publication Production Unit, pp. 1–13.

Leutz, W. N. 1999, 'Five laws for integrating medical and social services: Lessons from the United States and the United Kingdom', *The Milbank Quarterly* 77(1):77–110.

Lewis, D. 1996, 'Setting drinking water quality guidelines: Theory and practice', in *Economics and Health: 1995*, Sydney: School of Health Services Management, UNSW, pp. 61–71.

Lewis, J. 2000, 'From "fightback" to "biteback": The rise and fall of a national dental program', *Australian Journal of Public Administration* 59:84–96.

Lewis, J. and M. Considine 1999, 'Medicine, economics and agenda-setting', *Social Science & Medicine* 48:393–405.

Lexchin, J., L. A. Bero, B. Djulbergovic and O. Clark 2003, 'Pharmaceutical industry sponsorship and research outcome and quality: Systematic review', *British Medical Journal* 326(31 May):1167–77.

Liang, M. H., K. E. Cullen, M. G. Larson, J. A. Schwartz, C. Robb-Nicholson, A. H. Fossel, N. Roberge and R. Poss 1987, 'Effects of reducing physical therapy services on outcomes in total joint arthroplasty', *Medical Care* 25:276–85.

Liaw, S.-T., C. M. Pearce, P. Chondros, B. P. McGrath, L. Piggford and K. Jones 2003, 'Doctors' perceptions and attitudes to prescribing within the Authority Prescribing System', *Medical Journal of Australia* 178(3 March):203–6.

Lin, V. and C. King 2000, 'Intergovernmental reforms in public health', in A. L. Bloom (ed.) *Health sector reform in Australia and New Zealand*, Melbourne: Oxford University Press, pp. 251–63.

Lin, V. and S. J. Duckett 1997, 'Structural Interests and organisational dimensions of health system reform', in H. Gardner (ed.) *Health Policy in Australia*, Melbourne: Oxford University Press, pp. 64–80.

Löfgren, H. 1996, 'State supremacy in decline: The pharmaceutical industry and the Australian government', *Journal of Industry Studies* 3:87–103.

Löfgren, H. 1998, 'The Pharmaceutical Benefits Scheme and the shifting paradigm of welfare policy', *Australian Health Review* 21:111–23.

Löfgren, H. 2002, *Generic drugs: International trends and policy developments in Australia*, Working Paper No. 10, Melbourne: Centre for Strategic Economic Studies, Victoria University of Technology.

Loke, T. W., C. K. Fong and J. E. Ward 2002, 'Pharmaceutical advertisement claims in Australian medical publications', *Medical Journal of Australia*, 177(16 September):291–3.

Lokuge, K. and R. Denniss 2003, *Trading in our health system? The impact of the Australia-US Free Trade Agreement on the Pharmaceutical Benefits Scheme*, Discussion Paper No. 55, Canberra: The Australia Institute, ANU.

Lomas, J. 1998, 'Social capital and health: implications for public health and epidemiology', *Social Science & Medicine* 47:1181–8.

Lowenthal, R. M., A. Piaszczyk, G. E. Arthur and S. O'Malley 1996, 'Home chemotherapy for cancer patients: Cost analysis and safety', *Medical Journal of Australia* 165:184–7.

Lubalin, J. S. and L. D. Harris-Kojetin 1999, 'What do consumers want and need to know in making health care choices?', *Medical Care Research and Review* 56(Supp. 1):67–102.

Lubitz, J. and R. Prihoda 1984, 'The use and costs of Medicare services in the last 2 years of life', *Health Care Financing Review* 5:117–31.

Lubitz, J., J. Beebe and C. Baker 1995, 'Longevity and Medicare expenditures', *New England Journal of Medicine* 332:999–1003.

Lukes, S. 1974, *Power: A radical view*, Oxford: Macmillan Press.

Lupton, G. and J. M. Najman (eds) 1995, *Sociology of health and illness: Australian readings*, Melbourne: Macmillan Education Australia Pty Ltd.

Lyon, K. 2000, 'They said it couldn't be done: Contracting for veterans' hospital care in Australia', in A. L. Bloom (ed.) *Health sector reform in Australia and New Zealand*, Melbourne: Oxford University Press, pp. 223–34.

MacArthur, I. and X. Bonnefoy 1998, *Environmental health services in Europe 2: Policy options*, Copenhagen: WHO Regional Publications, European Series No. 77.

McCall, N., J. Korb, A. Petersons and S. Moore 2002, 'Constraining Medicare home health reimbursement: What are the outcomes?', *Health Care Financing Review* 24(2):57–76.

McCallum, J. and Mundy, G. 2002, *Australia's aged care service system: The need for an industry strategy*, Melbourne: The Myer Foundation.

McCaughan, B. C. and D. M. Piccone 1994, 'Devolved clinical management and casemix', *Medical Journal of Australia* 161:s20–3.

McClelland, A. and R. Scotton 1998, 'Poverty and health,' in R. Fincher and J. Nieuwenhuysen (eds) *Australian poverty: Then and now*, Melbourne: Melbourne University Press, pp. 185–202.

McDermott, F. T., S. M. Cordner and A. B. Tremayne 1996, 'Evaluation of the medical management and preventability of death in 137 road traffic fatalities in Victoria, Australia: An overview', *Journal of Trauma: Injury, Infection and Critical Care* 40:520–35.

McGuire, A., D. Parkin, D. Hughes and K. Gerard 1993, 'Econometric analyses of national health expenditures: Can positive economics help to answer normative questions?', *Health Economics* 2:113–26.

McGuire, T. E., J. A. Bender and C. Maskell 1995, *Casemix episodic payment for private health insurance*, Canberra: Australian Government Publishing Service.

Macinko, J., B. Starfield, and L. Shi 2003, 'The contribution of primary care systems to health outcomes within Organization for Economic Cooperation and Development (OECD) countries, 1970–1998', *Health Services Research* 38(3):831–65.

MacIntyre, C. R., C. W. Brook, E. Chandraraj and A. J. Plant 1997, 'Changes in bed resources and admission patterns in acute public hospitals in Victoria, 1987–1995', *Medical Journal of Australia* 167:186–9.

Mackenbach, J. and M. Bakker (eds) 2002, *Reducing inequalities in health. A European perspective*, London: Routledge.

McKie, J., H. Kuhse, J. Richardson and P. Singer 1996, 'Allocating healthcare by QALYs: The relevance of age', *Cambridge Quarterly of Healthcare Ethics* 5:534–45.

McKinlay, J. B. and S. M. McKinlay 1977, 'The questionable contribution of medical measures to the decline of mortality in the United States in the twentieth century', *The Milbank Memorial Fund Quarterly, Health and Society* Summer:405–28.

McKinlay, J. B., S. M. McKinlay and R. Beaglehole 1989, 'A review of the evidence concerning the impact of medical measures on recent mortality and morbidity in the United States', *International Journal of Health Services* 192:181–208.

McManus, P., N. Donnelly, D. Henry, W. Hall, J. Primrose and J. Lindner 1996, 'Prescription drug utilization following patient co-payment changes in Australia', *Pharmacoepidemiology and Drug Safety* 5:385–92.

McMichael, A. J. 1985, 'Social class (as estimated by occupational prestige) and mortality in Australian males in the 1970s', *Community Health Studies* 9:220–30.

McMichael, A. J. 1993, *Planetary overload: Global environmental change and the health of the human species*, London: Cambridge University Press.

McMillan, J. 1992, *Commonwealth Constitutional power over health*, Canberra: Consumers' Health Forum of Australia.

McNair, P. and S. J. Duckett 2002, 'Funding Victoria's public hospitals: The casemix policy of 2000-2001', *Australian Health Review*, 25(1):72–98.

Malcolm, L. 1994, 'Primary health care and the hospital: Incompatible organisational concepts?', *Social Science & Medicine* 39:455–8.

Malin, N., S. Wilmot and J. Manthorpe 2002, *Key concepts and debates in health and social policy*, Buckingham, UK: Open University Press.

Marjoribanks, T. and J. M. Lewis 2003, 'Reform and autonomy: Perceptions of the Australian general practice community', *Social Science & Medicine* 56:2229–39.

Marshall, S. and H. Swerissen 1999, 'A qualitative analysis of parental decision making for childhood immunisation', *Australian and New Zealand Journal of Public Health* 23:543–5.

Martin, C. M., R. G. Attewell, M. Nisa, J. McCallum and C. J. Raymond 1997, 'Characteristics of longer consultations in Australian general practice', *Medical Journal of Australia* 167:76–9.

Mason, C., L. Adamson, R. Cotton, M. Reid, H. Lapsley, E. Barrett and A. Rotem 1993, *General practitioners in hospitals*, Sydney: School of Medical Education, University of New South Wales.

Mathers, C. 1994, *Health differentials among adult Australians aged 25–64 years*, Canberra: Australian Institute of Health and Welfare.

Mathers, C. 1996, 'Trends in health expectancies in Australia 1981–1993', *Journal of Australian Population Association* 131:1–14.

Mathers, C. 1998, 'Health patterns of immigrants in Australia', *People and Place 4*.

Mathers, C., R. Penm, R. Carter and C. Stevenson 1998, *Health system costs of diseases and injury in Australia 1993/94*, AIHW Cat. No. HWE 5, Canberra: AIHW.

Mathers, C., T. Vos and C. Stevenson 1999, *The burden of disease in Australia*, AIHW Cat. No. PHE 17, Canberra: AIHW.

Mathers, C. D. 1999, 'International trends in health expectancies: Do they provide evidence for expansion or compression of morbidity?', in *Compression of morbidity workshop*, Canberra: Community Care Branch, Commonwealth Department of Health and Family Services.

Mathers, C. D., C. J. L. Murray, J. A. Saloman, R. Sadana, A. Tandon, A. D. Lopez, B. Ustün and S. Chatterji 2003, 'Healthy life expectancy: Comparison of OECD countries in 2001', *Australian and New Zealand Journal of Public Health*, 27(1):5–11.

Mathers, C. D. and J. M. Robine 1998, 'International trends in health expectancies: A review', *Australasian Journal on Ageing* 17:51–5.

Mathers, C. D. and D. J. Schofield 1998, 'The health consequences of unemployment: The evidence', *Medical Journal of Australia* 168:178–82.

Mathews, J. D. 1997, 'Historical, social and biological understanding is needed to improve Aboriginal health', *Recent Advances in Microbiology* 5:257–34.

Mathews, R. L. and W. R. C. Jay 1972, *Federal finance: Australian fiscal federalism from Federation to McMahon*, Melbourne: Thomas Nelson.

May, R. J. 1971, *Financing the small states in Australian federalism*, Melbourne: Oxford University Press.

Mayhew, C. and C. Peterson (eds) 1999, *Occupational health and safety in Australia: Industry, public sector and small business*, Sydney: Allen & Unwin.

Maynard, A. and K. Bloor 2003, 'Dilemmas in regulation of the market for pharmaceuticals', *Health Affairs* 22(3):31–41.

Mazur, A. 1981, *The dynamics of technical controversy*, Washington: Communications Press.

Mechanic, D. 1996, 'Changing medical organization and the erosion of trust', *The Milbank Quarterly* 74:171–89.

Mechanic, D. and M. Schlesinger 1996, 'The impact of managed care on patients' trust in medical care and their physicians', *Journal of the American Medical Association* 275:1693–7.

Mello, M. M., D. M. Studdert and T. A. Brennan 2003, 'The leapfrog standards: Ready to jump from marketplace to courtroom', *Health Affairs*, 22(2):46–59.

Milio, N. 1992, 'Keeping the promise of community health policy revival under Hawke 1983–1985', in F. Baum, D. Fry and I. Lennie (eds) *Community health; Policy practice in Australia*, Bondi Junction: Pluto Press Australia, pp. 28–47.

Millman, M. 1977, *The unkindest cut: Life in the backrooms of medicine*, New York: Morrow Quill Paperback.

Mitchell, A. 1996, 'Update and evaluation of Australian guidelines: Government perspective', *Medical Care* 34:DS216–25.

Moïse, P. and S. Jacobzone 2003, 'Population ageing, health expenditure and treatment: An ARD perspective', in OECD (ed.) *A disease-based comparison of health systems. What is best and at what cost?*, Paris: OECD, pp. 163–79.

Montalto, M. 1999, 'Hospital in the home; take the evidence and run: The time for apathy and cynicism towards home-based care is over', *Medical Journal of Australia* 170:148–9.

Moon, L. 1996, *Waiting for elective surgery in Australian public hospitals, 1995*, Health Services Series No. 7, Canberra: AIHW.

Mooney, G., L. Irwig and S. Leeder 1997, 'Priority setting in health care: Unburdening from the burden of disease', *Australian and New Zealand Journal of Public Health* 21:680–1.

Mooney, G. and R. Scotton (eds) 1998, *Economics and Australian Health Policy*, Sydney: Allen & Unwin.

Morgan, S., M. Barer and R. Evans 2000, 'Health economists meet the fourth tempter: Drug dependency and scientific discourse', *Health Economics*, 9:659–67.

Morrell, S. L., R. J. Taylor and C. B. Kerr 1998, 'Unemployment and young people's health', *Medical Journal of Australia* 168:236–40.

Morrison, A. L., U. Beckmann, M. Durie, R. Carless and D. M. Gillies 2001, 'The effects of nursing staff inexperience (NSI) on the occurrence of adverse patient experiences in ICUs', *Australian Critical Care*, 14(3):116–21.

Moss, J. 2002, 'Funding of South Australian public hospitals', *Australian Health Review* 25(1):156–72.

Mott, K., M. Kidd and D. Weller 2000, 'Quality and outcomes in general practice', in *General Practice in Australia: 2000*, Canberra: Department of Health and Aged Care, pp. 270–309.

Moulds, R. F. W. 1992, 'Promoting and advertising therapeutic goods: Trade Practices Commission report on self-regulation', *Medical Journal of Australia* 157:513–14.

Mount, C. D., C. W. Kelman, L. R. Smith and R. M. Douglas 2000, 'An integrated electronic health record and information system for Australia?', *Medical Journal of Australia* 172:25–7.

Moynihan, R. 2003, 'Who pays for the pizza? Redefining the relationships between doctors and drug companies. I: Entanglement', *British Medical Journal* 326(31 May):1189–92.

Moynihan, R., I. Heath and D. Henry 2002, 'Selling sickness: The pharmaceutical industry and disease mongering', *British Medical Journal* 324(13 April):886–91.

Mukamel, D. B., J. Zwanziger and A. Bamezai 2002, 'Hospital competition, resource allocation and quality of care', *BMC Health Services Research* 2(10):1–9.

Murray, C. J. L. and A. D. Lopez (eds) 1996, *The global burden of disease: A comprehensive assessment of mortality and disability from diseases, injuries and risk factors in 1990 and projected to 2020*, Cambridge, MA: The Harvard School of Public Health.

Murray, C. J. L., J. A. Salomon, C. D. Mathers and A. D. Lopez (eds) 2002, *Summary measures of population health. Concepts, ethics, measurement and applications*, Geneva: World Health Organisation.

Murray, J. F., N. A. Hanchak and N. Schlackman 1996, 'Health services research at U.S. Quality Algorithms, Inc.', *Medical Care Research and Review* 53:104–17.

Musgrove, P. 1999, 'Public spending on health care: How are different criteria related?', *Health Policy*, 47:207–23.

Myer Foundation (no date), *2020: A vision for aged care in Australia*, Melbourne: Myer Foundation.

Myers, B. 1965, *A guide to medical care administration: Concepts and principles*, Washington: American Public Health Association.

Najman, J. M. and A. A. Congalton 1979, 'Australian occupational mortality, 1965–67: Cause specific or general susceptibility', *Sociology of Health and Illness* 1:158–76.

National Centre for Epidemiology and Population Health 1992, *Improving Australia's health: The role of primary health care*, Canberra: NCEPH.

National Commission of Audit 1996, *Report to the Commonwealth government*, Canberra: Australian Government Publishing Service.

National Expert Advisory Group on Safety and Quality in Australian Health Care 1999, *Implementing safety and quality enhancement in health care: National actions to support quality and safety improvement in Australian health care*, Canberra: Ausinfo.

National Health and Medical Research Council 1994, *National framework for environmental and health impact assessment*, Canberra: Australian Government Publishing Service.

National Health and Medical Research Council 1995, *Promoting health in Australia*, Canberra: National Health and Medical Research Council.

National Health and Medical Research Council 1996a, *Guidelines for preventive interventions in primary health care: cardiovascular disease and cancer. A report of the assessment of Preventive Activities in the Health Care System Initiative*, Canberra: National Health and Medical Research Council.

National Health and Medical Research Council 1996b, *Promoting the health of Australians: A review of infrastructure support for national health advancement*, Canberra: Australian Government Publishing Service.

National Health and Medical Research Council 1997, *Guidelines for preventive interventions in primary health care: Cardiovascular disease and cancer*, Australian Government Publishing Service Cat. No. 970499X, Canberra: National Health and Medical Research Council.

National Health and Medical Research Council 2003, *Using socioeconomic evidence in clinical practice guidelines*, Canberra: Ausinfo.

National Health Strategy 1992, *Issues in pharmaceutical drug use in Australia*, Issues paper No. 4, Canberra: National Health Strategy.

National Occupational Health and Safety Commission 1998, *Compendium of Workers' Compensation Statistics Australia, 1996–97*, Canberra: Ausinfo.

National Occupational Health and Safety Commission 2002, *Compendium of workers' compensation statistics, Australia, 2000–01*, Canberra: National Occupational Health and Safety Commission.

National Review of Nursing Education 2002, *Our duty of care: Final Report of National review of nursing education*, Canberra: Ausinfo.

Navarro, V. and L. Shi 2001, 'The political context of social inequalities and health', *International Journal of Health Services* 31(1):1–21.

Needleman, J., P. I. Buerhaus, S. Mattke, M. Stewart and K. Zelevinsky 2002, 'Nurse-staffing levels and the quality of care in hospitals', *New England Journal of Medicine* 346(22):1715–22.

Nelson, M. R., J. J. McNeil, A. Peeters, C. M. Reid and H. Krum 2001, 'PBS/RPBS cost implications of trends and guideline recommendations in the pharmacological management of hypertension in Australia, 1994–1998', *Medical Journal of Australia* 174(4 June):565–8.

Nethercote, J. 2000, 'Departmental machinery of government since 1987', *Australian Journal of Public Administration* 59(3):94–110.

Neumann, P. J., E. A. Sandberg, C. M. Bell, P. W. Stone and R. H. Chapman 2000, 'Are pharmaceuticals cost-effective? A review of the evidence', *Health Affairs* 19:92–109.

Newhouse, J. 1996, 'Reimbursing health plans and health providers: Efficiency in production versus selection', *Journal of Economic Literature* XXXIV:1236–63.

Newhouse, J. P. 1993, 'An iconoclastic view of health cost containment', *Health Affairs* 12:152–71.

Newhouse, J. P. 1998, 'Risk adjustment: Where are we now?', *Inquiry* 35:122–31.

NHS Centre for Reviews and Dissemination 1995, *Review of the research on the effectiveness of health service interventions to reduce variations in health*, CRD Report 3, University of York.

NHS Modernisation Agency 2003, *Changing Workforce Programme Pilot Sites Progress*.

Nichol, W., K. McNeice and J. Goss 1994, *Expenditure on health research and development in Australia*, Canberra: AIHW.

Noseworthy, T. W., J. J. McGurran, D. C. Hadorn and Steering Committee of the Western Canada Waiting List Project 2003, 'Waiting for scheduled services in Canada: Development of priority-setting scoring systems', *Journal of Evaluation in Clinical Practice* 9(1):23–31.

Nutbeam, D. 1997, 'Creating health-promoting environments: Overcoming barriers to action', *Australian and New Zealand Journal of Public Health* 21:355–9.

Nutbeam, D. 1998, 'Health promotion glossary', *Health Promotion International* 13:349–64.

Nutbeam, D. and M. Wise 1996, 'Planning for Health for All: international experience in setting health goals and targets', *Health Promotion International* 11:219–26.

Oates, W. E. 1972, *Fiscal federalism*, New York: Harcourt Brace Jovanovich.

O'Connell, B. and P. Sharwood 1997, 'Casemix funding for emergency and other non-admitted patients?', in *The Ninth Casemix Conference in Australia*, Brisbane: Department of Health and Family Services.

O'Connell, J. M. 1996, 'The relationship between health expenditures and the age structure of the population in OECD countries', *Health Economics* 5:573–8.

OECD 1995, *New directions in health care policy*, Health Policy Studies No. 7, Paris: OECD.

OECD 2003, 'OECD Health data 2003: A comparative analysis of 30 countries', Paris: OECD.

Office of Regulation Review (Industry Commission) 1995, *Enforcing Australia's food laws: A survey and discussion of the practices of Australian food regulation enforcement agencies*, Canberra: Office of Regulation Review.

Office of the Australian Government Actuary 1995, *Australian Life Tables 1990–92*, Canberra: ABS.

Offredy, M. 2000, 'Advanced nursing practice: The case of nurse practitioners in three Australian states', *Journal of Advanced Nursing* 31:274–81.

O'Hara, D. A. and N. J. Carson 1997, 'Reporting of adverse events in hospitals in Victoria, 1994/1995', *Medical Journal of Australia* 166:460–3.

O'Loughlin, M. A. 2002, 'Conflicting interests in private hospital care', *Australian Health Review* 25(5):106–17.

Osborne, D. and T. Gaebler 1992, *Reinventing government: How the entrepreneurial spirit is transforming the public sector*, Reading, Mass.: Addison-Wesley.

Owen, A. and I. Lennie 1992, 'Health for all and community health', in F. Baum, D. Fry and I. Lennie (eds) *Community health: Policy and practice in Australia*, Sydney: Pluto Press, pp. 6–27.

Paalman, M., H. Bekedam, L. Hawken and D. Nyheim 1998, 'A critical review of priority setting in the health sector: The methodology of the 1993 world development report', *Health Policy and Planning* 13:13–31.

Page, A., S. Morrell and R. Taylor 2002, 'Suicide and political regime in New South Wales and Australia during the 20th century', *Journal of Epidemiological and Community Health* 56:766–72.

Palmer, G. 1996, 'Casemix funding of hospitals: Objectives and objections', *Health Care Analysis* 4:185–93.

Palmer, G., C. Aisbett, B. Reid and Y. Jayawardena 1986, 'The validity of Diagnosis Related Groups for use in Victorian public hospitals: Report to the Departments of Health and of Management and Budget, Victoria', Sydney: School of Health Administration, University of New South Wales.

Palmer, G. and S. Short 1994, *Health care and public policy: An Australian analysis*, South Melbourne: Macmillan Education Australia.

Palmer, G. R. 2000, 'Evidence-based health policy-making, hospital funding and health insurance', *Medical Journal of Australia* 172:130–3.

Parker, M. and M. Dent 1996, 'Managers, doctors and culture: Changing an English health district', *Administration & Society* 28:335–61.

Parkin, A. 2003, 'The states, federalism and political science: A fifty-year appraisal', *Australian Journal of Public Administration* 62(2):101–12.

Paterson, J. 1994, 'A new look at national medical workforce strategy', *Australian Health Review* 17:5–42.

Paterson, J. 1996, *National healthcare reform: The last picture show*, Melbourne: Department of Human Services.

Peacock, S. 1998, 'Setting priorities in community health: Experiences with PBMA in South Australia', in *Economics of Health: 1997, Proceedings of the Nineteenth Australian Conference of Health Economists*, Sydney: School of Health Services Management, University of New South Wales.

Pearse, J. (ed.) 1994, *The outcomes of the 1993 Medicare Agreements*, Sydney: Australian Studies in Health Service Administration.

Peckham, C. S. and C. Dezateux 1998, 'Issues underlying the evaluation of screening programmes', *British Medical Bulletin* 54:767–8.

Pegram, R., A. Sprogis and J. Buckpitt 1995, 'Divisions of general practice: A status review', *Australian Health Review* 18:78–94.

Pfaff, M. 1990, 'Differences in health care spending across countries: Statistical evidence', *Journal of Health Politics, Policy and Law* 15:1–24.

Pollitt, C. 1993, 'The struggle for quality: The case of the National Health Service', *Policy and Politics* 21:161–70.

Posnett, J. 2002, 'Are bigger hospitals better?', in M. McKee and J. Healy (eds) *Hospitals in a changing Europe*, Buckingham, UK: Open University Press, pp. 100–18.

Pritchard, P. and J. Hughes 1995, *Shared care: The future imperative?*, London: Royal Society of Medicine Press.

Private Health Insurance Administration Council 1999, *Annual Report 1998/99*, Canberra: Ausinfo.

Private Health Insurance Administration Council, June 1999 (and prior years), *Quarterly Statistics*, Canberra: Private Health Insurance Administration Council.

Productivity Commission 1997, *Private health insurance*, Inquiry Report, Canberra: Ausinfo.

Productivity Commission 1999, *Private hospitals in Australia*, Commission Research Paper, Canberra: Ausinfo.

Productivity Commission 2001, *International Pharmaceutical Price Differences*, Research Report, Canberra: Ausinfo.

Propper, C. 2003, 'Expenditure on healthcare in the UK: A review of the issues', in D. Miles, G. Myles and I. Preston (eds) *The economics of public spending*, Oxford: Oxford University Press, pp. 89–119.

Ranson, S., B. Hinings and G. Royston 1980, 'The structuring of organizational structures', *Administrative Science Quarterly* 25:1–17.

Rasmussen, B. 2002. *Implications of the business strategies of pharmaceutical companies for industry developments in Australia*, Melbourne: Centre for Strategic Economic Studies, Victoria University of Technology.

Reagan, M. D. 1972, *The new federalism*, New York: Oxford University Press.

Redman, S. 1996, 'Towards a research strategy to support public health programs for behaviour change', *Australian and New Zealand Journal of Public Health* 20:352–8.

Reid, B. A. 1991, *The effect of coding on the allocation of DRGs*, Sydney: School of Health Services Management, UNSW.

Reid, J. C. and R. A. Boyce 1995, 'Reconciling policy and practice: Australian multicultural health policy in perspective', *Policy and Politics* 23:3–16.

Reid, M. 1978, 'Women in health occupations', in *Women's health in a changing society*, Canberra: Commonwealth Department of Health, University of Queensland, pp. 169–75.

Renwick, M. and R. Harvey 1989, *Quality assurance in hospitals*, Canberra: Australian Government Publishing Service.

Renwick, M. and K. Sadkowsky 1991, *Variations in surgery rates*, Canberra: Australian Institute of Health, Health Services Series No. 2, Australian Government Publishing Service.

Restuccia, J. D., S. M. C. Payne, G. Lenhart, H. P. Constantine and J. P. Fulton 1987, 'Assessing the appropriateness of hospital utilization to improve efficiency and competitive position', *Health Care Management Review* 12:17–27.

Reynolds, C. 1995, 'Public health and the Australian Constitution', *Australian Journal of Public Health* 19:243–9.

Rice, T. 2002, 'Addressing cost pressures in health care systems', in Productivity Commission and Melbourne Institute of Applied Economic and Social Research (eds) *Health Policy Roundtable*, Melbourne: Productivity Commission and Melbourne Institute of Applied Economic and Social Research, pp. 67–119.

Richardson, G. and A. Maynard 1995, *Fewer doctors? More nurses? A review of the knowledge base of doctor-nurse substitution*, York: The University of York.

Richardson, J. 1998a, 'Economic evaluation of health promotion: Friend or foe?', *Australian and New Zealand Journal of Public Health* 22: 247–53.

Richardson, J. 1998b, 'Supplier induced demand reconsidered', in J. C. Baldry (ed.) *Economics and Health 1998*, Sydney: School of Health Services Management, UNSW, pp. 143–66.

Richardson, J. 1998c, 'The health care financing debate', in G. Mooney and R. Scotton (eds) *Economics and Australian Health Policy*, Sydney: Allen & Unwin, pp. 192–213.

Richardson, J. 2001a, 'A GODS analysis of Medicare: Goals, obstacles, deficiencies, solutions: Or, in what form should we adopt managed care', in G. Mooney and A. Plant (eds) *Daring to dream: The future of Australian health care*, Perth: Black Swan Press, pp. 159–68.

Richardson, J. 2001b, 'Supply and demand for medical care: Is the health care market perverse?', *Australian Economic Review* 34(3):336–52.

Richardson, J. 2003, *Financing health care: Short run problems, long run options*, Working Paper 138, Melbourne: CHPE, Monash University.

Richardson, J., K. Macarounas, F. Milthorpe, J. Ryan and N. Smith 1991, *An evaluation of the effect of increasing doctor numbers in their geographic distribution*, National Centre for Health Program Evaluation, Technical Report No. 2, Melbourne: NH&MRC.

Richardson, J. and S. Peacock 2003, *Will more doctors increase or decrease death rates? An econometric analysis of Australian mortality statistics*, Melbourne: Centre for Health Program Evaluation, Monash University, Working Paper 137.

Richardson, J. and I. Robertson 1999, *Ageing and the cost of health services*, Working Paper No. 90, Melbourne: Health Economics Unit, Monash University.

Ridolfo, B. and C. Stevenson 2001, *The quantification of drug-caused mortality and morbidity in Australia, 1998*, Cat. No. PHE 29, Canberra: AIHW.

Rigby, K., R. B. Clark and W. B. Runciman 1999, 'Adverse events in health care: Setting priorities based on economic evaluation', *Journal of Quality in Clinical Practice* 19:7–12.

Robertson, I. K. and J. R. J. Richardson 2000, 'Coronary angiography and coronary artery revascularisation rates in public and private hospital patients after acute myocardial infarction', *Medical Journal of Australia* 173(18 September): 291–5.

Robinson, J. C. 1994, 'The changing boundaries of the American hospital', *The Milbank Quarterly* 72:259–75.

Robinson, J. C. 2001, 'Theory and practice in the design of Physician Payment Incentives', *The Milbank Quarterly* 79(2):149–77.

Rodwin, M. A. 1995, 'Strains in the fiduciary metaphor: Divided physician loyalties and obligations in a changing health care system', *American Journal of Law & Medicine* XXI:241–57.

Rodwin, M. A. 1996, 'Consumer protection and managed care: issues, reform proposals and trade-offs', *Houston Law Review* 32:1319–81.

Ross, B., A. Hallam, J. Snasdell-Taylor, Y. Cass and L. Clarke 1999, *Health expenditure: Its managements and sources*, Health Financing Series Vol. 3, Canberra: Commonwealth Department of Health and Aged Care.

Roughead, E. E., A. L. Gilbert, J. Primrose and L. Sansom 1998a 'Coding drug-related admissions in medical records: Is it adequate for monitoring the quality of medication use?', *Australian Journal of Hospital Pharmacy* 28(1):7–12.

Roughead, E. E., A. L. Gilbert, J. G. Primrose and L. N. Sansom 1998b 'Drug-related hospital admissions: A review of Australian studies published 1988–1996', *Medical Journal of Australia* 168(20 April):405–8.

Roughead, E. E., K. J. Harvey and A. L. Gilbert 1998c 'Commercial detailing techniques used by pharmaceutical representatives to influence prescribing', *Australian and New Zealand Journal of Medicine* 28:306–10.

Roughead, E. E., A. L. Gilbert, J. G. Primrose, K. J. Harvey and L. N. Sansom 1999, *Report of the national indicators: Evaluating the quality use of medicines component of Australia's national medicines*, Canberra: Publication Production Unit, Commonwealth Department of Aged Care.

Royal College of Physicians of London 1962, *Smoking and health: Report on smoking in relation to cancer of the lung and other diseases*, London: Pitman Medical.

Runciman, W. B. and J. Moller 2001, *Iatrogenic injury in Australia: A report prepared by the Australian Patient Safety Foundation*, Adelaide: Australian Patient Safety Foundation.

Runciman, W. B., R. K. Webb, et al. 2000, 'A comparison of iatrogenic injury studies in Australia and the U.S.A. II: Reviewer behaviour and quality of care', *International Journal for Quality in Health Care* 12(5):379–88.

Russell, L. B. 1986, *Is prevention better than cure?*, Washington, D.C.: Brookings Institution.

Russell, L. B. 1987, *Evaluating preventive care: Report of a workshop*, Washington, D.C.: Brookings Institution.

Russell, L. B. 1994, *Educated guesses: Making policy about medical screening tests*, Berkeley: University of California Press.

Saffer, H. and F. Chaloupka 2000, 'The effect of tobacco advertising bans on tobacco consumption', *Journal of Health Economics* 19:1117–37.

Saggers, S. and D. Gray 1991, *Aboriginal health and society: The traditional and contemporary Aboriginal struggle for better health*, Sydney: Allen & Unwin.

Sakr, M., J. Angus, J. Perrin, C. Nixon, J. Nicholl and J. Wardrope 1999, 'Care of minor injuries by emergency nurse practitioners or junior doctors: A randomised control trial', *The Lancet* 9187:1321–6.

Salisbury, J. and L. Ferrari 1997, *Ozone: National environmental health forum monographs*, Rundle Hall, South Australian Health Commission.

Salkeld, G. 1998, 'What are the benefits of preventive health care?' *Health Care Analysis* 6:106–12.

Salkeld, G., A. Mitchell and S. Hill 1999, 'Pharmaceuticals', in G. Mooney and R. Scotton (eds) *Economics and Australian Health Policy*, Sydney: Allen & Unwin, pp. 115–36.

Saltman, R. B. and O. Ferroussier-Davis 2000, 'The concept of stewardship in health policy', *Bulletin of the World Health Organization* 78(6):732–9.

Saltman, R. B. and J. Figueras 1997, *European health care reform: Analysis of current strategies*, Copenhagen: WHO Regional Publications, European Series No. 72.

Saltman, R. B. and J. Figueras 1998, 'Analyzing the evidence on European health care reforms', *Health Affairs* 17:85–108.

Saltman, R. B. and C. von Otter 1989, 'Public competition vs mixed markets: An analytic comparison', *Health Policy* 11:43–55.

Saltman, R. B. and D. W. Young 1981, 'The hospital power equilibrium: An alternative view of the cost containment dilemma', *Journal of Health Politics, Policy and Law* 6:391–418.

Saturno, P. J., R. H. Palmer and J. J. Gascon 1999, 'Physician attitudes, self-estimated performance and actual compliance with locally peer-defined quality evaluation criteria', *International Journal for Quality in Health Care* 11:487–96.

Saunders, P. 1996, 'Poverty, income distribution and health: an Australian study', Report No. 128, Reports and Proceedings, Social Policy Research Centre, Sydney: University of New South Wales.

Sax, S. 1972, *Medical Care in the melting pot: An Australian review*, Melbourne: Angus & Robertson.

Sax, S. 1978, *Report of the Committee on Application and Costs of Modern Technology in Medical Practice*, Canberra: Australian Government Publishing Service.

Sax, S. 1984, *A strife of interests: Politics and policies in Australian health services*, Sydney: Allen & Unwin.

Scherer, F. M. 2000, 'The pharmaceutical industry', in A. J. Culyer and J. P Newhouse (eds) *Handbook of health economics: Volume 1B*, Amsterdam: Elsevier, pp. 1297–336.

Schlesinger, M. 2002, 'On values and democratic policy making: The deceptively fragile consensus around market-oriented medical care', *Journal of Health Politics, Policy and Law* 27(6):889–925.

Schoen, C. 2003, 'Ageing and health policy: The value of international comparisons and the potential of surveys to add a missing perspective', *A disease-based comparison of health systems. What is best and at what cost?* Paris: OECD, pp. 339–50.

Schofield, D. 1997, *The distribution and determinants of private health insurance in Australia, 1990*, Discussion Paper No. 17, Canberra: National Centre for Social and Economic Modelling, University of Canberra.

Schofield, D. 1998, *Re-examining the distribution of health benefits in Australia: Who benefits from the Pharmaceutical Benefits Scheme*, Discussion Paper No. 36, Canberra: National Centre for Social and Economic Modelling, University of Canberra.

Schofield, D. 1999, 'Ancillary and specialist health services: The relationship between income, user rates and equity or access', *Australian Journal of Social Issues* 34:79–96.

Schofield, D., S. Fischer and R. Percival 1997, *Behind the decline: The changing composition of private health insurance in Australia, 1983–95*, Discussion Paper No. 18, Canberra: National Centre for Social and Economic Modelling, University of Canberra.

Schon, D. A. 1971, *Beyond the stable state: Public and private learning in a changing society*, London: Temple-Smith.

Schulz, J. A. 1998, 'The economics and financing of long-term care', *The Australasian Journal on Ageing* 17(1(Supp)):82–4.

Scitovsky, A. A. 1988, 'Medical care in the last twelve months of life: The relation between age, functional status and medical care expenditures', *The Milbank Quarterly* 66:640–60.

Scott, A. 2000, 'Economics of general practice', in A. J. Culyer and J. P. Newhouse (eds) *Handbook of health economics: Volume 1B*, Amsterdam: Elsevier, pp. 1175–200.

Scott, M. 1997, 'Equity in the distribution of health care in Australia', in *18th Annual Conference of the Australian Health Economics Society*, Coffs Harbour Health Economics Unit, Centre for Health Program Evaluation Centre for Health Program Evaluation, pp. 1–24, A1–3, and B1–3.

Scotton, R. 1995, 'Managed competition: Issues for Australia', *Australian Health Review* 18:82–104.

Scotton, R. 1999, 'Managed competition: The policy context', *Australian Health Review* 22:103–21.

Scotton, R. B. 1977, 'Health costs and health policy', *Australian Quarterly* 492:5–17.

Scotton, R. B. 1980, 'Health insurance: Medibank and after', in R. B. Scotton and H. Ferber (eds) *Public Expenditures and Social Policy in Australia*, Melbourne: Longman Cheshire, pp. 145–75.

Scotton, R. B. and C. R. Macdonald 1993, *The making of Medibank*, Sydney: School of Health Services Management, University of NSW.

Scotton, R. B. and H. J. Owens 1990, *Case payment in Australian hospitals: Issues and options*, Melbourne: Public Sector Management Institute, Monash University.

Segal, L. 1998, 'Health funding: The nature of distortions and implications for the health service mix', *Australian and New Zealand Journal of Public Health* 22:271–3.

Segal, L. and J. Richardson 1994, 'Economic framework for allocative efficiency in the health sector', *Australian Economic Review* 2nd quarter: 89–98.

Selby-Smith, C. and S. Crowley 1995, 'Labor force planning issues for allied health in Australia', *Journal of Allied Health* 24:249–65.

Senate Community Affairs References Committee 1995, *The tobacco industry and the costs of tobacco-related illness*, Canberra: Senate Printing Unit.

Senate Community Affairs References Committee 1998, *Report on public dental services*, Canberra: Senate Printing Unit, Parliament House.

Senate Community Affairs References Committee 2002, *The patient profession: Time for action. Report on the Inquiry into Nursing*, Canberra: Senate Printing Unit.

Sergison, M., B. Sibbald and S. Rose 1999, *Skill mix in primary care: A bibliography*, Manchester: National Primary Care Research and Development Centre (NPCRDC), University of Manchester.

Seshamani, M. and A. Gray 2003, 'Health care expenditures and ageing: An international comparison', *Applied Health Economics and Health Policy* 1:9–16.

Sharman, C. 1991, 'Executive federalism', in B. Galligan, O. Hughes and C. Walsh (eds) *Intergovernmental relations and public policy*, Singapore: Allen & Unwin, pp. 23–39.

Shenfield, G. M. and J. L. Tasker 1997, 'History in the making: The evolution of Consumer Product Information (CPI)', *Medical Journal of Australia* 166:425–8.

Shepard, D. S., M. J. Larson and N. G. Hoffman 1999, 'Cost-effectiveness of substance abuse services', *Addictive Disorders* 22:385–400.

Shepperd, S. and S. Iliffe 2003, 'Hospital at home versus in-patient hospital care (Cochrane Review)', *The Cochrane Library*, Oxford: Update Software Issue 1.

Shiell, A. 1997, 'Health outcomes are about choices and values: An economic perspective on the health outcomes movement', *Health Policy* 39:5–15.

Short, S. 1998, 'Community activism in the health policy process: The case of the Consumers' Health Forum of Australia, 1987–96', in A. Yeatman (ed) *Activism and the policy process*, St Leonards, NSW: Allen & Unwin, pp. 122–45.

Siahpush, M. and G. K. Singh 1999, 'Social integration and mortality in Australia', *Australian and New Zealand Journal of Public Health* 23:571–7.

Silagy, C., B. Pekarsky, J. Leigh, B. Fagg, R. Quigley, G. Masters, C. Southwell, J. King, P. Tyler, A. Church, A. Esterman and M. Pradham 1999, *The Australian Coordinated Care Trials: Interim national evaluation summary*, Canberra: Commonwealth Department of Health and Aged Care.

Sindall, C. 1992, 'Health promotion and community health in Australia: An overview of theory and practice', in F. Baum, D. Fry, and I. Lennie (eds) *Community health: Policy and practice in Australia*, Sydney: Pluto Press Australia, pp. 277–95.

Singh, B. S. and P. D. McGorry 1998, 'The Second National Mental Health Plan: An opportunity to take stock and move forward', *Medical Journal of Australia* 169:435–7.

Single, R. 1997, *The National Drug Strategy: Mapping the future: an evaluation of the National Drug Strategy 1993–1997: a report*, Canberra: Australian Government Publishing Service.

Siskind, V., J. M. Najman and P. C. Veitch 1992, 'Socioeconomic status and mortality revisited: An extension of the Brisbane area analysis', *Australian Journal of Public Health* 16:315–20.

Sloan, C. 1995, *A history of the Pharmaceutical Benefits Scheme 1947–1992*, Canberra: Commonwealth Department of Human Services and Health.

Smallwood, R. A. and H. M. Lapsley 1997, 'Clinical practice guidelines: To what end?', *Medical Journal of Australia* 166:592–5.

Smith, J. 1997, 'The journey towards a national food safety policy', in H. Gardner (ed.) *Health Policy in Australia*, Melbourne: Oxford University Press, pp. 154–66.

Smith, J. 2001, 'Tax expenditures and public health financing in Australia', *The Economic and Labour Relations Review* 12(2):239–62.

Sochalski, J. 2002, 'Nursing shortage redux: turning the corner on an enduring problem [comment]', *Health Affairs* 21(5):157–64.

South Australian Health Commission 1997, *Casemix funding for health—hospitals—1997/98*, Adelaide: South Australian Health Commission.

Spencer, A. J. 2001, *What options do we have for organising, providing and funding better public dental care?*, Sydney: Australian Health Policy Institute, University of Sydney.

Stamp, K. M., S. J. Duckett and D. A. Fisher 1998, 'Hospital use for potentially preventable conditions in Aboriginal and Torres Strait Islander and other Australian populations', *Australian and New Zealand Journal of Public Health* 22:673–84.

Starfield, B. and L. Shi 2002, 'Policy relevant determinants of health: An international perspective', *Health Policy* 60:201–18.

State of the Environment Advisory Council 1996, *Australia: State of the environment 1996*, Collingwood: CSIRO Publishing.

Steering Committee for the Review of Commonwealth/State Service Provision 1998, *Implementing reforms in government services 1998*, Canberra: Ausinfo.

Steering Committee for the Review of Commonwealth/State Service Provision (SCRCSSP) 2003, *Report on government services 2003*, Canberra: Ausinfo.

Steiner, A. and A. Robinson 1998, 'Managed care: US research evidence and its lessons for the NHS', *Journal of Health Services Research and Policy* 3(3):173–84.

Stockigt, J. R. 1996, 'The commercialisation of public teaching hospitals is a fundamental error', *Medical Journal of Australia* 165:482–4.

Stoelwinder, J. U. and M. A. Abernethy 1989, 'The design and implementation of a management information system for Australian public hospitals', *Health Services Management Research* 2:176–90.

Street, A. and S. Duckett 1996, 'Are waiting lists inevitable?', *Health Policy* 36:1–15.

Stuart, B. and B. Briesacher 2002, 'Medication decisions—right and wrong', *Medical Care Research and Review* 59(2):123–45.

Susser, M. and E. Susser 1996, 'Choosing a future for epidemiology: I. Eras and paradigms', *American Journal of Public Health* 86:668–73.

Sweeny, K. 2002, *Trends in the use and cost of pharmaceuticals under the Pharmaceutical Benefits Scheme*, Centre for Strategic Economic Studies, Victoria University of Technology, Working Paper No. 5, Melbourne.

Swerissen, H., J. Macmillan, et al. 2001, 'Community health and general practice: The impact of different cultures on the integration of primary care', *Australian Journal of Primary Health* 7(1):65–70.

Syrett, K. 2003, 'A technocratic fix to the "legitimacy problem"? The Blair government and health care rationing in the United Kingdom', *Journal of Health Politics, Policy and Law* 28(4):715–46.

Szreter, S. 1988, 'The importance of social intervention in Britain's mortality decline c.1850–1914: A re-interpretation of the role of public health', *The Society for the Social History of Medicine* 1:1–41.

Szreter, S. 1995, *Rapid population growth and security: Urbanisation and economic growth in Britain in the nineteenth century. Population and security*, Cambridge: Centre for History and Economics, Kings College.

Tallis, G. and J. I. Balla 1995, 'Critical path analysis for the management of fractured neck or femur', *Australian Journal of Public Health* 19:155–9.

Taylor, M. C., D. C. Hadorn and Steering Committee of the Western Canada Waiting List Project 2002, 'Developing priority criteria for general surgery: Results from the Western Canada Waiting List Project', *Canadian Journal of Surgery* 45(5):351–7.

Taylor, R., M. Lewis and J. Powles 1998, 'Australian mortality decline: Cause-specific mortality 1907–1990', *Australian and New Zealand Journal of Public Health* 22:37–44.

Taylor, R., S. Quine, D. Lyle and A. Bilton 1992, 'Socioeconomic correlates of mortality and hospital morbidity differentials by local government area in Sydney, 1985–1988', *Australian Journal of Public Health* 16:305–14.

Technological Change in Health Care (TECH) Research Network 2001, 'Technological change around the world: Evidence from heart attack care', *Health Affairs* 20(3):25–42.

Tengs, T. O., G. Meyer, J. E. Siegel, J. S. Pliskin, J. D. Graham and M. C. Weinstein 1996, 'Oregon's Medicaid ranking and cost-effectiveness', *Medical Decision Making* 16:99–107.

Tesh, S. N. 1988, *Hidden arguments: Political ideology and disease prevention policy*, New Brunswick: Rutgers University Press.

Thomas, E. J., D. M. Studdert, W. B. Runciman, R. K. Webb, E. J. Sexton, R. M. Wilson, R. W. Gibberd, B. T. Harrison and T. A. Brennan 2000 'A comparison of iatrogenic injury studies in Australia and the U.S.A. I: Context, methods, casemix, population, patient and hospital characteristics', *International Journal for Quality in Health Care* 12(5):371–8.

Thomas, E. J., E. J. Orav and T. A. Brennan 2000, 'Hospital ownership and preventable adverse events', *Journal of General Internal Medicine* 15(4):211–19.

Thompson, S. C., R. E. Goudey and T. Stewart 1994, 'Legislation for school entry immunisation certificates in Victoria', *Australian Journal of Public Health* 18:261–6.

Treweek, S. 2003, 'The potential of electronic medical record systems to support quality improvement work and research in Norwegian general practice', *BMC Health Services Research* 3(10):1–9.

Tuohy, C. H. 1999, *Accidental logics: The dynamics of change in the health care arena in the United States, Britain and Canada*, New York: Oxford University Press.

Turner, L. and S. D. Short 1999, 'George Rupert Palmer—DRG carrier and champion', *Australian Health Review* 22:86–102.

Turner, V. F., P. J. Bentley, S. A. Hodgson, P. J. Collard, R. Drimatis, C. Rabune and A. J. Wilson 2002, 'Telephone triage in Western Australia', *Medical Journal of Australia* 176(4 February):100–3.

Twaddle, A. C., L. Eisenberg and A. Kleinman 1980, *'Sickness and the sickness careers: Some implications.' The relevance of social sciences for medicine*, Dordrecht, Holland: D. Reidel Publishing, pp. 111–33.

Vaithianathan, R. 2002, 'Will subsidising private health insurance help the public health system?', *The Economic Record* 78(242):277–83.

van Konkelenberg, R. V. and A. McAlindon 1993, 'Hospital non-specialist medical workforce survey 1993', Canberra: Australian Government Publishing Service.

Viney, R., M. Haas, M. Shanahan and I. Cameron 2001, 'Assessing the value of hospital-in-the-home: Lessons from Australia', *Journal of Health Services Research and Policy* 6(3):133–8.

Wagstaff, A., E. van Doorslaer, H. van der Burg, S. Calonge, T. Christiansen, G. Citoni, U.-G. Gerdtham, M. Gerfin, L. Gross, U. Hakinne, J. John, P. Johnson, J. Klavus, C. Lachaud, J. Lauritsen, R. Leu, B. Nolan, E. Peran, J. Pereira, C. Propper, F. Puffer, L. Rochaix, M. Rodriguez, M. Schellhorn, G. Sundberg and O. Winkelhake 1999, 'Equity in the finance of health care: Some further international comparisons', *Health Economics* 19:263–90.

Waitzkin, H. 1991, *The politics of medical encounters: How patients and doctors deal with social problems*, New Haven: Yale University Press.

Walker, A. and A. Abello 2000, *Changes in the health status of low income groups in Australia, 1977–78 to 1995*, Discussion Paper No. 52, Canberra: National Centre for Social and Economic Modelling, University of Canberra.

Walker, A. and A. Maynard 2003, 'Managing medical workforces: From relative stability to disequilibrium in the UK NHS', *Applied Health Economics and Health Policy* 2(1):25–36.

Walker, A., R. Percival and A. Harding 1998, *The impact of demographic and other changes on expenditure on Pharmaceutical Benefits in 2020 in Australia*, Discussion Paper No. 31, Canberra: National Centre for Social and Economic Modelling, Faculty of Management, University of Canberra.

Wan, T. T. H. and A. M. Connell 2003, *Monitoring the quality of health care: Issues and scientific approaches*, Norwell, Massachusetts: Kluwer Academic Publishers.

Wang, A., S. Hall, H. Gilbey and T. Ackland 1997, 'Patient variability and the design of clinical pathways after primary total hip replacement surgery', *Journal of Quality Clinical Practice* 17:123–9.

Waring, M. 1988, *If women counted: A new feminist economics*, San Francisco: Harper & Row.

Waring, M. 1999, *Counting for nothing: What men value and what women are worth*, Wellington: Allen & Unwin.

Watts, J. 2002, in J. R. G. Butler and L. B. Connelly (eds) *2001 Proceedings of Twenty-third Australian Conference of Health Economists*, Sydney: AHES, pp. 399–425.

Wennberg, J. E., E. S. Fisher and J. S. Skinner 2002, 'Geography and the debate over Medicare reform', *Health Affairs*, Web Exclusive (13 February) W96–W114.

Wheare, K. C. 1963, *Federal Government (4th edn)*, London: Oxford University Press.

Wheelwright, K. 1994, 'Controlling pathology expenditure under Medicare – a failure of regulation', *Federal Law Review* 22:92–115.

White, J. 1995, *Competing solutions: American health care proposals and international experience*, Washington, D.C.: Brookings Institution.

White, J. 1999, 'Targets and systems of health care cost control', *Health Politics, Policy and Law* 24:1–44.

White, K. and F. Collyer 1998, 'Health care markets in Australia: Ownership of the private hospital sector', *International Journal of Health Services* 28:487–510.

White, K. N. 2000, 'The state, the market, and general practice: The Australian case', *International Journal of Health Services* 30(2):285–308.

WHO 2000, *The World Health Report 2000: Health systems: Improving performance*, Geneva: World Health Organization.

WHO 1986a, 'A discussion document on the concept and principles of health promotion', *Health Promotion International* 1:73–6.

WHO 1986b, *Ottawa Charter for health promotion*, Ottawa: World Health Organization.

WHO 2001, *International classification of functioning, disability and health*, Geneva: World Health Organization.

Wiggers, J. H. and R. Sanson-Fisher 1997, 'Duration of general practice consultations: association with patient occupational and educational status', *Social Science & Medicine* 44:925–34.

Wiktorowicz, M. E. 2003, 'Emergent patterns in the regulation of pharmaceuticals: Institutions and interests in the United States, Canada, Britain, and France', *Journal of Health Politics, Policy and Law* 28(4):615–58.

Wilkinson, R. 1996, *Unhealthy societies: The afflictions of inequality*, London: Routledge.

Willcox, S. 1991, 'A healthy risk? Use of private insurance. Background Paper No. 4', Melbourne National Health Strategy.

Williams, A. 1999a, 'Calculating the global burden of disease: Time for a strategic reappraisal?', *Health Economics* 8:1–8.

Williams, A. 1999b, 'Commentary on the Acheson Report', *Health Economics* 8:297–9.

Williamson, O. E. 1975, *Markets and hierarchies: Analysis and antitrust implications*, New York: The Free Press.

Williamson, O. E. 1986, *Economic organization: Firms, markets and policy control*, Hemel Hempstead: Wheatsheaf Books Ltd.

Willis, E. 1994, *Illness and social relations: Issues in the sociology of health care*, Sydney: Allen & Unwin.

Wilson, J. M. C. and G. Junger 1968, *Principles and practice of screening for disease*, Geneva: World Health Organization.

Wilson, R. McL., W. B. Runciman, R. W. Gibberd, B. T. Harrison, L. Newby and J. D. Hamilton 1995, 'The quality in Australian health care study,' *Medical Journal of Australia* 163:458–71.

Wingert, T. D., J. E. Kralewski, T. J. Lindquist and D. J. Knutson 1995, 'Constructing episodes of care from encounter and claims data: Some methodological issues', *Inquiry* 32:430–43.

Winstanley, M., S. Woodward and N. Walker 1995, *Tobacco in Australia: Facts and Issues*, Melbourne: Quit Victoria.

Wise, M. and L. Signal 2000, 'Health promotion development in Australia and New Zealand', *Health Promotion International* 15(3):237–48.

Wyke, S., N. Mays, A. Street, G. Bevan, H. McLeod and N. Goodwin 2003, 'Should general practitioners purchase health care for their patients? The total purchasing experiment in Britain', *Health Policy* 65:243–59.

Yeatman, H. 2002, 'Australia's food regulations – challenges for public health advocacy', *Australian and New Zealand Journal of Public Health* 26(6):515–17.

Yen, I. H. and S. L. Syme 1999, 'The social environment and health: A discussion of the epidemiologic literature', *Annual Review of Public Health* 20:287–308.

Young, D. W. and R. B. Saltman 1985, *The hospital power equilibrium: physician behaviour and cost control*, Baltimore: Johns Hopkins University Press.

Zajac, J. D. 2003, 'The public hospital of the future', *Medical Journal of Australia* 179:250–2.

Zarilli, S. and C. Kinnon (eds) 1998, *International trade in health services: A development perspective*, Geneva: Joint publication UNCTAD-WHO.

Zhang, J. X., T. J. Iwashyna and N. A. Christakis 1999, 'The performance of different look-back periods and sources of information for Charlson Comorbidity Adjustment in Medicare claims', *Medical Care* 37:1128–39.

Zines, L. 1989, 'A legal perspective', in Brian Galligan (ed.) *Australian Federalism*, Melbourne: Longman Cheshire, pp. 16–44.

Zipser, B. 1999, 'Professionals and the standard of care', *Torts Law Journal* 7:167–83.

Zweifel, P., S. Felder and M. Meier 1999, 'Aging of population and health care expenditure: A red herring?', *Health Economics* 8:485–96.

Useful Web Sites

Aged Care Standards and Accreditation Agency:
<www.accreditation.aust.com> 17 December 2003

Analysis Section Pharmaceutical Benefits Branch, PBS Expenditure and Prescriptions:
<www.health.gov.au/pbs/general/pubs/pbbexp/index.htm> 17 December 2003

ANCI National Competency Standards for the Registered Nurse and Enrolled Nurse:
<www.anc.org.au/02standards/competency.php#StandardsRN> 17 December 2003

Australian Institute of Health and Welfare:
17 December 2003

Australian Institute of Health and Welfare Knowledgebase:
<www.aihw.gov.au/knowledgebase/index.html> 17 December 2003

Australian Medical Workforce Advisory Committee:
<www.healthworkforce.health.nsw.gov.au/amwac/> 17 December 2003

Communicable Disease Network of Australia & New Zealand:
<www.cda.gov.au/cdna/index.htm> 17 December 2003

Department of Health and Aged Care: Medicare Benefits Schedule:
<www.health.gov.au/pubs/mbs/#nov03> 17 December 2003

Department of Health and Aged Care, useful ACC Data:
<www.health.gov.au/acc/stat/> 17 December 2003

Guidelines for the Pharmaceutical Industry on preparation of submissions to the Pharmaceutical Benefits Advisory Committee, including major submissions involving economic analyses:
<www.health.gov.au/pbs/general/pubs/pharmpac/gusubpac.htm> 17 December 2003

Medicare Statistics:
<www.health.gov.au/haf/medstats/index.htm> 17 December 2003

National Public Health Partnership; the Memorandum of Understand-
ing for the Partnership may be accessed at:
<http://hna.ffh.vic.gov.au/nphp> 17 December 2003
Worksafe Australia Statistics:
<www.worksafe.gov.au/Statistics/OverviewDataPolicyAnalysis/> 17
December 2003

Index